Immunosuppression and Human Malignancy

Contemporary Immunology

Immunosuppression and Human Malignancy, by *David Naor, Benjamin Y. Klein, Nora Tarcic,* and *Jonathan S. Duke-Cohan*

Clinical Cellular Immunology, *Molecular and Therapeutic Reviews,* edited by *Albert A. Luderer* and *Howard H. Weetall*

The Lymphokines: *Biochemistry and Biological Activity,* edited by *John W. Hadden* and *William E. Stewart II*

Immunosuppression and Human Malignancy

Foreword by

Marc Feldmann

By

David Naor, Benjamin Y. Klein, Nora Tarcic, and Jonathan S. Duke-Cohan

*The Lautenberg Center for General
and Tumor Immunology
The Hebrew University, Jerusalem, Israel*

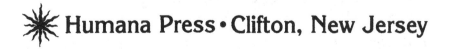 Humana Press • Clifton, New Jersey

© 1989 The Humana Press Inc.
Crescent Manor
PO Box 2148
Clifton, NJ 07015

Printed in the United States of America

Library of Congress Cataloging-in-Publication Data

Immunosuppression and human malignancy / by David Naor .. [et al.] ;
   foreword by Marc Feldmann.
   p.   cm. -- (Contemporary immunology)
   Bibliography: p.
   ISBN   0-89603-149-7
   1. Cancer--Immunological aspects. 2. Immunossuppression.
3. Cancer cells. 4. Suppressor cells. I. Naor, David.
II. Series.
   [DNLM: 1. Immune Tolerance. 2. Killer Cells, Natural--immunology.
3. Neoplasms--immunology. 4. Suppressor Cells--immunology.
5. Suppressor Cells--physiology.   QW 568 I339]
RC268.3.I4629   1989
616.99'4079--dc20
DNLM/DC   89-7474
for Library of Congress   CIP

"We shall require a substantially new manner of thinking if mankind is to survive"

Albert Einstein

.

Contents

Foreword

The immune system can deal effectively with the majority of viruses and bacteria, less effectively with parasites, and very poorly with cancer. Why is this so? Why are McFarlane Burnet's and Lewis Thomas' predictions that the immune system is involved in ridding the body of cancer cells, encapsulated in the catchy phrase "immunologic surveillance," so difficult to experimentally establish?

Cancer differs from infectious agents in being derived from the host. Hence, it has been postulated that cancer cells lack antigens that the immune system can recognize. They are not "immunogenic." However, this argument is seriously weakened by the existence of numerous human autoimmune diseases, in which the immune system effectively recognizes and attacks a variety of self tissues. Thus, the potential clearly exists for recognition of the surfaces of tumor cells.

Professor Naor and his colleagues have written a book that explores another possible reason: cancer cells are recognized by the immune system—but is it possible that the consequence of recognition is inhibition of the immune system—by suppressor T cells or macrophages? The evolution of the malignant state may only occur in individuals who develop this suppression.

This book reviews the evidence that suppressor cells, poorly characterized and difficult to study, may be of fundamental importance in cancer. In fact, our incapacity to understand the nature of suppressor cells and their mode of action is one of the major problems in immunology research today.

Clearly, further work is needed in this area to complete the analysis of suppressor phenomena in cancer, and the book by Prof. Naor and his colleagues will greatly assist all those who wish to push their explorations more deeply into its intricacies.

Marc Feldmann
The Charing Cross Sunley Research Centre
Hammersmith, London, UK

Introduction

If one reviews the literature dealing with the function of suppressor macrophages and suppressor T cells in experimental animals confronted with malignancy (1,2), one may reach a conclusion that increased suppressor-cell function is frequently associated with the immunodepression observed in many tumor-bearing hosts (TBH). It is difficult, however, to evaluate the genuine extent of immunodepression in experimental models of malignancy, and its relationship to concurrent suppressor cell function, simply because negative results are not always reported.

A separate question is how much the immunodepression mediated by suppressor cells is associated with the initial transformation event of malignancy and with the promotion of tumor growth. Again, it is impossible to make any generalization: at one extreme, we may observe in animals tumor progression despite normal immunocompetence (3–5), and at the other extreme, there is clear evidence that immunodepression mediated by suppressor cells is associated with the progression of cancer or even with the carcinogenic process itself (1,2). These latter experimental models further imply that the immune system may control tumor progression, if excessively active suppressor cells do not interfere. Indeed, our previous review articles (1,2) present many examples of experimental cancer prevention, or even therapy, that were dependent on the eradication of suppressor cells and the subsequent establishment of an efficient immune response against the tumors.

In order to assess the association of suppressor cells with the human malignant process, one must first demonstrate the existence of increased suppressor-cell activity in patients with malignant diseases and, secondly, must correlate the function of the suppressor cells with the immunocompetence and the pathological status (stage of disease, remission, or relapse) of the patients. From experimental models, we have learned that suppressor-cell function presented in vitro does not necessarily indicate a general depression of the immune response (4). Even if an association between the in vitro function of suppressor cells and in vivo immunodeficiency has been convincingly demonstrated in a clinical presentation of malignancy, it is still necessary to show that immunodepression is associated with either carcinogenesis or tumor progression.

Clearly, the relative ease of assessing such associations in experimental models cannot be extended to studies in humans. In the classical animal experiments, an association between immunodeficiency mediated by suppressor cells and malignancy has been evidenced by the eradication of suppressor cells or their precursors, using specific experimental manipulations (1,2). Under such circumstances, it is then possible to observe whether or not the increase in the immune function is associated with tumor regression. Ideally, the elimination of suppressor cells from the TBH and resultant induction of antitumor immunity should be assayed by the adoptive transfer of TBH immune cells to naive tumor-bearing recipients. These cells may slow the progression of the recipient tumor cells or may even impose complete regression on them. The reciprocal experiment of transferring suppressor cells to suppressor-cell-deficient animals may result in providing conditions for reestablishment of tumor growth. Clearly, such approaches are not feasible for human studies, in which suppressor cells can be detected by in vitro tests only.

The heterogeneity of the immunodeficiency seen in experimental models of TBH and the further heterogeneity of the suppressor cells themselves (*see* the conclusion of our previous article; 1) makes any attempt to extrapolate conclusions from experiments in animals to human studies hazardous. Furthermore, except in the instance of spontaneously arising tumors, the majority of laboratory-induced tumors present tumor-specific transplantation antigens (TSTA), implying that they are able to stimulate immunological rejection of the tumor. We do not know, however, whether human malignancies express such TSTA, simply because we have no in vivo assay to test them. Thus, human tumors may express entirely different antigenic properties than laboratory-induced tumors, and any attempt to compare the two may be misleading.

Even if fundamental differences between experimental and human tumors do exists, that fact does not necessarily suggest that human tumors do not employ a distinct mechanism to induce the appearance of suppressor cells. On the contrary, such tumors may induce efficient suppressor-cell activity in an attempt to avoid an autoimmune response against their own antigens, which may be normal components of the cellular differentiation process rarely presented by the normal mature cells.

In assessing immunocompetence and its relationship to malignancy, factors specific to each patient must be taken into account. For instance, if certain drug regimens cause regression of a tumor and this effect is accompanied by acquisition of immunocompetence (as indicated by a positive skin test) and disappearance of suppressor cells (as indicated by an in vitro assay), we may suggest that the suppressor cell activity is associated with the malignancy. This notion may gain support from direct experiments in animals, proving that the same drug eliminates suppressor cells under controlled conditions. Reappearance of the suppressor cells upon relapse would further support the suggestion that the suppressor-cell activity is associated with the malignant state.

Such careful analysis of the available facts may enable formulation of an objective concept concerning the association between an excessive function of suppressor cells and human malignancy. If such an association does exist, at least in some human malignancies, one may go further in planning a rational immunotherapy strategy based on the elimination of suppressor cells that are preventing an immune reaction against the tumor.

Such approach is, however, practical only if the same immunosuppression mechanism operates in all or most patients exhibiting the same disease. If not (as happens in few animal models; 1), application of a treatment protocol to all patients may be useless or even hazardous.

Before discussing the interrelationships between suppressor cells and malignancy in humans, we shall describe some related subjects in experimental animals that are essential for evaluating the data of the human studies, but have not been previously reviewed (1). We shall describe certain immunomodulators, used in cancer therapy, that under defined conditions induce the appearance of suppressor cells rather than facilitate antitumor immunity. The relationship between suppressor cells and natural killer (NK) cells is another aspect that will be discussed in detail, because of the possible contribution of NK cells to cancer defense (reviewed in 6). Some malignant cells coexpress antagonistic immunogenic and suppressogenic entities (7). Suppressor cells, induced by the suppressogenic entities of the tumors, may downregulate the antitumor activity of other cells that had been induced by the immunogenic entities of the same tumor. It is possible that the apparent lack of immunogenicity of spontaneous tumors, including many human tumors, may be associated with the coexistence of such antagonistic immunoreactive cellular components. This interesting aspect of tumor immunology will also be discussed before focusing our attention upon human malignancy.

Finally, we shall briefly review in a separate chapter recent publications dealing with suppressor cells and malignancy in experimental animals, most of which appeared after the printing of an earlier review (1). The reader is advised to examine previous reviews (1,2) especially for their introductory and concluding remarks. Additional information on similar, or related, subjects may be found in other review papers (8–17), and in a collection of symposium papers that appeared in *Suppressor Cells in Human Cancer* (1981) (Serrou B. and Rosenfeld C. eds.), Amsterdam: Elsevier/North-Holland.

Induction of Suppressor Cells by Immunostimulants

1. Introduction

Bacillus Calmette-Guérin (BCG; *18,19*), a viable attenuated strain of *Mycobacterium bovis*, and *Corynebacterium parvum* (*C. parvum, 20*), a gram-negative bacterium, are widely employed as immunostimulants though their precise mechanism of action is unknown. Functionally, BCG enhances antigen clearance and phagocytosis, augments cellular and humoral immune responses, and increases resistance to infection (*18,19*). In addition, activation of thymus-derived cells (T cells) by BCG has been reported (*21*), but this may only occur in the presence of small levels of macrophages (*19*). Both BCG (*19*) and *C. parvum* (*20,22*) activate the macrophages, and consequently, an efficient killing capacity may be found in these cells. Humoral and cellular immune responses may be enhanced in animals treated with BCG (*19*) or *C. parvum* (*20*) because of the ability of these immunostimulants to augment the capacity of macrophages to process and present antigen to lymphocytes. In addition, *C. parvum* and BCG can augment the activity of NK cells (*23*).

The impressive immunological augmenting effect of BCG and *C. parvum* has encouraged several investigators to explore their ability to enhance immunological antitumor responses. Although BCG (or its methanol extract residue, MER, *24*) and *C. parvum* potentiated immunological activity to such an extent that tumors were rejected in animal models (*18–20,25*), their ability to control human malignancy has not yet been firmly established (*19,26*). Intralesional injections of the immunostimulants have so far proved to be the most efficient route for an efficient response against localized tumors (*18–20,26,27*), but this strategy does not affect metastases and may even enhance their development (*19*).

The positive antitumor effects of BCG and *C. parvum* may be antagonized by their ability to stimulate the appearance of non-specific suppressor cells. Consequently, under certain circumstances, these immunostimulants may enhance tumor growth rather than retard its progression (19). Such an undesirable event deserves special attention and will be discussed briefly in the following sections.

2. Induction of Suppressor Cells by BCG

Enhancement of tumor growth associated with BCG (28,29) or MER (30) treatment was observed in several early experiments, but only in more recent studies have attempts been made to elucidate the mechanism of action of these particulate adjuvants. Orbach-Arbouys and colleagues (31–35) demonstrated that spleen cells or nylon-wool-purified T cells derived from C57BL/6 mice injected intravenously with BCG proliferated much less intensively than the corresponding normal cells when stimulated by allogeneic cells (mixed lymphocytes culture, MLC; 31). The proliferative responses of these splenocytes to phytohemagglutinin (PHA), concanavalin A (Con A), or lipopolysaccharide (LPS) were also considerably reduced in comparison with normal cells. Incubating spleen cells of BCG-injected mice with normal nylon-wool-purified T cells or with normal spleen cells inhibited the mitogenic responses (32) and the MLC (34) of the normal cells, indicating that BCG induces suppressor cells. The suppressor cells were plastic-adherent, and they were effective after incubation at 56° for 30 min or exposure to X-irradiation of 900–1500 rad (32–34). Treatment with anti-Thy-1 and complement (C) did not affect the suppressor-cell activity, and purified T cells from BCG injected mice were totally ineffective suppressors (35). It was concluded, therefore, that the suppressor cells were macrophages (35), and the possible coexistence of suppressor T cells (32) was excluded.

The detection of the suppressor by the in vitro assays is very much dependent upon the dose of BCG used for injection and the time chosen for assay. Intravenous injection of 1 mg BCG induced the appearance of efficient suppressor cells, which could be detected 14 d later, but not 7 d later. Injection of 3 mg BCG was required in order to detect the suppressor cells on the seventh day (32). Other authors have confirmed these observations by showing that low doses of BCG (e.g., 0.05 mg or 10^3 microorganisms) failed to induce suppressor cells (28,36,37).

The BCG-stimulated macrophages also inhibited the proliferation of methylcholanthrene (MCA)-induced fibrosarcoma (35). Furthermore, injection of BCG into mice inoculated with the tumor 7 d previously resulted in tumor regression in about 50% of the mice (35). Apparently, BCG induces the appearance of suppressor macrophages that inhibit proliferation of both mitogen-stimulated cells and tumor cells (*see also* ref. 38). This dual effect of the macrophages may support the tumor growth (by inhibiting proliferating antitumor immune cells) or cause tumor regression (by blocking the tumor proliferation). The balance between the two forces may determine the fate of the tumor. In the last-mentioned experimental model, BCG caused tumor regression, but under different circumstances, as will be discussed further on, it may enhance the tumor growth.

The ability of intravenously administered BCG to augment the suppressor-cell activity of normal bone marrow cells was demonstrated by Mitchell and his colleagues (39–42). Bone marrow cells of C57BL/6 mice inhibited the allogeneic antitumor (P815-Y) cytotoxic response of normal syngeneic spleen cells when the responder cells, the stimulator cells, and the bone marrow cells were cultured together. Bone marrow cells from mice intravenously injected with viable BCG exerted a stronger suppressive effect than their normal counterparts. The augmented suppressive activity of the bone marrow cells appeared 2 d after the BCG injection and on the seventh day, such activity also appeared among spleen cells (40). A course of cylophosphamide (CY; 60 mg/kg/d) given during the 4 d preceding or following the administration of BCG potentiated the induction of suppressor cells by BCG (41). The authors suggest that BCG not only augments the normal suppressor cell activity of the bone marrow, but also induces the migration of these cells into the spleen (40). Both macrophage-granulocyte-committed stem cells and suppressor cells were increased in the spleens by Tice BCG (but not by Phipps NC 734 BCG), and both were included in the same cellular subpopulation (42), suggesting that the suppressor cells were macrophages. This possibility was supported by the fact that the suppressor cells were found in the nylon wool-adherent cellular population (39,40) and were resistant to antithymocyte serum (ATS) and C (39). The appearance of suppressor cells in the spleens of BCG-injected mice was associated with an elevation of the number of splenic macrophages (from 0.5 to 12%; 42), suggesting that the suppressive effect may be attributed to both the macrophage population expansion and its activation.

Wepsic and colleagues (43–50) explored the effect of BCG cell walls (BCGcw) on the immune response of rats and mice and their ability to induce tumor rejection. They found that BCGcw enhanced the growth of Morris hepatoma (induced with N-2-fluorenyldiacetamide) in inbred rats (43). The effect of tumor enhancement was observed when BCGcw was injected 7 d before, at the same time, or 7 d after tumor inoculation (45). BCGcw prevented the induction of antitumor immunological rejection, but it failed to affect the rejection of tumor from rats that were immunized against this tumor before the BCGcw inoculation (45). The enhancement of the tumor growth was attributed to induction of suppressor macrophages by BCGcw.

Plastic-adherent cells from the spleens of rats injected with BCGcw suppressed, upon cocultivation, the Con A induced-proliferative response of normal spleen cells. In addition, removal of adherent cells enabled splenocytes of BCGcw-injected rats to mount an increased MLC (44,48). The MLC and the Con A mitogenic responses of rats injected with BCGcw and inoculated with tumor (which developed at an accelerated rate) were also markedly depressed. In such animals, restoration of the MLC activity by removal of the adherent cells was less effective than in animals injected with BCGcw alone (44).

The dualistic effect of BCG is clearly illustrated in the instance where BCGcw enhanced the subcutaneous growth of B16 melanoma in C57BL/6 mice, but diminished the number of tumor colonies after intravenous injection of the tumor. In addition, as in rats, BCGcw induces suppressor macrophages in mice, characterized as plastic-adherent, radiation-resistant (1300 rad), and insensitive to anti-T serum plus C. The suppressive activity was detected by the ability of the cells to inhibit the PHA mitogenic response of cocultivated normal spleen cells (49). The ability of suppressor macrophages induced with BCGcw (49) or viable BCG (38) respectively to inhibit the in vitro PHA (49) or Con A (38) mitogenic responses was further supported by experiments in vivo. X-irradiated (1000 rad) BCGcw-induced suppressor cells could inhibit, upon their adoptive transfer, splenomegaly (indicating graft v host reaction, GVHR) caused by the inoculation of normal parental C57BL/6 cells into (C57BL/6 × CBA)F$_1$ mice (47). Injection of indomethacin or aspirin, both inhibitors of prostaglandin (PG; usually referring to PGE_2) synthesis, restored the GVHR in mice transplanted with BCGcw-induced suppressor cells, suggesting that PG mediates the suppressive effect. The fact that BCGcw induces both the appearance of suppressor cells and an enhancement of tumor growth, and that the suppressor cells appear at the time when maximal immunological lymphoproliferation is observed, if tumor cells are inoculated alone, suggests a cause–effect relationship between the two phenomena (44).

The mechanism by which BCG-induced suppressor macrophages operate has been explored by Klimpel and colleagues (51–53). They found that the suppressor cells (macrophage-like adherent cells, 53) could inhibit not only the mitogen-induced proliferative responses and the primary and secondary allogeneic cytotoxic responses (51,52), but also the proliferation-independent differentiation of memory cells into effector cells. Mitomycin C (MMC)-treated spleen cells of mice injected with allogeneic cells developed a cytotoxic activity, after incubation with the homologous allogeneic cells, which was suppressed when spleen cells from BCG-injected mice were added into the culture (52). In contrast to the results of Wepsic and colleagues (44,48,49) discussed above, Klimpel and coworkers (53) found that membrane preparations of BCG did not induce appearance of suppressor cells. The suppressive activity could be induced by viable BCG that was injected intraperitoneally (51). The suppression was reversible, was not mediated by a suppressor factor (SF), and was effective only when the suppressor cells were added during the induction phase of the allogeneic cytotoxic response (53).

Spleen cells from BCG-injected mice suppressed the ability of normal spleen cells to produce or release a helper/amplifying factor when incubated with inactivated allogeneic cells (the activity of the helper/amplifying factor was measured by its ability to support the allogeneic cytotoxic response of responder T cells stimulated with ultraviolet-treated allogeneic cells). The ability of BCG-induced suppressor cells to inhibit the allogeneic cytotoxic response of cocultivated normal spleen cells could be overcome by addition into the culture of helper/amplifying factor, further supporting the notion that the suppressor macrophages inhibit the production or the release of this factor. Another possibility is that the BCG-induced macrophages modify the factor activity after its secretion from the helper cells, because helper/amplifying factor that was incubated at 37°C with a large number of BCG-induced suppressor cells lost its activity (53).

Whereas Klimpel and colleagues (53) found that killed BCG failed to induce suppressor cells, Allen and Moore (54) claimed that killed lyophilized BCG in an oil in saline emulsion stimulated the appearance of suppressor macrophages in C57BL/6 mice, but not in CBA mice (possibly because of genetic control). They found that plastic-adherent splenocytes [Thy-1 negative; immunoglobulin (Ig) negative] from C57BL/6 mice injected iv with killed BCG suppressed the PHA and the LPS mitogenic responses of cocultivated normal spleen cells (54,55). In addition, C57BL/6 mice reconstituted with such adherent cells failed to generate a delayed-type hypersensitivity (DTH) response against sheep red blood cells (SRBC, 55).

Again, in contrast to the findings of Klimpel and associates (53), Allen et al. (56) demonstrated that supernatants of the killed BCG-induced macrophages contained SF that inhibited the PHA mitogenic response, DTH response to SRBC, and the inflammation associated with the BCG injection. This last observation may represent a feedback control mechanism mediated by the suppressor macrophages. Whereas CBA spleen cells failed to produce or release SF, the PHA mitogenic response of their spleen cells was inhibited by SF derived from C57BL/6 splenocytes (56).

Despite the numerous reports demonstrating induction and activation of suppressor macrophages by BCG, others have shown that BCG stimulated the activity of suppressor T cells. Collins and Watson (36) found that iv injection of viable BCG induced in B6D2 mice suppressor cells that inhibited both antigen-specific and PHA mitogen-nonspecific proliferative responses. The suppressor cell activity was attenuated by MMC or anti-Thy-1 serum, and C treatments indicting that proliferating suppressor T cells are involved with the inhibition (36).

Payelle and colleagues (37) demonstrated that iv injection of viable BCG (1 mg, but not 0.05 mg) induced the appearance of suppressor T cells that inhibited the ability of immune T cells to neutralize MCA-induced fibrosarcoma (MC B6-1) in the Winn assay (the mixing of the suppressor cells with the immune T cells and their coinjection into recipient mice prevented the immune cells from inhibiting tumor growth in the recipients). The immune T cells were induced by injecting C57BL/6 mice with hybrid cells derived from fusion of MC B6-1 tumor cell with A9 C3H allogeneic fibroblastic cells or by surgical resection of the MCA tumor. T cells obtained from mice reconstituted with BCG-induced suppressor T cells (Thy-1$^+$, Lyt-1$^+$) and immunized against the tumor, were ineffective in the Winn assay. Injection of IL-2 into BCG treated mice partially reduced the suppressive activity induced by the microorganism, since immunization of such mice with the hybrid cells yielded relatively effective tumor-neutralizing cells (37). This experiment suggests, therefore, that cells producing IL-2 may be one of the targets for the BCG induced suppressor cells.

In another study (57), it was found that both T cells and macrophages of viable BCG-injected CBA mice produced SF (in contrast to the findings of Moore and colleagues, who failed to find a suppressive activity in the splenocytes of BCG-injected CBA mice; 54,56). Both SFs inhibited the Con A mitogenic responses of normal splenocytes, but they differed in their molecular weights and their biological properties. The T cell SF (mw 50,000–70,000) inhibited the Con A mitogenic responses only when added at the initiation of the culture, whereas the macrophages' SF (mw 10,000–30,000) was effective when added at any time during the culture. It was further found that the T cell SF suppressed the production or the release of IL-2 by Con A-stimulated splenocytes (57).

3. Induction of Suppressor Cells by *C. parvum* and Other Immunostimulants

Injection of *C. parvum*, particularly by an intravenous route, enhanced in certain instances the growth of either syngeneic MCA-induced tumors (58) or even allogeneic tumors, which are normally rejected (59), suggesting that *C. parvum* may induce a suppressive mechanism. The induction of nonspecific suppressor cells by *C. parvum* was reported in 1972 by Scott (60,61). He demonstrated that glass-adherent splenocytes, obtained from CBA mice iv injected with formalin-killed C. parvum (1.4 mg) 7 d beforehand, inhibited the PHA mitogenic response of cocultured normal splenocytes. Suppressor factor was not detected in the supernatants of the unstimulated or the PHA-stimulated splenocytes derived from *C. parvum*-injected mice (61), suggesting cell-to-cell contact as the mechanism of suppression. Injection of C. *parvum* also suppressed the murine DTH response to SRBC (62), as well as the ability to resist tumor growth after immunization with irradiated tumor cells (*25*). *C. parvum* injected into unimmunized mice conferred, however, various degrees of protection against different tumors (*25*).

The suppressive effect of *C. parvum* was confirmed by Kirchner and colleagues (*63*), who found that spleen cells from C57BL/6N mice injected ip with 2.1 mg formalin-killed *C. parvum* inhibited the mitogenic response of cocultivated normal splenocytes stimulated with PHA. The suppressor spleen cells could be removed by rayon columns and could engulf particulate iron or carrageenan (CAR; a sulfated polygalactans extract of algae that inactivates macrophages), but were not sensitive to anti-Thy-1 and C, indicating that they were macrophages (*63*). The *C. parvum*-induced suppressor macrophages also inhibited the growth in vitro of tumor cells (*63*) and the ability of stimulated splenocytes to produce migration inhibitory factor (MIF, *64*) and macrophage activating factor (MAF, *65*), as well as the ability to synthesize proteins (*66*). In addition, such macrophages exerted a direct cytotoxic effect against tumor cells (*65*), stressing again the dual effect of the suppressor cells induced with the immunostimulants. Lotzová (*67*) and Milisauskas et al. (*68*) demonstrated, in contrast to the findings of Ojo et al. (*69*), that *C. parvum* could induce suppressor cells with anti-NK cell activity. The suppressor cells of Lotzová (*67*) lacked the properties of macrophages or bursal-equivalent derived cells (B cells), and their T-cell characteristics were not completely defined. The discrepancy between Lotzová (*67*), Milisauskas et al. (*68*), and Ojo et al. (*69*) may be explained to some extent by the fact that the former groups injected formalin-killed bacteria, whereas the latter used heat-killed microorganisms.

Other studies found that cells, presumably macrophages obtained from *C. parvum*-injected mice, produced more PG than their similar normal counterparts (*70,71*), suggesting a mechanism of action for at least some of the *C. parvum*-induced suppressor cells. Other adjuvants that have been used in an attempt to augment immunological rejection of tumors may also induce suppressor cells. Mitogen-induced proliferation of mouse T and B lymphocytes was suppressed by plastic adherent cells (macrophages) derived from the peritoneal exudate cells (PEC) of pyran copolymer (a synthetic polyamine) treated mice. Corresponding normal PEC produced a less effective suppression (*72*). Similarly, nylon wool adherent Fc-receptor-bearing cells (presumably macrophages) from spleens, but not lymph nodes of mice treated with a precipitate of aluminum hydroxide suppressed the PHA mitogenic response of cocultured normal splenocytes (73). It should be stressed that the ability of adjuvant-injected mice to mount an anti-SRBC plaque forming cells (PFC) response or a cytotoxic response to allogeneic cells was enhanced rather than suppressed (73), implying that the detection of suppressor cells in vitro does not always reflect the immunological status of the animal. The widely used immunostimulator, complete Freund's adjuvant (CFA) may also enhance nonspecific suppressor cells in mice. Thus, spleen cells of CBF_1 mice injected with CFA enhanced, upon their adoptive transfer, the growth of SV40 transformed cells in the recipient mice, which otherwise generated an immune response and rejected the tumor. The suppressor cells did not adhere to nylon wool and were sensitive to anti-Thy-1 plus C treatment, indicating that they were T cells. This fact was confirmed in thymectomized mice treated with CFA, which in contrast to similarly treated sham-thymectomized mice rejected the inoculated tumor (74).

In contrast, spleen cells from A mice injected with CFA did not suppress in culture syngeneic antitumor cytotoxic cells generated against the MCA-induced S1509a fibrosarcoma (75). Suppressor cells were found, however, in spleen cells of mice inoculated with S1509a tumor and simultaneously injected with CFA. In fact, the activity of these suppressor cells was considerably greater than that of suppressor cells derived from TBH not injected with CFA. The suppressor cells lost their activity after treatment with anti-Thy-1 and C, and they failed to inhibit the cytotoxic cells induced with another syngeneic MCA tumor (Sal), indicating their thymic origin and specificity.

Whereas mice injected with MMC-treated S1509a tumor rejected a subsequent challenge of the homologous viable tumor, the growth of the tumor was enhanced in similarly treated mice that were also injected with CFA (75). These results emphasize not only the enhancement of the tumor growth associated with the CFA-potentiated suppressor cells, but more importantly, clearly demonstrate the lack of uniformity of the action of CFA, in one instance being immunostimulatory, and in another being immunosuppressive.

In contrast to CFA, injection of BCG-cw did not enhance the suppressor-cell activity in the spleen and the lymph nodes of A mice simultaneously inoculated with viable S1509a tumor. Injection of this immunomodulator, rather, augmented the cytotoxic activity of spleen and lymph node cells of mice simultaneously immunized with MMC-inactivated S1509a cells (76). Conflicting results demonstrating the ability of BCGcw to enhance suppressor-cell activity can be found in refs. 44, 48, and 49.

4. Conclusions

The inconsistent effect of the immunostimulants on the immune response and/or the fate of a tumor is probably the dominant feature of the reports reviewed in this section. Although under certain circumstances the immunostimulants activate or augment the immune responses, under different conditions they may induce a suppression. This variability in immune modulation reflects well, however, the clinical results utilizing immunostimulants where reports of beneficial effects are balanced by reports of inefficacy (19,26).

The physical properties of the immunostimulants, internal and external environmental factors, and the genetic background of the animal may determine the type of the immunological activity induced by the immunomodulators. Injection of the immunostimulant by an intravenous route and at relatively high doses increases, in certain instances, the tendency to enhance suppressor-cell activity in experimental animals. However, in many other instances, it is almost impossible to confidently predict how the immunostimulants would affect the tumor, and its enhancement rather than regression must be always taken into account.

In this respect, it should be indicated that certain drugs such as busulfan or mitomycin partially blocked in an experimental model the ability of BCGcw to enhance suppressor-cell activity or to accelerate tumor growth (50). Indomethacin, the PG synthetase inhibitor, reduced both the in vivo (47) and in vitro (50) activity of BCGcw-induced suppressor cells (see also ref. 77) and antagonized the BCGcw tumor enhancement effect (50), suggesting that PGs are the effector elements of the suppressor cells (for support, see ref. 78). Thus, combining such drug therapy with immunostimulants treatment may aid elimination of the suppressor cells activated by the immunostimulants, and consequently, their antitumor positive effects may dominate.

Control of Natural Killer
Cells by Suppressor Cells

1. Introduction

NK cells may develop cytotoxic activity against a variety of tumor cells, as well as against fetal fibroblasts, thymus cells, bone marrow cells, and microorganisms or microbially infected cells (6,23,79–81). Their activity has been observed mostly in vitro, detecting their ability to kill radiolabeled target cells in a short-term assay. Nevertheless, tests in vivo for NK-cell activity do exist; for example, the restoration of NK-cell activity in Cy-treated mice by systemic transfer of normal spleen cells may be detected by the ability of the recipient mice to clear radiolabeled tumor cells (82). The NK cells may have an important role in controlling the development of both normal and neoplastic cells (81). Since induction signals are not required for NK activity, they exert a rapid effect upon their target cells. As a result of this property, NK cells are considered as a first line of defense against malignancy. The validity of such a proposal remains, however, in doubt until it can be shown that NK cells are as effective against naturally occurring spontaneous tumors as they are against laboratory-induced tumors or their derivative cell lines.

Although NK cells are considered to be a distinct category of lymphocytes, they exhibit considerable heterogeneity. They do not carry distinctive B cell, T cell, or macrophage markers (see ref. 79, p. 277), (although the human NK cells may belong to T-cell lineage; 83), and do express receptors for the Fc portion of IgG (83). Human NK-cell activity is associated with a population of large lymphocytes exhibiting an indented nucleus and prominent cytoplasmic azurophilic granules (hence their designation as large granular lymphocytes, LGL; 23). In addition, human NK cells (84,85) and other cells (86) present the HNK-1 differentiation antigen. Other markers of the human NK cells are the HTLA and gp120, which are also presented on human T cells. Most murine

NK cells present the asialo-GM-1 marker, which appears also on some murine T cells (*see* ref. *79*, p. 278).

The function of the NK cells is regulated by both positive and negative signals. The activity of NK cells is augmented by interferon (INF; ususally referring to α-INF), INF inducers such as polyinosinic–polycytidilic acid (poly I:C), viruses, BCG or C. *parvum*, or by tumor cells susceptible to NK activity. Other factors that augment NK activity include diethylthiocarbamate, OK432, and ethanol (reviewed in *23*). NK activity may be reduced by PGs, phosphodiesterase inhibitors, or choloera toxin, probably by elevating the cyclic AMP level within the cells. The tumor promoter, phorbol myristate acetate (PMA), and human or rabbit monomeric IgG also provide negative signals for NK cell reactivity (reviewed in *23*). In addition to these various inhibitory direct effects, suppressor cells have been found also as down regulators of NK activity. Such suppressor cells will be the focus of interest in the following sections.

2. Activity of Anti-NK Suppressor Cells in Normal Animals

Since NK cells might play a role in regulating the development of normal haemopoietic and lymphoid tissues (*87–89*), it is not surprising that suppressor cells that perhaps control such NK-cell activity are found in normal infant and adult animals. Cudkowicz and Hochman (*81*) found that infant (8–15 d old) spleen cells of the mouse failed to develop NK-cell activity in contrast to spleen cells of adult (40 d old or more) mice. By mixing the infant spleen cells with adult spleen cells at ratios of 2:1 to 4:1, they showed that the former blocked the ability of the latter to cytolyze radiolabeled YAC-1 cells in a 4 h ^{51}Cr-release assay, suggesting that suppressor cells populate the infant spleen (*81*). These results were confirmed by Santoni et al. (*90*), who demonstrated that infant mice (9 or 11 d old) contain anti-NK nylon-adherent and nonadherent suppressor cells. Nasrallah et al. (*91*) failed to find anti-NK suppressor cells in infant mouse spleen, but they used a suppressor cell to NK cell ratio of 1:1, which may not be sufficient to detect suppressive activity (a ratio of 2:1 to 4:1 is usually required; *81,90*). The low NK-cell activity of aged mice cannot be attributed to suppressor cells (*90,91*), suggesting that other mechanisms are responsible for the depression of the NK function.

Some strains of mice (e.g., SJL/J, A/Hen, or ASW) develop a low level of NK-cell activity in comparison with other strains (e.g., C57BL/6, BD2F1, or CBA/J). The low NK-cell activity of SJL mice (and presumably of A/Hen and ASW mice) is associated with a suppressor-cell activity found in the spleen and the PEC of these mice (90,92). The SJL suppressor cells were characterized as Thy-1 negative adherent cells (92), but after in vitro cultivation, they were replaced by nonadherent cells (93). The activity of the SJL suppressor cells, assessed by their ability to inhibit C57BL/6 or BD2F1 NK cells, could be replaced by a soluble factor that they released (90,92). The possible role of SJL suppressor cells in inhibiting the NK-cell activity was supported by in vivo experiments (94). Cyclophosphamide-injected SJL mice failed to clear ^{125}IUdR-labeled YAC-1 cells from their lungs after reconstitution with CBA splenocytes expressing high NK-cell activity. In contrast, CY-injected BD2F1 or CBA mice (82,94) and 850 rad-irradiated CBA mice (94) were able to clear, at least partially, the radiolabeled tumor cells and expressed a higher NK-cell activity, after reconstitution with homologous spleen cells. These experiments suggest that suppressor cells of SJL mice antagonize the NK activity of the reconstituting cells. Indeed, SJL nylon adherent splenocytes blocked the ability of CBA spleen cells to reconstitute the clearance capacity of CY-treated CBA mice when both cellular populations were transplanted into the recipients (94). However, both the SJL and the CBA cells received mutual allogeneic antigenic stimuli, a fact that complicates the interpretation of the results.

The thymus (95,96) and the lymph nodes (96) of normal rats and mice develop low or negligible levels of NK-cell activity. However, removal of relatively high-density cells by Percoll density fractionation allowed expression of a moderate NK activity in the remaining low density cells (96,97), suggesting that suppressor cells reside in the high density cellular fractions of these organs. This assumption was confirmed by direct mixing experiments. Using the ^{51}Cr-release assay as a measure of cytotoxicity, the suppression of NK cells by high-density cells could be shown in both mice and rats by mixing high density cells, derived from the thymus and the lymph nodes, with low-density spleen cells containing the NK activity (96,97). High-density suppressor cells were found also in the spleen and the bone marrow of rats, but not in their PEC and the peripheral blood lymphocytes (PBL), explaining why these two latter organs exhibit relatively high NK-cell activity (96,97). It was further found that the suppressor cells, which were cortisone resistant, inhibited their target cells in a reversible manner, presumably via a cell-mediated contact mechanism (98). The results of earlier experiments (95) support the above mentioned finding. On velocity sedimentation of murine thymocytes, one of the relatively fast sedimenting fractions (4–5 mm/h) suppressed the ability of the spleen NK cells to kill radiolabeled YAC-1 or RL♂1 target cells. These suppressor cells, similarly to the Percoll fractionated suppressor cells (97,98), resisted 2000 rads and were genetically unrestricted (95). In contrast to the above findings, Brooks and Flannery (99) found that rat thymus and lymph nodes do not contain cells capable of suppressing NK cells, but since they did not test enriched cellular fractions (such as high-density cells) for suppressive activity, the basis for their conclusion may be doubted.

Although anti-NK suppressor cell activity was not found in the peritoneum of rats (96,97), such activity was detected in the peritoneal cavity of mice. The cells, which exhibited characteristics of macrophages, were found in the PEC of both normal and thymusless mice, indicating that the thymus is not the origin of the suppressor cells. A soluble factor released from the peritoneal macrophages may mediate the suppressive effect (90).

When the PEC suppressor cells are tested for their ability to prevent the killing of the ^{51}Cr-labeled YAC-1 cells in the standard [51]CR-release assay, high proportions (2:1–4:1) of suppressor cells to NK cells are required. However, prior inoculation (18 h) of nylon-wool-nonadherent spleen cells, expressing NK activity, with the peritoneal macrophages resulted in a more efficient suppressor-cell activity (100–103), which was expressed even using a suppressor to NK cell ratio of 1:30 (102,103). Such suppressor cells were observed even if INF was present during the 18 h preincubation in order to activate the NK cells. In contrast, 18 h preincubation of alloimmune cytolytic T cells with peritoneal macrophages did not affect their activity (101–103). It was further found that the suppressor cells were genetically unrestricted as indicated by their ability to suppress NK-cell activity of allogeneic cells (90,100,103). Injection of *C. parvum* into high NK reactive mice caused an augmentation of the peritoneal NK-cell activity, which was associated with a profound reduction in peritoneal NK-suppressor macrophage activity (90,102,103), indicating that under normal conditions the NK-suppressive function may exert a strong immunoregulatory activity. Normal thymus (*87,90*), bone marrow (*87*), and peritoneal cells (*104*), but not spleen cells (*87*), are sensitive targets for NK-cell activity. Therefore, it could be suggested that the cells in these organs are protected, to some extent, by suppressor cells.

3. Activation of Anti-NK Suppressor Cells by Irradiation or Treatment with Estrogen

Total body irradiation of animals, their total lymphoid irradiation (*105*), or local irradiation of their bone marrow with the bone-localizing isotope strontium-89 (^{89}Sr, *106*) may cause partial or complete destruction of the hemopoietic and the lymphoid areas exposed to the treatment. The gradual renewal of the lymphohematopoietic tissue in the irradiated areas may generate an environment similar to the developing immune system of the newborn. Indeed, such irradiated animals, like neonates (*81,107*), express a relatively high, nonspecific suppressor cell activity in lymphopoietic tissues (*81,106–109*). Concerning the local bone marrow irradiation with ^{89}Sr, it was suggested that such treatment may eliminate regulatory cells (M cells) that control the activity of suppressor cells (*110*).

Cudkowicz, Hochman, and Dausset (*81,107,111*) found that the splenocytes of ^{89}Sr-injected mice (*81,107*) or of 700 rad-γ-irradiated mice (*81,107,111*) contain, like splenocytes of newborn mice (*81,107*), reduced or negligible levels of NK cell activity 7–14 d after such treatments. One may speculate that the lack of NK-cell activity is associated with the expression of anti-NK suppressor cells. Indeed, suppressor cells in the spleens of the ^{89}Sr injected mice (*81,107*) and the γ-irradiated (*81,107,111*) mice could be detected by their ability to inhibit the anti-YAC-1 NK cell cytotoxicity of cocultivated normal splenocytes. However, since the restoration of the NK-cell activity of spleen cells from newborn, ^{89}Sr injected, or γ-irradiated mice was not demonstrated by separating away T cells or adherent macrophages (*81,107*), the existence of suppressor function in vivo is still a matter of debate. One possibility is that the irradiation procedures may eliminate precursors of NK cells in vivo and simultaneously induce suppressor cells that express their function in in vitro testing. The irradiation-induced-suppressor cells have been defined as "null" cells, since they neither displayed characteristics of B cells, T cells, nor of macrophages, and they were found in the nude mouse, indicating their thymus independency. In addition, the suppressor cells were insensitive to 2000 rad irradiation and genetically unrestricted (they suppressed NK-cell activity of allogeneic cells; *81,107*).

In contrast to Cudkowicz and Hochman (*81,107*), Kumar, Bennett, and associates (*112–117*) failed to find in (C57BL/6 × DBA/2)F1 (BD2F1) hybrid mice (the same strain used by Cudkowicz and Hochman) ^{89}Sr-induced anti-NK suppressor cells using both in vitro (mixing experiments) and in vivo tests and YAC-1 targets. For the in vivo test, spleen cells from ^{89}Sr treated mice, when adoptively transferred with normal splenocytes, failed to inhibit the ability of the normal cells to clear radiolabeled YAC-1 cells from the lungs of the recipient mice (*117*). [89]Sr injection induced, however, the appearance of suppressor cells capable of inhibiting the in vitro antibody response to SRBC (*108*). Although ^{89}Sr treatment failed to induce suppressor cells inhibiting anti-YAC-1 NK cells (NK-YAC-1 cells), it was found that such treatment induced the appearance of suppressor cells inhibiting natural cytotoxic (NC) cells directed against EL4 or FLD3 tumor cells. (FLD3 is a Friend-virus transformed erythroleukemia cell line.) However, the NK-YAC-1 cell differs from the NC cells directed against EL4 or FLD3 (designated NC-EL4 and NC-FLD3 cells, respectively) in that it is sensitive to radiation delivered by bone-localized [89]Sr (*118–120*). Hence, the cells directed against EL4 and FLD3 are termed natural cytotoxic cells rather than NK cells (*120*), and this may form the basis of differences in their sensitivities to suppressor cells.

The resistance of BD2F1 hybrid mice to the growth of a parental EL4 tumor may be attributed to the high level of NC-EL4 cells found in these mice (*119*). Injecting the hybrid mice with irradiated or viable EL4 cells, *C. parvum* or poly I:C elevated the level of the NC cells in their spleens. Interestingly, combining these treatments with prior ^{89}Sr-injection caused a considerable reduction in the NC-cell activity. Splenocytes of BD2F1 mice subjected to the combined treatment of ^{89}Sr and *C parvum* inhibited the NC-cell activity of cocultivated syngeneic normal spleen cells in the ^{51}Cr release assay (*119*). Injection of BD2F1 with the ^{89}Sr alone resulted in the loss of ability of these mice to reject parental

EL4 tumor cells (*119*). Together, these results suggest that ^{89}Sr-sensitive bone-marrow cells downregulate suppressor cells induced with *C. parvum* or EL4 cells. Elimination of these cells by ^{89}Sr injection released the suppressor cells from their arrest, and they could express their function against the NC-EL4 cells, resulting in the enhancement of tumor growth. If the suppressor cells are arrested (as in normal mice), the same stimulators (e.g., *C. parvum*) induce NC cell activity rather than suppression. Further support for this idea is provided by experiments demonstrating the activation of suppressor cells in ^{89}Sr-injected mice that suppressed the generation of anti-E14 cytotoxic cells in EL4 sensitized spleen cells (*119*). ^{89}Sr-activated suppressor cells expressing activity against NC-FLD3 cells were found also in mice injected with ^{89}Sr and infected with Friend virus (*114,120*).

Treatment with the female hormone estrogen also causes local changes in the marrow expressed by its replacement with bone (*121*). Such changes are associated with a decrease of NK-cell activity in the spleen (*120,122,123*) and the appearance of anti-NK suppressor cells (*123*). Nevertheless, results of a separate group (*122,124*) failed to demonstrate suppressor cells in the spleen of NZB/NZW and C57BL/6 mice after administration of estrogen.

4. Activation of Anti-NK Suppressor Cells by External Stimulators

Should the hypothesis that NK cells are a first line of defense against malignancy prove to be true, then investigation will clearly concentrate upon the use of externally introduced agents to augment NK-cell activity. *C. parvum* (an immunostimulator and possibly INF inducer; *20,125*) may enhance or inhibit (*67–69*) the NK-cell activity depending upon the interval between injection and assay (*67,68*), which organ was tested (*67,69*), and the route of the injection used (*69*). Intravenous injection of *C. parvum* inhibited NK-cell activity in CBA/H mice spleens, although intraperitoneal injection of this immunostimulator markedly enhanced the PEC natural cytotoxic response (*69*). The possibility that suppressor cells mediate the inhibitory effect of *C. parvum* has been investigated by several groups.

Milisauskas et al. (*68*) found that spleen cells from (C57BL/6 × C3H/He)F$_1$ (B6C3F1) mice injected with *C. parvum* inhibited the

NK-cell activity of cocultivated syngeneic splenocytes in the ^{51}Cr-release assay. The nature of the suppressor cells was not conclusively characterized in this study, although it was found that depletion of adherent phagocytic cells neither removed suppressor cell nor enriched NK-cell activity. However, the possibility cannot be ruled out that the suppression of NK activity observed in vitro does not function in vivo, and that C. parvum directly affects the activity of NK cells.

The anti-NK suppressor could be induced by C. parvum even after 500 rad total body irradiation or after neonatal thymectomy (68), suggesting that the suppression was not of T cell origin. These suppressor cells (68), as well as suppressor cells found in lymph nodes of normal mice (126), could also inhibit effector cells mediating antibody-dependent cellular cytotoxicity (ADCC), which are possibly identical with NK cells (127). The possibility that NK cells and cells mediating ADCC are, however, distinct populations is discussed elsewhere (128).

Santoni and colleagues (125) found in the spleens of C. parvum-injected mice two types of anti-NK-YAC-1 suppressor cells: macrophage-like cells expressing adherent and phagocytic properties and nylon and plastic nonadherent cells lacking Thy-1 and GM-1 markers (GM-1 is an NK cell marker; 129,130). This latter type of cells was designated "null" cells. In addition, the supernatant of C. parvum-induced suppressor cells contained an SF, inhibiting the NK-cell activity (125). Conflicting with the results described before (68), it was found that the suppression was thymus dependent, as indicated by the fact that adherent suppressor cells were not detected in the spleens of athymic nude mice injected with C. parvum (125). Although C. parvum activates suppressor cells in the spleens, it reduces the normal anti-NK suppressor-cell function in the peritoneum (90), an event associated with elevated NK-cell activity in PEC (125).

In agreement with the observation that the suppressor cells are thymus dependent, Lotzová (67) provides some evidence that the anti-NK suppressor cells induced by C. parvum are T cells. The suppressor cells were found in the nylon-wool-nonadherent fraction, and they were partially inactivated with anti-Thy-1 and C. Finally, in contrast to all the previous reports, Ojo et al. (69) and Brunda et al. (103) failed to find any anti-NK suppressor cells in the spleens of C. parvum-injected mice, in spite of the low level of NK-cell activity. In the experiment described by the former of these negative reports (69), however, much lower doses of C.

parvum (0.1 mg) were injected into the mice than was used by other groups (0.4–2.1 mg), and the spleen cells tested for suppressive activity, although H-2 compatible, were allogeneic to the NK cells, possibly explaining the conflicting results. In the experiment described in the second of these reports (*103*), only the adherent splenocytes were tested for suppression, although it is possible that suppressive activity was located in the nonadherent cells.

BCG, like *C. parvum*, exerts a dual effect upon NK cells, enhancing (*131*; maybe via induction of INF, *132,133*) or inhibiting (*see below*) NK cell activity. Intraperitoneal injection of BCG into mice caused a decrease in splenic NK cell activity against YAC-1, the appearance of splenic anti-NK plastic-adherent suppressor cells, and an elevation of NK-cell activity in the peritoneum. Migration of NK cells from the spleen into the peritoneum could not account for the altered NK-cell distribution, because splenectomy did not affect the augmentation of peritoneal NK activity after administration of BCG. The inhibition of NK cells was not mediated by cells bearing receptors to the Fc portion of Ig, as indicated by the fact that elimination of cells formed rosettes with SRBC coated with IgG anti-SRBC (EA-rosettes) did not affect the suppression (*128*).

Pyran copolymer, a synthetic polyamine, is both a powerful stimulator of the reticuloendothelial system (*134*) and an inducer of INF production (*135*), and clearly affects the regulation of NK cells. In general, it enhances the NK-cell activity in instances where such activity is weak and depresses NK activity in instances where NK function is strongly expressed (*136*). Thus, pyran enhances the splenic NK function of young (3–4-wk-old) or old (over 12-wk-old) mice, which develop a low level of NK-cell activity, but it inhibits the splenic NK function of young adult (4–8-wk-old) mice, which present an efficient NK-cell activity (*136–138*). Similarly, pyran enhances the weak NK-cell activity of the peritoneum of young and aged mice. The depression of splenic NK-cell activity by pyran copolymer is found in mouse strains expressing a high NK-cell activity, but not in strains (e.g., SJL) of low NK-cell activity (*136,138*). The enhancement or depression of NK-cell activity induced by pyran injection correlates with the ability of pyran-injected mice to clear radiolabeled tumors from their lungs (*136*).

The depression of NK-cell activity induced in young adult (4–8-wk-old) mice by pyran copolymer is associated with the acti-

vation of macrophages expressing an antitumor cytostatic effect
in vitro (*139*). These activated macrophages may be responsible
for the suppression of the NK-cell function, particularly as the NK
activity of splenocytes derived from pyran-injected 8-wk-old mice
is improved after removal of nylon-wool-adherent cells (*139*).
Similarly, splenocytes from pyran-injected young adult mice depressed the anti-YAC-1 NK activity of cocultivated syngeneic normal spleen cells in a ^{51}Cr-release assay. The suppressor cells were
characterized as being plastic-adherent, phagocytic, resistant to
5000 rad, and Thy-1 negative, supporting the notion that they
were macrophages (*136,137,140,141*). The suppression of the NK
cells may be mediated by released factors rather than direct cell-
to-cell contact, since it could also be achieved using soluble factors
released from the suppressor cells (*140*). The adherent suppressor
cells induced by pyran disappear by 2 wk after injection, but the
NK-cell activity remains depressed for a considerably longer period (*136*). Thus pyran may also directly affect NK cells or NK accessory cells (*139*). An alternative possibility is that the suppressor cells may not only block mature NK cells, but also their
precursors. Thus, there is a lag between disappearance of suppressor cells and reappearance of mature NK cells. A low level of
suppressor cells that are not detected by the in vitro assay, but are
still active in vivo may be another explanation for the late suppression of the NK cells.

Since pyran copolymer may exert antagonistic effects, depending on the status of the NK cells, it may be affecting a general
regulatory mechanism of NK cell function. High NK activity is
sensitive to suppressor cells, but resistant to the NK stimulatory
effects mediated by agents such as INF (*136*). In contrast, low NK
activity is quite sensitive to stimulating mediators, but resistant to
suppressive effects (as mentioned before, pyran copolymer can
stimulate both INF production and the appearance of suppressor
cells).

Adriamycin, a potent antitumor chemotherapeutic agent, enhanced the NK-cell activity in the peritoneum, the bone marrow,
and the lymph nodes, but inhibited NK-cell activity in the spleen
(*136,142*). Maximal inhibition was found 3 d after the drug injection, and on the ninth day, the levels of NK activity returned to
normal level (*142*). Removal of nylon-adherent cells from
splenocytes of adriamycin-injected mice enhanced their NK-cell
activity, suggesting that adherent cells mediate the suppressive
effect. Indeed, plastic adherent (presumably macrophages)

splenocytes of mice injected 3 d earlier with adriamycin inhibited the NK-cell activity of normal syngeneic spleen cells when incubated with them during the ^{51}Cr release assay (*136,142*).

Cudkowicz and associates (*81,107,143*) reported that CAR and hydrocortisone (*107,144*; anti-inflammatory steroid) induced in B6C3F1 mice suppressor cells that inhibited NK-cell activity when mixed with them at ratios of 2:1–4:1 during the ^{51}Cr-release assay. The supernatants of the incubated suppressor cells also inhibited the NK-cell activity (*143,144*). In vitro incubation of spleen cells with CAR induced appearance of nonspecific suppressor cells inhibiting, in the cytotoxic assay, both NK cells (*145*) and cytotoxic T cells (*146*). The NK-cell activity of splenocytes from CAR- or hydrocortisone-treated mice was restored by removing with a magnet cells that had phagocytosed carbonyl iron (*107,143,144*) or by removing glass wool-adherent cells (*143*). These experiments suggest that macrophage-like cells mediate both the in vivo and in vitro suppressive effects.

Although INF under normal conditions delivers positive signals to NK cells (*147*), it can induce under other circumstances negative signals that are possibly mediated by T cells (*148*). Preincubating normal spleen cells or spleen cells from nude athymic mice with INF, washing the cells, and then culturing them for 7 d with IL-2 and feeder cells increases the frequency of NK preeffector cells as measured by the limiting dilution assay (LDA). However, addition of INF directly into the cultures (containing IL-2 and homologous feeder cells) decreases the frequency of NK cell preeffectors among normal splenocytes, but increases the frequency of NK cell preeffectors among nude mouse splenocytes. Addition of irradiated feeder thymocytes from normal mice into cultures of nude mice splenocytes decreases, in the presence of INF, the frequency of NK preeffector cells, similar to the effect of INF upon normal splenocytes (*148,149*). Thus INF delivers, in the in vitro culture, negative signals to NK cells when T cells are present.

The effect of Friend virus infection on the induction of anti-NK suppressor cells has been explored in the murine system. Early reports indicated that inoculation of Friend leukemia virus (FLV) into DBA/2 mice induced in the mice appearance of suppressor cells inhibiting the ability of cocultured normal splenocytes to respond to Con A (*150*), whereas inoculation of its polycythemic variant (FLV-P) activated suppressor cells inhibiting the ability of normal cells to generate cytotoxic cells in vitro against allostimulator cells (*151*). The suppressor cells induced by FLV-P were characterized as macrophages (*151*).

In subsequent, studies Migliorati and colleagues (*152,153*) found that FLV-P induced in DBA/2 mice suppressor cells that inhibited splenic NK cell activity, but such suppression was only evident 14 d after virus inoculation. Initially, splenic NK-cell activity was elevated. The NK-cell activity of normal BALB/c-nu/nu splenocytes was markedly reduced when they were cocultivated during the ^{51}Cr release assay with spleen cells from FLV-P infected mice, expressing depressed NK-cell function. The cells suppressing the NK-cell activity were operationally defined as "null" cells, since they were insensitive to treatment with anti-Thy-1 and C, or to γ-irradiation, and they adhered to nylon and sephadex G-10, but did not adhere to plastic (*153*). The possibility that the suppression seen in the ^{51}Cr-release assay is an artifact mediated by unlabeled target cells (derived from the virus-infected mice) competing with the labeled target cells was excluded. The pattern of inhibition developed by splenocytes from FLV-P-infected mice was quite different from that generated by unlabeled YAC-1 cells competing with labeled YAC-1 cells as targets for NK cells. Furthermore, the splenocytes of infected mice underwent minimal lysis during a 4-h ^{51}Cr-release assay, suggesting they were not acting as "cold" competitors (*153*).

Pettey and Collins (*154*) demonstrated that DBA/2 mice passively protected against FLV-induced leukemia by administration of heterologous antisera against disrupted virion did not develop anti-NK suppressor cells after virus infection. However, the splenic NK cells of these mice, as those of normal mice, were susceptible to the suppressive effect of cocultured splenocytes of FLV-infected, but not protected mice. Exogenous FLV added into the mixture of NK cells and their YAC-1 targets did not inhibit the lysis of the target cells, indicating that the virus is not directly responsible for the suppressive effect. Antisera against T cells, B cells, macrophages, and gp71 failed to abolish the activity of the FLV-induced anti-NK suppressor cells. In addition, the suppressor cells did not adhere to Sephadex G-10 and were distributed among both nylon-wool-adherent and nonadherent cells. Since the suppressor cells did not fit with any previously defined cell category, they were defined as "null" cells. In contrast to the above-mentioned authors (*153,154*), Moody and coworkers (*155,156*) claimed that FLV activated in BALB/c mice anti-NK suppressor macrophages (nylon wool-, Sephadex G-10-, and plastic-adherent) that were sensitive to indomethacin treatment (*156*), suggesting that PG mediate the suppressive effect.

5. Activity of Anti-NK Suppressor Cells in TBH

The serum concentrations of PG are elevated in mice bearing Lewis lung carcinoma (LLC;*157*), suggesting that either the tumor itself secretes this potentially immunosuppressive factor or it stimulates other cells to produce it. Leung and associates (*158*) found that spontaneous production of PG by plastic adherent human monocytes is remarkably enhanced after their incubation with the K562 tumor cell line, which itself does not produce PGs. Other human tumor lines also enhanced the production of PG by monocytes when cocultured with them, but not to such a great extent. A supernatant from a K562 tumor cell culture was capable of inducing monocytes to synthesize PG, while a supernatant from a culture of monocytes failed to induce K562 tumor to produce PG, indicating that the monocytes but not the tumor cells are the major source of PG. The PG production was suppressed by cyclooxygenase inhibitors (indomethacin, aspirin, and eicosatetraynoic acid) and protein synthesis inhibitors (cycloheximide, puromycin, and emetine). The authors suggest that this model elucidates a possible escape route for the tumor cells, subverting the host immunosurveillance.

Young and colleagues (*157*) described the interrelationships between the rise of circulating PG in the TBH and the fall of NK-cell activity in these animals, in association with the tumor (LLC) progression. The concentrations of plasma PG were elevated as the LLC progressed (*157,159*) and the NK-cell activity simultaneously declined (*157*). Both tumor cells (*157,159*; and *see also* ref. *160*) and TBH macrophages produced the PG. Depletion of plastic-adherent macrophages from the TBH splenocytes restored the NK cell activity, and their addition to normal spleen cells resulted in suppression of the NK cells. This suppression could be prevented if indomethacin was added to the cellular mixture. Oral administration of indomethacin to the TBH prevented the elevation of the plasma PG and the suppression of NK-cell activity (*157*). This treatment slowed the progression of the tumor, especially during the initial stages (*157,159*). When the tumor attained a large size, the mechanism of suppression underwent a change. The plasma PG concentrations declined, indomethacin treatment no longer prevented the suppression of NK cell activity, and depletion of splenic macrophages did not restore NK cytotoxicity (*157*).

It should be stressed, however, that the NK-cell activity was measured in this study on YAC-1 target cells rather than on the LLC target. As a result, it was not determined whether the enhanced NK-cell activity induced with indomethacin also reflects enhanced NK-cell activity against LLC or if this treatment also induced an alternative immunological mechanism that independently affected the tumor. In conclusion, it is possible that, at least in some cases, the progression of the tumor in the animal is associated with an elevation of PG concentration, which causes depression of various functions of the immune system, including the NK-cell activity. The PGs are produced either by the tumor itself (*160*) or by tumor-stimulated monocytes (reviewed in *161,162*). Treatment of such tumor hosts, especially at an early stage of tumor progression, either with PG synthetase inhibitors or with agents toxic to macrophages may permit destruction of the tumor by reactivated effector cells including the NK cells.

Gerson and colleagues (*163–165*) found that the systemic and *in situ* NK-cell activities were considerably depressed in CBA and C57BL/6 mice bearing progressively growing murine sarcoma virus (MSV)-induced tumors. Removal of plastic-adherent cells or iron-ingesting cells (with a magnet) from the cellular population of the tumor significantly increased the NK cell activity, suggesting that suppressor macrophages are responsible for the inhibitory effect. In agreement with this proposal, it was found that the NK activity of splenocytes from normal CBA mice was inhibited when they were mixed at 4:1 ratio with plastic-adherent cells derived from progressive tumors of CBA mice. The suppressor cells resisted anti-Thy-1 serum plus C, but they were eliminated by plastic adherence or by magnetic removal of iron-ingesting cells, confirming that they were macrophages (*164,165*). A different study (*166*) reported that TBH systemic suppressor cells inhibiting natural cytotoxicity displayed similar characteristics. In contrast to the results in mice, NK-cell activity was not found in human tumor sites even after removal of adherent cells or in vitro incubation with INF, although such activity was detected in the patients' peripheral blood (*163*).

6. Mechanisms

Although the activity of NK cells against sensitive target tumor lines has been demonstrated by experiments in vivo (*82*), the hypothesis that NK cells may be important as effectors in surveillance against malignancy (*6*) is not yet supported by solid experimental findings. The NK cells are exceedingly heterogeneous in their properties, and therefore, demonstration of in vivo NK cell activity against, for example, YAC-1, does not necessarily imply that a similar activity exists against a relevant tumor. In fact, just the reverse has been reported; whereas NK activity was detected against YAC-1, no NK activity against the tumor actually growing in the animal (FLV-P-induced leukemia, in this instance) could be found in DBA/2 mice (*153*). As a result, tumor progression (in this instance induced by FLV-P infection), even if followed by a decrease of anti-YAC-1 NK-cell activity, cannot be attributed to NK cell disfunction. On the other hand, the failure to detect NK-cell activity against standard tumor cell targets (e.g., YAC-1) does not necessarily indicate that a different NK-cell population with, perhaps, different specificities and properties is not active against the growing tumor. Consequently, it is still not known if NK-cell activity is an important defense system against malignancy, or if it is an expression of limited function only detected under experimental conditions.

How the suppressor cells recognize their target NK cells remains in question, and our knowledge of the mechanism of inhibition is very limited (*see* ref. *167*). The anti-NK suppressor cells are quite heterogeneous with regard to their cellular lineage and their sensitivity to various treatments. Some of them have been characterized as macrophages, whereas others were defined as T cells or "null" cells. Some suppressor cells release suppressor factors, and others require cell-to-cell contact in order to exert their function. Clearly, heterogeneity of NK cells is the basis for heterogeneity in inhibitory mechansism.

Proving the suppressive activity of macrophages and planning their elimination in order to augment the NK-cell activity, we must remember that macrophages are also required to maintain both the endogenous and the INF-induced NK-cell activities (*168*). Thus, they manifest a dual effect, maintenance and suppression of NK cells. The final outcome is possibly determined by quantitative and qualitative factors. It should not be surprising, however, if removal of marcophages causes reduction in the NK activity rather than the expected augmentation.

The possibility that the inhibition of the NK-cell activity is not mediated by suppressor cells, but rather the cells compete with the NK cell by binding to the target cells without lysing them has been proposed (*93*). Cudkowicz and Hochman (*81,107*) suggested that the "null" suppressor cells of infant or irradiated mice are immature pre-NK cells that possess receptors capable of recognizing and binding to the target cells without causing their lysis. Thus, the immature pre-NK cells may competitively inhibit cytolysis normally caused by mature NK cells. If correct, it might be possible to show that such pre-NK "suppressor cells" form conjugates (*169*) with their target cells, or that anti-NK cell serum (asialo GM-1, for example) and C inhibit the "suppressor-cell" function (such a treatment failed, however, to inhibit anti-NK suppressor cells induced with estrogen, *123*; or with FLV, *154*). Competition as a mechanism gains no support from the observation that the inhibition pattern of NK cells by suppressor cells is different from the inhibition pattern expressed by cotarget competition (*153*).

It is possible that, rather than suppressing, the suppressor cells eliminate NK cells. Zöller and Wigzell (*98*) demonstrated, however, that the suppressor cells do not kill the NK cells, but rather exert a reversible inhibition. When high-density thymic suppressor cells were mixed with low-density splenic NK cells, suppression of NK-cell activity was observed. However, refractionation of this cellular mixture on Percoll and removal of the high-density fraction allowed the low-density cells to reexpress their cytotoxic activity against target cells.

Prostaglandins may play a role in the suppression of NK cells (reviewed in *161*). Prostaglandin increases the intracellular level of cyclic AMP, which in turn may inhibit phospholipase activity, leaving the cell refractory to further activation. In addition to the many immunological functions that are inhibited by PGs, including allograft rejection, the primary in vitro antibody response to SRBC, the proliferative responses initiated by antigens or mitogens as well as the production of MIF (reviewed in *161,170,171*), prostaglandins may also inhibit NK cells (*172–176*).

Since macrophages can synthesize and release PGs (*177–181*) and macrophages inhibit NK-cell activity (*102,140,142*), it is possible that their suppressive effect is mediated by PGs. Anti-NK suppressor macrophages found in mice bearing MSV-induced tumors (*165*) may be included in this category, because it was reported that such mice produce increased amounts of PG (*182,183*) and express low levels of NK activity (*184,185*). Administration of PG synthetase inhibitors (e.g., indomethacin or aspirin) to mice bearing the MSV-induced tumors restored partially or completely their NK-cell activity (*175,176*). Moreover, supplementing drinking water with indomethacin prevented tumor progression in mice inoculated with MSV (*176*). The experimental evidence presented above, however, is based upon an overall summation of findings gathered from diverse sources, but a real association of macrophages, PGs, and depressed NK function remains to be demonstrated in a single system.

Further support for the possible role of PG released from suppressor macrophages in inhibiting NK-cell activity was presented by Parhar and Lala (*186*). These authors demonstrated that spleen cells of CBA/J mice inoculated with Ehrlich ascites tumor or C3H/HeJ mice bearing spontaneous mammary tumors or transplanted with syngeneic mammary tumor line of recent origin contained suppressor macrophages with anti-NK-cell activity. Splenocytes from such TBH, when mixed with normal spleen cells for 20 h, abolished the NK-cell activity of the latter cells. The suppressor-cell activity was found in the plastic-adherent population of the TBH spleen cells, which were further characterized by the ability to phagocytose latex particles and to bind Mac-1 monoclonal antibody (Mac-1 is a marker of murine macrophages). Addition of indomethacin into the cellular mixture of the normal and the TBH splenocytes restored its NK-cell activity. Similarly, Young and colleagues (*157*) demonstrated that macrophages of LLC-bearing mice suppressed the NK-cell activity of cocultivated normal spleen cells. Administration of indomethacin to the TBH prevented both the appearance of PG in the serum and the depression of NK-cell activity. These last two experimental models highly suggest that the suppression of the NK-cell activity is mediated by PG released from macrophages. Nevertheless, natural cytotoxicity downregulated by suppressor cells is not always completely restored by PG synthetase inhibitors, and sometimes it is not affected by them at all (*187*), indicating that PG released from suppressor macrophages is not the only mediator of the suppressive effect.

7. Suppression or Artifact?

Studying anti-NK suppressor cells, Hochman and Cudkowicz (*144*) carefully investigated various sources of errors. Invariably, the assay of NK activity used is the ^{51}Cr-release from cytolysed cells. One possibility investigated was that supposed suppressor cells were simply reutilizing released ^{51}Cr, giving artificially low cytotoxicities. However, reutilization of released ^{51}Cr could not be demonstrated when the radioactive label was added to the suppressor cells. Furthermore, factors released by the suppressor cells were shown not to reduce release of ^{51}Cr from target cells, indicating that the target cell membranes were not stabilized by these factors. The "crowding effect" was excluded by showing that thymocytes incubated with NK cells instead of suppressor cells failed to affect the NK-cell activity.

The conclusion that the TBH cellular population does not contain suppressor cells just because these cells failed to suppress the NK-cell activity when administered to the short NK-cell assay might be wrong. Parhar and Lala (*186*) clearly demonstrated that administration of the suppressor cells to the NK-cell assay did not inhibit the lysis of the target cells above the dilution effect, whereas preincubation of the suppressor cells with the NK cellular population for 20 h abolished its ability to lyse the target cells in the subsequent short cytotoxicity assay. These results suggest that the suppressor cells should be activated under the culture conditions before expressing their effector function, or alternatively, that the precursors of the NK cells, and not the mature NK cells, are sensitive to the suppressor-cell activity. Mixing preincubated suppressor cells with unincubated NK cellular populations in the ^{51}Cr release assay, or, conversely, mixing preincubated NK cellular populations with unincubated suppressor cells may resolve this question.

8. Suppressor Cells Controlling NK-Cell Activity in Human Beings

The blood of healthy individuals contains suppressor cells, which may regulate NK-cell activity, but their function is hardly detected unless they are enriched by various purification procedures. Percoll gradient separated blood small lymphocytes of some healthy donors suppressed the NK-cell activity of cocultivated autologous blood LGL. Higher proportions of individuals with suppressor-cell function were found if the small lymphocytes were further fractionated with antibody-coated erythrocytes (EA rosettes), and the resultant Ig-Fc receptor-bearing cells were tested for suppressive activity. Several individuals presented suppressor cells not bearing Fc-Ig receptors. Most of the EA$^+$ suppressor cells bore the OKT-3 phenotype marker indicting their T cell origin. These suppressor cells lost, however, at least part of their activity after preincubation with INF (*188*). A similar type of EA$^+$ small lymphocyte with anti-NK-cell suppressive activity was found in the umbilical-cord blood (*189*). Most importantly, the proportions of peripheral blood anti-NK suppressor cells among patients with epidermoid carcinomas of the upper respiratory tract, adenocarcinomas of the kidney, and ovarian carcinomas were somewhat lower than among healthy donors, suggesting that in these cases the depression of NK-cell activity by suppressor cells was not associated with the malignant state (*188*). An alternative way of purifying peripheral blood cells capable of suppressing NK cells is to absorb them on monolayers of the bacteria *Bacillus globigii*. The cells released from the monolayers (designated T_2 cells) suppressed the NK-cell activity of cocultivated autologous PBL. The activity of the NK cells was not changed when they were cocultivated with nonviable lymphocytes, autologous red blood cells (RBC), or cellular subpopulations depleted of T_2 cells, indicating that dilution or crowding effects were not associated with the reduced NK-cell activity. It was further evidenced that the decrease in NK-cell activity was not the result of contamination by small numbers of bacteria or of a simple competition by T_2 cells for the binding sites of the target cells (*190*).

Normal individuals' granulocytes isolated from the top of the red cells pellet after separation of a buffy coat over a Ficoll-

Hypaque gradient also suppressed the NK cell activity of cocultivated autologous or allogeneic PBL. The suppression was effective if granulocytes were added to lymphocytes-K562 conjugates immediately after their formation or for up to 60 min afterwards, but if added after more than 60 min had elapsed, then there was no suppression of NK cell activity, estimated by the chromium release assay. This latter finding, indicating that the suppression mediated by granulocytes was not artifactual resulting from their ingestion of released chromium, was further supported by the observation that addition of granulocytes directly to the radiolabeled target cells did not alter their spontaneous chromium release. The inhibition was not the result of competition with NK cells for binding sites on the target cells, since granulocytes killed by heating maintained their capacity to inhibit NK-cell activity despite losing their ability to adhere to surfaces. Moreover, since NK cells did not develop any cytotoxicity against chromium-labeled granulocytes, nor could they bind to heat-treated granulocyte targets, it is unlikely that the granulocytes were acting as an alternative target for the NK cells. Apparently, structurally intact granulocytes were required for the suppression, since potential granulocytic products such as PGs, oxygen radicals, proteases, and ferroproteins could not reproduce the suppressive effect (*191–193*).

Suppressor cells inhibiting autologous or allogeneic NK-cell activity were found among unfractionated PBL cultured alone for 72 h prior to their addition to the NK cell cytotoxic assay. The presence of Con A during the PBL preincubation further augmented their suppressive activity (*194*). A complicating factor that often needs to be taken into account during such precultures is the possibility that the fetal calf serum (FCS) used in the culture may activate suppressor cells, as has been shown previously (*195*). The inhibition of NK-cell activity by the cultured induced suppressor cells was not, however, associated with crowding, cell death, steric hindrance, generation of cytotoxic cells against the effector cells, or competition between the cultured cells and the target cells for interaction with the effector cells (*194*).

In contrast to the peripheral blood, bone marrow does not contain an appreciable NK-cell activity. The bone marrow collected from the ribs of patients undergoing thoracotomy contains, however, plastic adherent cells, suppressing the INF-induced NK-cell activity of cocultured autologous PBL. The noninducible NK-cell activity of PBL was not suppressed by the adherent cells

(196,197). Interestingly, the bone marrow of patients with myeloma contains a high NK activity and does not contain suppressor cells with anti-NK-cell function *(197,198)*, this being the reverse of the situation found in normal bone marrow. The strong suppressor function directed against NK cells in normal bone marrow may be aimed at preventing local natural cytotoxicity against normal cells. If this concept is correct, autoreactivity mediated by NK cells may be detected in the bone marrow of patients with myeloma.

Lung mononuclear cells, similarly to bone marrow cells, express very low levels of natural cytotoxicity. Removal of plastic- and nylon-adherent cells or carbonyl iron-ingesting cells significantly enhanced the NK-cell activity of the lung cells and, to an even greater extent, augmented the natural cytotoxicity induced with INF *(199)*, suggesting that macrophages control these cellular functions. In agreement with this prediction, it was further found that bronchoalveolar macrophages suppressed the NK-cell activity of cocultivated autologous PBL. The suppressive effect was revealed even at a suppressor–effector ratio of 1:8, indicating its efficiency. The INF-induced NK-cell activity of the PBL was suppressed by the alveolar macrophages to the same extent as the noninducible NK-cell activity *(200,201)*. Peripheral blood NK cells, suppressed by a low concentration of alveolar macrophages, could have their NK-cell activity restored if carbonyl iron-ingesting cells were subsequently removed by a magnet. In contrast, the activity of NK cells suppressed by a high concentration of macrophages could not be restored by removal of carbonyl iron-ingesting cells *(200)*. The alveolar macrophages could not be killed by NK cells *(201)*, indicating that the macrophages were not acting as alternative targets and thus reducing the activity against chromium-labeled target cells.

A possible association between malignancy and expression of suppressor cells with anti-NK cell-activity has been suggested by De Boer and associates *(202)*, who found that cancer patients with disseminated disease expressed lower levels of blood NK-cell activity than normal individuals or patients with local diseases. The low level of NK-cell activity could be associated with suppressor cell activity, since removal of glass-adherent cells from the blood cellular population improved the level of natural cytotoxicity *(202)*. Surprisingly, Uchida and Micksche *(203)* found that the level of anti-NK suppressor cells (plastic adherent) is raised after tumor surgery.

The possibility that soluble factors released from the suppressor cells (or from the tumors themselves, 204) mediate the inhibition of NK cell function has been explored by several groups. Blood mononuclear cells (MNC) of normal individuals incubated for 4 d in serum-free medium released into the supernatant an SF that inhibited the NK-cell activity of allogeneic blood lymphocytes. Removal of monocytes from the MNC did not affect the release of the SF from the residual lymphocyte population (205). The SF exerted maximal suppression, not a cytotoxic effect, 72 h after its incubation with effector lymphocytes. Gel filtration of the SF on Sephacryl S-200 revealed that the suppressive activities were associated with two molecular sizes, one between 13,700 to 25,000 daltons and the other smaller than 13,700 daltons. NK cells suppressed by the factor could have their activity restored by a 24-h incubation with INF. The monosaccharides α-methyl-D-mannoside and L-fucose coincubated with SF and effector lymphocytes blocked in a dose-dependent fashion the inhibitory activity of the factor (205), from which it could be deduced that the SF and the sugars compete for the same receptors on the NK cells. An independent study (206) found that preincubation of blood MNC for 18 h was not sufficient to obtain a high level of SF with anti-NK-cell activity. However, preincubation of monocytes, isolated by plastic adherence, with ploy-I:C stimulated a secretion of a high amount of SF that suppressed the NK-cell activity in the chromium release assay. In this system, the SF was identified as PG by radioimmunoassay, corroborated by the observation that monocytes preincubated with poly-I:C and indomethacin failed to produce the SF. In contrast, the nonadherent cells incubated with poly-I:C released into the supernatant an INF that, on preincubation with effector cells, increased their NK activity. In fact, the poly-I:C could not induce maximal NK activity, since it induced not only a release of INF-potentiating NK activity, but also a production of PGs antagonizing the INF effect. The potentiating effect of poly-I:C-induced INF could be fully expressed if the release of PG was blocked by addition of indomethacin to the culture. These results suggest that poly-I:C or INF treatment of cancer patients may achieve greater efficacy if indomethacin is also added to the treatment protocol.

This study (206) emphasizes a further point of interest. Removal of monocytes from the blood MNC population enhanced the NK-cell activity of the residual nonadherent cells. This effect was associated, however, with the enrichment of the effector population, rather than with the removal of cells with suppressive potential. Readdition of monocytes to the nonadherent cells did not inhibit their NK-cell activity. The monocytes express their suppressive activity only when exposed to a stimulator such as poly-I:C (*206*).

Addition of PG to assays of human NK cells inhibited the cytotoxic activity of the effector cells, but pretreatment of the cellular population containing the NK-cell activity with INF (for 3 h) or poly-I:C partially prevented this effect. Similarly, spleen cells from mice injected with poly-I:C expressed partial resistance to the in vitro anti-NK-cell effect of PG (*207,208*), indicating again that external manipulations may change the balance between positive and negative signals affecting NK-cell activity.

The kinetics of PG effect on INF-induced NK-cell activity was explored in an independent study (*209*). Addition of PG 5, 10 and 20 min after the addition of INF not only prevented the enhancing effect of INF, but also inhibited the residual NK-cell activity. If the addition of the PG was delayed until 40 min after the addition of INF, the NK-cell activity was once again enhanced. These results suggest that the initial processing phase induced by INF is sensitive to the inhibitory signal of PG (*209*).

In the absence of INF in the NK-cell assay system, the mechanism of action of PG is entirely different. It inhibits the lytic process at a very later phase, or even when the lysis program has been already completed and target killing is no longer dependent upon the physical presence of the killer cell (killer-cell independent phase). It has been suggested that PG increases the membrane fluidity of the programmed target cell and, consequently, antagonizes the physical nature of the lethal hit (*210*).

The finding that PG affects the target cell conflicts with two other reports (*204,211*). The first of these (*204*) found that PG-pretreated effector cells rather than PG-pretreated target cells are sensitive to the PG inhibition effect. The second study (*211*) demonstrated that, after removal of T cells from the effector cellular population, a suppressive restraint was lifted, and effector cells were able to develop an NK-cell activity even in the presence of PG. Neither of these reports support the notion that PG rescues the target cells during the killer-independent phase. The lack of agreement may be explained by the use of different target cells (K562, refs. *204,211* vs Molt-4, ref. *210*) in the above-mentioned studies, which may be sensitive to differing mechanisms of killing. In addition, high (10^{-4}–$10^{-5}M$, refs. *210,211*) or low

(10^{-6}–$10^{-8}M$, ref. *204*) concentrations of PG were used in the different studies, and finally, the culture conditions of one experimental system were not identical with those used in other systems.

NK-cell activity may also be suppressed by addition of 12-0-tetradecanoylphorbol-13-acetate (TPA) or opsonized zymosan (yeast cell walls) to the NK-cell assay system (*212,213*). These reagents stimulate the production of superoxide anion (0^-_2) and hydrogen peroxide (H_2O_2) by monocytes and polymorphonuclear leukocytes (PMN). Hydrogen peroxide in particular mediates, either directly or indirectly, the inhibition of NK-cell activity. Addition of catalase, which inactivates H_2O_2, to the assay system prevented the inhibition of NK-cell activity by TPA (*213*). Similarly, removal of monocytes from the effector cell population prevented an efficient production of H_2O_2 after addition of TPA or zymosan, and consequently, the NK-cell activity could be expressed (*212,213*). Readdition of monocytes or PMN to the monocyte-depleted effector cell population restored the TPA or the zymosan-induced suppression (*213*).

It has been suggested that the antagonistic responses of human lymphocytes to high and low doses of histamine are associated with two subsets of cells expressing opposing functions. Those cells that bear the H_1-receptor are stimulated by relatively low doses of histamine and enhance the proliferative responses induced by mitogens. In contrast, lymphocytes bearing H_2-receptors are stimulated by relatively high doses of histamine and suppress the mitogen-induced proliferative responses. Diphenhydramine, an H_1-receptor blocker, inhibits the enhancing effects of low doses of histamine, whereas cimetidine, an H_2-receptor blocker, prevents the suppressive effects of high doses of histamine (*214*). Rocklin and colleagues (*215*) demonstrated that the H_2-receptor-bearing suppressor T cells are stimulated not only by histamine, but also by Con A or specific antigen, and consequently, they release an SF. The release of the SF may, however, be prevented by administration of cimetidine.

As for other cells of the immune system, NK cells may also be downregulated by suppressor cells bearing H_2 receptors. This possibility was explored by Nair and Schwartz (*216*), who demonstrated that PBL precultured with histamine ($10^{-3}M$) suppressed the NK-cell activity of cocultivated autologous effector cells. Peripheral blood lymphocytes precultured with histamine and subsequently killed at 56° C were not able to exert any significant suppression, indicating that this inhibition was not associated with crowding or steric hindrance effects. The level of T8$^+$ cells among the histamine ($10^{-3}M$)-incubated PBL was higher than among untreated PBL, suggesting that at least part of the anti-NK suppressor cell function is associated with the T8$^+$ subclass of T cells.

If H$_2$-receptor-bearing suppressor T cells downregulate the NK-cell activity, preincubation of the effector cells with cimetidine may augment their NK-cell activity. In agreement with this notion, Flodgren and Sjögren (*217*) demonstrated that cimetidine (10^{-4}–$10^{-5}M$), as did indomethacin, slightly enhanced the NK-cell activity of PBL from melanoma and colorectal carcinoma patients or normal individuals, but on comparison with INF, their enhancing effects were nowhere near as efficient. In contrast, other authors (*216,218*) found that the above-indicated concentrations of cimetidine did not affect the NK-cell activity, whereas lower ($10^{-7}M$, *218*) or higher (10^{-2}–$10^{-3}M$; *216,218*) concentrations had an inhibitory effect. Perhaps such variation in results is expected, since cimetidine may affect NK cells directly through the H$_2$ receptors that they carry (*216*). Thus, cimetidine may either block the NK cells or the anti-NK suppressor cells, and the net natural cytotoxicity is determined by the balance between the two effects, which may vary from one experiment to another. The suppressor activity of glass-adherent cells may also be blocked by cimetidine ($10^{-5}M$), but the mechanism of this effect has not been elucidated (*218*).

If NK cells are essential in the immune surveillance against malignancy, a concept that has not yet been convincingly demonstrated, then knowing the "off" and "on" signals that regulate these cells may help to design more effective protocols for immunotherapy of cancer. We have learned from this and the previous sections that reagents such as cimetidine, indomethacin, or catalase block the activity of anti-NK suppressor cells or their products, whereas other reagents such as INF directly potentiate the NK cells. Sophisticated and careful use of such reagents, perhaps in mutual combinations or in combinations with other therapeutic protocols, may help us to determine if this approach is advantageous or not in a clinical setting.

Antigenic Entities of the Tumor That Induce Suppressor Cells May Prevent the Potentiation of Coexpressed Immunogenic Entities

The apparent inactivity of the immune system in the face of antigenic stimuli delivered by tumor cells appearing spontaneously in man and animal, has been used as a major argument against the immune surveillance hypothesis (219), claiming that malignant transformation is continuously regulated by immunocompetent cells (220). The lack of an immune response against a spontaneous tumor does not, however, negate the possibility that the tumor antigens can, under the right circumstances, induce an immune response. As an example, tumors may express both moieties that induce suppressor cells (suppressogenic entities) and those that induce immune cells (immunogenic entities). The resultant dominant function of the suppressor cells may result in a restraint of the immune response against the tumor. If this conception is correct, we may consider the possibility of blocking or altering the suppressogenic moieties, thus preventing their function and allowing the other entities to express their immunogenicity. This concept has been considered in a previous review written by one of us (7); as a result, we shall discuss this issue briefly, referring only to new findings.

The search for suppressogenic and immunogenic entities in malignant cells has received encouragement from the findings of such antagonistic epitopes in several macromolecules. Direct and circumstantial evidence implies the coexistence of immunogenic and suppressogenic epitopes in lysozyme (221,222), β-Galactosidase (223), cytochrome C (224), SRBC (225), bovine serum albumin (226), human mixed lymphocyte reaction (MLR)-stimulating antigen (227), and myelin basic protein (MBP; 228). It has been found that the first three amino acids at the N-terminal of the lysozyme contain the suppressogenic entity of this protein (221), and in this segment, the phenylalanine at position 3 is critical for the induction of the suppressor cells (229). The suppressogenic entity of the MBP was located in a peptide containing amino acids 44–89. Guinea pigs primed with peptide 44–89, obtained by limited pepsin digestion and purified by column chromatography, were significantly protected against experimental allergic encephalomyelitis induced by sensitization with MBP emulsified in CFA (228), the 44–89 peptide thus overcoming the immunogenicity of the complete MBP.

Biochemical excision of the suppressogenic epitope of some antigens (lysozyme, β-galactosidase, cytochrome C; 221–224) revealed an innate immunogenicity that was normally masked by the induction of suppressor cells. The interrelationship between the antagonistic epitopes of the antigen, the products of the major histocompatibility complex (MHC) of the antigen presenting cell (APC), and the cell receptors recognizing the antigen were described by Goodman and Sercarz (230). It was further demonstrated that suppression can be induced only when the antigen determinants recognized by helper cells, suppressor cells, and B cells are covalently linked on the same molecules (231). The distance between the different epitopes of the antigen must, however, be sufficiently short, in order to ensure safe transfer of regulatory signals between the cells that are bound to the antigen (223). Alternatively, binding of the suppressor cells to the suppressogenic site of the antigen may block (by steric hindrance) or modify (allosteric inhibition) the epitope recognized by the helper cells.

Circumstantial evidence for the coexistence of immunogenic and suppressogenic entities in tumor cells has been inferred from several studies. Although mice immunized against the MCA-induced S1509a tumor could also reject the similarly induced SAI tumor, the suppressor cells induced by either tumor were specific. The implication is that the entities that act as immunogens and those that act as suppressogens are distinct entities, the former being shared by S1509a and SAI, whereas the latter are specific for each tumor (232–234). For an evaluation of the experimental data, refer to the section on "Mechanism of Action" in our previous review paper dealing with suppressor cells and malignancy (1).

Ultraviolet (UV)-induced tumors may also express antagonistic antigens activating either immune cells or suppressor cells. This conclusion is indirectly inferred from the fact that the immune responses against UV tumors are distinctively regulated by specific antitumor effector cells (which are possibly activated by helper T cells recognizing specific immunogens on the UV tumors, 235) and nonspecific suppressor T cells induced by UV, and recognize determinants shared by all UV-tumors (236). It has been suggested (235) that the helper T cells are the target of the UV-induced suppressor T cells, as indicated by the finding that naive mice transplanted with syngeneic UV-induced suppressor cells failed to generate specific helper T cells after immunization. Note that the immunogenic entities on chemically induced tumors are nonspecific and their suppressogens are specific (232–234), whereas the reverse is true for the UV-induced tumors (235,236).

The expression of distinct immunogenic and immunosuppressive antigens in a rat colon carcinoma induced by 1,2-dimethylhydrazine was suggested by exploring the immunological properties of regressor and progressor sublines derived from the original tumor (the sublines were selected and isolated according to their susceptibility to trypsin-mediated detachment from a plastic surface). The regressor tumor inhibited the growth of the progressor tumor when injected before or simultaneously with the progressor tumor. A mixture of lymph node and splenic lymphocytes from rats having rejected the regressor tumor also inhibited the progressor tumor growth in syngeneic recipients. On the other hand, the regressor tumor is not rejected in rats bearing an established progressor tumor, and the lymphocytes of the progressor tumor host will enhance the growth of the regressor tumor in syngeneic recipients (237). These results suggest that the regressor tumor preferentially expresses immunogenic entities that induce an immunological rejection of the tumor, whereas the progressor tumor preferentially expresses suppressogenic entities that induce the appearance of suppressor cells, enhancing the tumor growth.

EL4 cells may also coexpress antagonistic antigens: nonself-tumor-associated antigens inducing antitumor immune responses and self-antigens stimulating appearance of suppressor cells. This conclusion was inferred from the observation that some clones of

EL4 induced appearance of suppressor cells inhibiting the proliferation of autoreactive clone cells after stimulation with syngeneic spleen cells, whereas a different clone induced the appearance of either suppressor cells recognizing normal antigens or immune cells recognizing tumor antigens (*238*).

The above evidence, however, is implicit rather than direct, since the function of the tumor antagonistic entities has not been demonstrated by isolated immunogens or suppressogens. The biochemical separation of immunogenic and suppressogenic entities from tumor homogenates and the demonstration of their opposing functions have been demonstrated in three different experimentally induced tumors: MCA induced fibrosarcoma of the mouse (*239,240*), adenovirus type 12 induced tumor of the hamster (*241*), and Moloney virus induced tumor (YAC) of the mouse (*7*). The biochemical separation procedures used to isolate the antagonistic entities and the immunological assays used to prove their contrasting functions have been described in a review previously written by one of us (*7*); thus, the subsequently published data, particularly concerning the MCA and YAC tumor systems, will be the main focus of attention.

Pellis and colleagues (*239,240*) subjected 3M KCl extracts of MCA tumors to preparative Isoelectric Focusing (pIEF). The focused slabs were sectioned into 30 zones by means of a steel-cutting grid, after which the gels were removed from each zone, eluted with NaCl, and injected into different groups of mice in order to test their ability to stimulate either antitumor activity or immunosuppression. Injection of strongly acidic (pI 2.5–3.6) proteins into mice enhanced the growth of subsequently inoculated tumor, whereas injection of mildly acidic (pI 5.8–6.0) proteins resulted in antitumor resistance (*239*). The isolated antagonistic entities did not affect the growth of an unrelated tumor, indicating their specificity. Spleen cells from mice injected with the pIEF-isolated immunogens or suppressogens transferred protective or enhancing activities, respectively, to naive recipients (*239*), indicating that a cellular mechanism regulates the tumor-related immunological activities. The pIEF-isolated immunogen was also shown to be effective in an immunotherapy protocol (*242*). Eighty percent of the mice that were first subjected to tumor resection and then injected with the pIEF-isolated immunogenic fraction survived, whereas the survival rate of mice subjected to tumor resection only was 50%.

Nevertheless, intact cells of MCA tumor are highly immunogenic. Mice primed with 10^5-10^6 irradiated tumor cells completely rejected a subsequent viable tumor challenge (243). In contrast, the injection of the pIEF-isolated immunogenic fraction of the tumor extract (243,244), the pIEF fraction sequentially purified by a preparative isotachophoresis (pITP, 243,244), or the pIEF fraction first separated by pITP and sequentially by a high-performance gel permeation chromatography (HPGPC; 243) delayed the neoplastic outgrowth, but never caused complete rejection. The superior immunogenicity of intact tumor cells over purified immunogens isolated from these cells may be explained by the necessity for presentation of the immunogen in the context of other cellular products destroyed by the separation procedure.

The mechanism of induction of suppression by pIEF acidic fraction has been examined and described in several reports (245–247). Normal spleen cells incubated for 1–6 h with the suppressogenic pIEF acidic (ph < 2.9) fraction of MCA-F tumor supernatant (246) or its 3M KCl extract (245–247) gained suppressive activity as indicated by their ability to enhance tumor growth (247) and inhibit the DTH response to dinitrochlorobenzene (DNCB; 245,246) or specific tumor antigen (247) after their transfer to appropriate recipients. The pIEF acidic fractions of other tumors such as UV-induced fibrosarcoma, LLC (245), spontaneous fibrosarcoma (246), and human colonic adenocarcinoma (245) also induced suppressor cells that inhibit the DTH to DNCB, whereas the mildly acidic fractions of these tumors failed to stimulate such cells (245); thus, the mechanism of suppression is not limited to the MCA tumors. Interestingly, the pIEF acidic fraction of an UV-induced tumor failed to induce the appearance of suppressor cells enhancing tumor growth or inhibiting the DTH to the tumor antigens (247), whereas it induced a suppressor cell function that inhibited the DTH to DNCB (245). The UV-induced tumor, in contrast to the MCA-induced tumor, is a regressor tumor that is spontaneously rejected from the recipient mice. Thus, the difference between a progressor tumor (such as MCA-F) and a regressor tumor may be associated with the ability of the former to express suppressogens, which induce inhibition of the antitumor immune responses.

The ability of the pIEF acidic fraction to induce suppressive activity in a normal cell population may indicate that the inhibitory effect is mediated by suppressor cells induced by the fraction, and is not exerted directly by the suppressogens themselves. However, the possibility that the incubated cells or subpopulation of cells carry over the suppressogenic entity to the tested recipient mice was not completely ruled out.

The suppressogenic pIEF acidic fraction was sensitive to treatment with heat and RNase, partially sensitive to treatment with trypsin, but resistant to treatment with DNase, pronase, and neuraminidase (245,246). High-performance permeation chromatography revealed that the apparent molecular weight of the MCA-F pIEF-isolated suppressogen was greater than 300,000 daltons (246). Thus, the initial biochemical characterization of the suppressogenic pIEF acidic fraction suggests that it is a large complex of RNA and protein (245,246).

Spleen cells from DNCB-sensitized mice injected with suppressor cells induced by the pIEF acidic fraction transferred normal DTH activity to naive recipients, implying that, although the donor mice were suppressed, their spleen cells were fully capable of mediating the DTH. It is possible that the suppressor cells inhibit the effector phase of the DTH, whereas cells stimulated during the induction phase remain unaffected and are capable of transferring the DTH to naive recipients. This proposal received some confirmation from the observation that the Lyt-1$^+$,2$^-$ effector cells of DNCB-sensitized mice failed to transfer the DTH to naive recipients if cotransplanted with the suppressor cells (Lyt-1$^-$,2$^+$ cells or macrophages) induced by the pIEF acidic fraction from the MCA-F tumor. The pIEF acidic fraction induced, however, suppressor-cell activity in both syngeneic and allogeneic cells, as well as in both T cells (Lyt-1$^+$,2$^-$ and Lyt-1$^-$,2$^+$) and macrophages (246), indicating that the effect is neither genetically restricted nor limited to certain subpopulations of cells (observations that may support the alternative notion that the cells just carry over the pIEF-isolated suppressogen to the recipient animals).

Suppressor cells obtained from mice bearing MCA-F tumor and suppressor cells induced by incubation of normal spleen cells with pIEF acidic fraction extracted from MCA-F tumor demonstrate several similar characteristics. Both types of cells facilitate the growth of MCA-F tumor, but not that of MCA-D tumor, and both inhibit the DTH to the MCA-F tumor antigens, but not to MCA-D tumor antigens, indicting the specificity of the cells (247). Consequently, one possibility is that the tumor cells of the TBH release suppressogens into the blood that may be similar to those obtained by the pIEF fractionation of the tumor extract.

A similar approach for isolating immunogens and suppressogens from various tumors, including the nonimmunogenic YAC tumor, has been used in our laboratory. The YAC tumor, in contrast to the MCA-induced tumors, is not immunogenic in the syngeneic host. Therefore, it may be an appropriate model for testing the hypothesis of coexistence of immunogenic and suppressogenic entities in nonimmunogenic tumors.

YAC is a Moloney virus-induced tumor originating in A mice (248). Such mice injected with the irradiated or MMC-treated tumor will not generate any immune response against the tumor (249,250), and they will be killed after a relatively short period by low doses (10^1–10^2 cells) of viable tumor (251). After incubation in vitro, however, the properties of the YAC tumor have changed substantially. A short period of culture, from a few hours up to a few days, results in a tumor, designated YAC-1, that is now immunogenic in the syngeneic hosts (250,251). Thus, the YAC-1 viable cells, in contrast to the YAC cells, are rejected by the unimmunized host even if inoculated with relatively high doses of tumor (10^4 cells; 251).

Assays in vitro show that the in vivo YAC tumor and the in vitro YAC-1 tumor induce cells with different functions. Spleen cells from mice injected with inactivated YAC-1 differentiated into anti-YAC cytotoxic cells when cultured for 6 d either in the presence or the absence of YAC-1 cells (250). Spleen cells from mice injected with inactivated YAC inhibited the ability of cocultured YAC-1 primed splenocytes to differentiate into anti-YAC cytotoxic cells (252). These experiments demonstrate that the in vitro tumor YAC-1 induces the appearance of memory cells that differentiate into cytotoxic cells under the in vitro culture conditions, whereas the in vivo tumor YAC induces the appearance of suppressor cells. This conclusion was supported by a separate in vivo assay where A mice injected with inactivated YAC-1 rejected a viable challenge of YAC tumor that would otherwise kill the host, whereas tumor growth was enhanced in mice inoculated with inactivated YAC tumor (251).

These findings may be explained by postulating that the YAC tumor simultaneously expresses both immunogenic and suppressogenic entities. The dominant suppressor cells induced by the suppressogenic entities could block the activity of the antitumor reactive cells induced by the immunogenic entities, masking the effect of the latter. During the in vitro culture, the YAC tumor may shed or internalize the suppressogenic entities leaving the immunogenic entities free to stimulate the antitumor immune responses. Physical separation of the antagonsitic immunoreactive entities and testing the ability of each one of them to induce either immune cells or suppressor cells was undertaken to test the above hypothesis.

In order to establish the technical procedures under optimal conditions, we first subjected the immunogenic Rauscher virus-induced tumor of C57BL/6 mice (designated RBL5) to the separation technique. The RBL5 tumor homogenate (treated with 2% SDS and 1% triton X-100) was exposed to sodium dodecyl sulfate polyacrylamide gel electrophoresis (SDS-PAGE) under nonreduced conditions. At the end of the electrophoresis, the gels were sliced into small pieces (4 mm each), each of which was injected into a separate group of syngeneic C57BL/6 mice. We found that certain SDS-PAGE isolated molecular entities induced in the animals antitumor reactive cells that, after further incubation in vitro, could kill RBL5 tumor cells but not syngeneic unrelated tumor cells, demonstrating the specificity of the cytotoxic response (253).

Having successfully established a technique for the separation of immunogenic entities from RBL5 tumor and from a Moloney virus-induced tumor of CBA mice (YBA; 254), the methodology was then applied to YAC in order to test if this tumor contains the predicted immunogens and suppressogens (255–257). A YAC tumor homogenate solubilized with 2% SDS and 1% triton X-100 was subjected to nonreduced SDS-PAGE. At the end of the electrophoresis, the gel slices were injected in sequential order into various groups of A mice. It was found that, whereas intact YAC cells failed to stimulate any cytotoxic activity, some of the gel slices [usually less than 100,000 daltons (100 Kdaltons, e.g., 80 or 11 Kdaltons] induced antitumor reactive cells. Spleen cells from mice injected with these gel slices differentiated in in vitro cultures into anti-YAC cytotoxic cells. Other gel slices (usually with a molecular weight of about 150 Kdaltons) induced the appearance of supressor cells. Spleen cells from mice injected with these gel slices blocked the ability of YAC-1-primed splenocytes to differentiate into cytotoxic cells when both cellular populations were mixed together. Similarly, certain gel slices induced cells that inhibited the in vivo tumor growth, whereas others induced cells that enhanced the in vivo tumor growth (in the Winn assays). Effector cells induced with a molecular entity of 11 Kdaltons were characterized as T cells (and not as NK cells) bearing the Lyt-2$^+$ surface marker. The suppressor cells induced with the 150-Kdalton molecular entity were also characterized as T cells bearing the I-J^k surface marker (257).

The ability of the antagonsitic immunoreactive entities of the tumor to induce either immunological resistance to the tumor or enhancement of the tumor growth was subsequently explored (258). In a preliminary study the SDS-PAGE, isolated molecular entities were injected into separate groups of mice. Only the gel slices containing a molecular entity of 80–90 Kdaltons induced a significant immunological resistance to tumor growth in the mice. About 10% of the mice immunized with this molecular fraction rejected entirely the challenge of viable YAC cells. Although a complete protective effect was evident in only a small proportion of the mice, the molecular fraction of 80–90 Kdaltons was selected for further study, since the effect was significant and repeatable (258). The results of a representative experiment demonstrating the ability of SDS-PAGE isolated 80–90 Kdalton fraction to induce in vivo resistance to tumor growth are presented in Fig 1. The protective effect induced with the immunogenic entity was mediated by helper T cells, since spleen cells of mice injected with monoclonal antibody against nonspecific helper T-cell factor together with the 80–90 Kdalton molecular entity failed to neutralize tumor growth in Winn assay (viable YAC cells mixed with these splenocytes grew progressively in naive recipients and eventually killed the host, whereas viable YAC cells mixed with splenocytes derived from A mice injected with 80–90 Kdaltons molecular entity and control serum were rejected). It was further found that the helper T-cell function induced with 80–90 Kdalton fraction of YAC homogenate activated both T- and non-T-effector cells, which mediated the neutralizing effect indicated in a Winn assay.

The specificity of the immune response induced by immunogenic moieties present in SDS-PAGE gel slices of RBL5 tumor was explored in C57BL/6 mice challenged with viable syngeneic RBL5 cells or unrelated syngeneic tumor cells. C57BL/6 mice injected with the SDS-PAGE isolated 20 Kdalton molecular fraction of a RBL5 tumor homogenate resisted the growth of homologous viable tumor cells, whereas this fraction did not prevent the subsequent growth of another syngeneic tumor (B16 melanoma), indi-

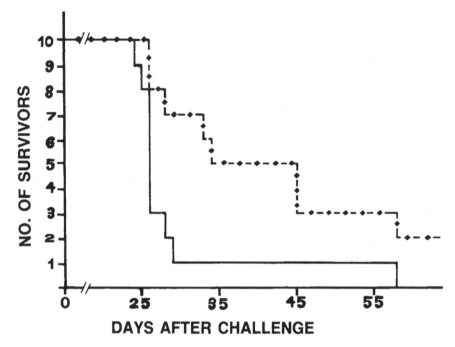

Fig. 1. SDS-PAGE isolated 80–90 K fraction of a YAC tumor homogenate induces in vivo resistance against YAC tumor growth. Strain A mice were injected with the 80–90 K fraction isolated by SDS-PAGE (—♦—; 10 mice) or left untreated (_____; 10 mice). Two weeks after the immunization, all mice were challenged with 20 viable YAC cells, and the survival time was recorded. In a separate experiment, we found that mice injected with blank gel slices or with blank gel slices and YAC tumor honogenate died at the same time as the control group of mice receiving viable tumor only (results are not shown).

cating the specific nature of the resistance induced by the 20 Kdalton fraction, as well as showing that the antigen was not destroyed by the isolation procedure (258).

In a different experiment, Dr. Sharon from our group has found that A mice injected with a 150 Kdalton fraction of a YAC tumor homogenate isolated by SDS-PAGE enhanced the tumor growth of a subsequent challenge of viable YAC cells. Fractions of other sizes, isolated from the same gel, failed to induce any similar enhancing effect, confirming our previous results, which showed that 150 Kdalton molecular fraction could induce the appearance of suppressor cells (257). Figure 2 presents the results of an experiment showing the ability of the 150 Kdalton fraction of a

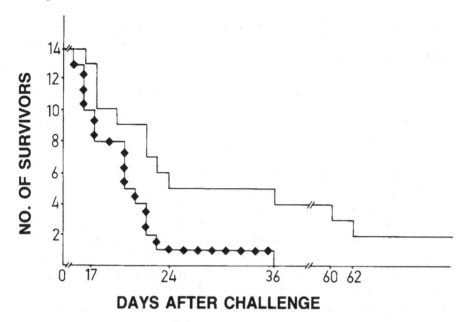

DAYS AFTER CHALLENGE

Fig. 2. SDS-PAGE isolated 150 K fraction of YAC tumor homogenate induces in vivo enhancement of YAC tumor growth. Strain A mice were injected with 150 K fraction isolated by SDS-PAGE (—♦—; 14 mice) or left untreated (____; 14 mice). Two weeks later, all mice were challenged with 20 viable YAC cells, and the survival time was recorded.

YAC tumor homogenate to induce the enhancement of tumor growth, where mice of the A strain injected with this fraction died significantly faster after challenge with the viable YAC tumor than mice that received the challenge dose alone.

In conclusion, using SDS-PAGE, we have succeeded in isolating two antagonistic molecular entities from the YAC tumor; first, an immunogenic entity of apparent molecular weight of 80–90 Kdaltons and, secondly, a suppressogenic entity of apparent molecular weight of 150 Kdaltons. Although the effects induced by these two molecular entities are not strong, they are significant and reproducible, and provide a basis for the principle of our approach: removal of suppressogenic entities from a nonimmunogenic tumor homogenate may reveal underlying immunogens that, when used alone, may induce an immunological resistance to tumor growth.

This prediction was further tested by subjecting the PIR-2 tumor homogenate to the SDS-PAGE protocol (259). PIR-2 is another nonimmunogenic tumor that was induced in C57BL/6 mice by X-irradiation. This primary tumor does not contain serologically detected viral antigens (*260*). Using the SDS-PAGE protocol, we succeeded in isolating from PIR-2 tumor an immunogenic entity of 10 Kdaltons that induced specific anti-PIR-2 tumor cytotoxic cells. The same immunogenic entity also induced in vivo resistance against 1,000 viable PIR-2 cells (*259*). Other SDS-PAGE isolated molecular entities of PIR-2 induced an in vivo enhancement of tumor growth.

Using a different biochemical separation procedure, we (*261*) have succeeded in isolating from a B16 melanoma tumor extract immunogenic entities that stimulated a specific primary antimelanoma B16 cytotoxic response in spleen cells of syngeneic normal mice. The 0.2% Triton X-100 tumor extract was applied to an Ultrogel AcA 34 column for separation by molecular weight, and a few fractions obtained from the column induced specific cytotoxic responses in the cultures (*261*). In contrast, B16 melanoma cells and the unfractionated tumor extract failed to stimulate such immunological responses, suggesting the possibility that suppressogens antagonize the immunogenic potential of the tumor. This approach is more suitable for extrapolation to human tumors than the SDS-PAGE protocol, since the test can be completed in a relatively short time and it uses an in vitro system to assay the immunogenicity of the isolated fractions.

Whereas the Meth A-induced tumor is immunogenic, the cytosol fraction of this tumor induced, upon its injection into the syngeneic host, a considerable enhancement of a subsequent tumor challenge, suggesting that the fraction may contain suppressogens (*262*). Although evidence for suppressogenic entities in the cytosolic fraction has not yet been presented, Srivastava and colleagues (*262*) have succeeded in isolating a relatively pure immunogen from the cytosol, using sequential fractionation procedures, including chromatography on Con A-Sepharose, diethylaminoethyl (DEAE)-Sepharose, and Mono Q column of Fast Protein Liquid Chromatography (FPLC) system. The final product was subjected to SDS-PAGE. A band of 96 Kdaltons eluted from the gel induced in syngeneic mice the ability to reject a viable challenge of the homologous tumor, which otherwise was fatal to the animals. Careful scrutiny with broadly reacting serological and molecular probes failed to reveal murine leukemia virus (MuLV)-related antigens or transcripts in the

MCA-induced tumor, indicating that the tumor antigen described here is not a component of murine leukemia virus.

If it can be shown in the instance of a particular tumor that its lack of immunogenicity is associated with the expression of suppressogens antagonizing the immunogens of the same tumor, it may be possible to use a rational strategy in an attempt to establish an antitumor immune response. One may try to change the immunological balance by injecting the TBH with isolated immunogens, or even better, with monoclonal antibodies against the suppressogens. Such antibodies may neutralize the suppressogenic entities, leaving the immunogens free to stimulate immunological rejection of the tumor.

Another approach that could also be used in the immunotherapy of cancer is based on a different consideration, implying that the suppressor cells may express distinct idiotypic structures not carried by other regulatory cells, as has actually been observed in the lysozyme experimental system (263). If factors obtained from the suppressor cells carry the same distinct idiotype as the receptors of the suppressor cells or if they carry other distinct structural markers, they may be injected to syngeneic or allogeneic animals in order to stimulate production of antibodies specific to the suppressor cells or their products. These antibodies may be injected later into the original TBH in order to eliminate the suppressor cells and subsequently to establish an immunological balance that will cause tumor rejection. Support for this approach has been provided by an experimental model developed by Maier and colleagues (264). Suppressor cells were induced in DBA/2J mice by injecting them with an extract of P815 mastocytoma. The nylon-wool-purified splenocytes of these mice contained specific suppressor T cells. The suppressor factor that was extracted from these suppressor T cells was purified by passage over an immunoabsorbent carrying P815 membrane components. Antibodies raised against the suppressor factor in syngeneic and allogeneic mice killed, in the presence of complement, the suppressor cells, but not cytotoxic cells specific to the P815 tumor. These results suggest that the P815 tumor extract contains distinct antigens capable of activating suppressor cells. The antibody against the extracts of these suppressor cells were used later in order to selectively eradicate the suppressor cells.

It should be remembered that the induction of effective immunological responses by isolated immunogens is dependent on the ability of the immunogen to be presented to the cells of the immune system via the APCs. For instance, if the separation procedure causes damage to the agretope of the fractionated antigen (the structure that combines the antigen with the APC MHC, 230), it may fail to stimulate the immune system.

We don't know yet if coexpression of immunogens and suppressogens is associated with the failure of spontaneous tumors in stimulating the immune system. If it proves to be the case, it may be possible to use the above-described classical biochemical separation procedures, as well as new approaches from the field of molecular biology (e.g., transfection of the separated genes of the immunogens and the suppressogens into normal fibroblasts) in order to open new avenues for the immunotherapy of cancer.

Suppressor Cells
in Human Malignant
Diseases

1. Introduction

In principle, the mechanisms of the immune response and its regulation are no different in humans than in mice. Thus, details pertinent to the operation of human suppressor cells may be found in the introduction to our previous review paper (1). However, since the terminology used in the description of the human immune system is different than the one used for the mouse, and since minor differences between the systems may still exist, there follows a brief overview of mechanisms in the human immune response. It should be borne in mind that much of the apparent mechanisms in human immunity are extrapolated from the findings in mice, where the various arms of the immune system may be manipulated experimentally, and where, by judicious use of pure strains and their recombinants or transgenic derivatives, the contributions of various entities to cellular communication in the immune system may be evaluated.

The description that follows (Fig. 3) is based on the model of Ballieux and Heijnen (265), which describes the cellular communications after stimulation with antigen. The model, depicted in Fig. 3, may be altered slightly to take account of mitogenic or other sources of stimulation (e.g., refs. 266,267). It should be borne in mind, however, that the cellular interactions described in Fig. 3 are a schematic representation of the current understanding of the immunoregulation system. Furthermore, this scheme has not yet been accepted by all immunologists, and even those who agree with the Fig. 3 description must realize that this research field is most dynamic and changes in the general model should be expected.

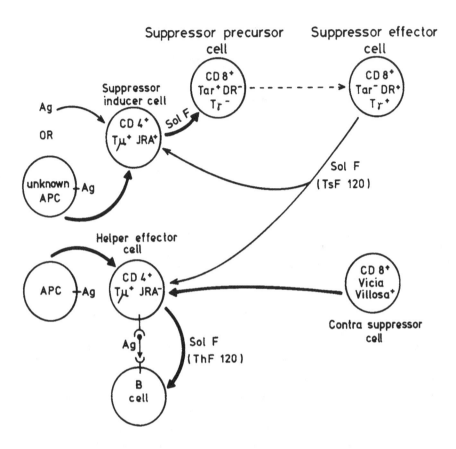

Fig. 3. Schematic description of the regulation of the immune response in humans based on data provided by refs. *265, 266, 270,* and
276. For a detailed explanation, *see* text. An unbroken arrow indicates
the effect of one cell on another; a broken arrow indicates induction of
differentiation; a broad line indicates a positive signal; a thin line indicates a negative signal. Ag, antigen; APC, antigen presenting cell;
$CD4^+$, T cells bearing the marker $T4^+$ or $Leu-3^+$; $CD8^+$, T cells bearing
the marker $T8^+$, $T5^+$, or $Leu-2^+$; DR^+, positive class II antigen expression; JRA^+, T cell that reacts with autoantibody found in the sera of patients with juvenile rheumatoid arthritis; Sol F, soluble factor; Tar^+, T
cell that expresses affinity for autologous erythrocytes; T_γ^+, T cell bearing receptor for the Fc portion of IgG; $T\mu^+$, T cell bearing receptor for
the Fc portion of IgM; unknown APC, nonphagocytic, nonadherent
antigen-presenting cell; Vicia villosa$^+$, T cell which binds vicia villosa
lectin.

Macrophages process the antigen and present its residual components to a subset of thymus-derived cells, which react with the monoclonal antibodies OKT4 or Leu-3 (designated T4$^+$, Leu-3$^+$, or CD4$^+$). During the interaction between the macrophage and the T4$^+$ cell, a soluble factor (perhaps, colony-stimulating factor, CSF; 268) is released from the T cells and the macrophage is activated. The interaction between the macrophage and the T4$^+$ cell will be productive if both cells express the same class II product (DR, DP, DQ) of the MHC. As a consequence of this interaction, the macrophage releases the monokine interleukin-1 (IL-1), which is accepted by the partner or other T4$^+$ cells, thus delivering to them a signal to initiate production of the lymphokine interleukin-2 (IL-2) (269). The IL-2 released from T4 cells binds to the IL-2 receptor expressed on various target cells (e.g., precursors of helper T cell or precursors of cytotoxic cell) already activated by the interaction with antigen. As a result, IL-2 does not stimulate all T cells to proliferate, only those which have been activated by antigen to express IL-2 receptor, thus generating the exquisite specificity of the immune response. Stimulated by IL-2, the preeffector cells will proliferate and differentiate into mature helper or cytotoxic effector T cells (*see* schematic model in ref. *268*). The cytotoxic effector T cell reacts with the monoclonal antibodies OKT5, OKT8, or Leu-2 (designated T5$^+$, T8$^+$, Leu2$^+$, or CD8$^+$). The T cell will not kill its cellular target unless both cells express the same class I (HLA A, B, or C) genetic product of the MHC. The helper effector T cell (phenotypically T4$^+$ or Leu-3$^+$) interacts with a B cell specific for the same antigen. It appears that both cells use the antigen as a bridge that may connect their receptors. The T4$^+$ helper effector cell delivers a factor (possibly ThF-120; *270*) that supports the differentiation of the B cell into antibody-producing cells (*see* Fig. 3 and schematic model in ref. *268*). In this instance, identity at class II (DR, DP, DQ) is required for successful interaction between the helper T cell and the B cell.

By a separate pathway, the T4$^+$ helper effector cell delivers, upon activation with the specific antigen, lymphokines that attract and activate the macrophages (*271*). These activated macrophages may destroy the target antigen by an inflammatory process known as DTH. The function of the T4$^+$ cells is not limited only to the immune system. These cells have been implicated in hematopoietic differentiation (*272*), osteoclast activation, and collagen production by fibroblasts (*273*).

The activity of the T4$^+$ helper cell is regulated by a cascade of suppressor cells (Fig. 3). The first cell in this cascade is the suppressor-inducer cell. This cell also expresses the T4$^+$ (Leu-3$^+$) marker, and like the T4$^+$ helper cell, it is radioresistant (265). In contrast to the T4$^+$ helper cell, the suppressor-inducer cell can interact with antibody found in the serum of patients with active juvenile rheumatoid arthritis (JRA). The T4$^+$ JRA$^+$ suppressor-inducer cell is activated either by free antigen or by APC, which are not amenable to the separation techniques used normally for the isolation of monocytes or macrophages (265). The activated suppressor-inducer cell interacts with the suppressor-precursor cell expressing T8$^+$ (T5$^+$, Leu-2$^+$, or CD8$^+$) marker. Unlike the cytotoxic T cell, the suppressor-precursor cell does not express the T20 differentiation antigen (274), although they are phenotypically similar in most other respects. The interaction between the suppressor-inducer cell and the suppressor-precursor cell, possibly mediated by a soluble factor, leads to the differentiation of the suppressor-precursor into a suppressor-effector cell. The differentiated suppressor-effector cell (T8$^+$, T5$^+$, Leu-2$^+$, or CD8$^+$) releases a suppressor factor (possibly TsF 120; 265) that downregulates the helper cell activity and, consequently, the activity of the effector cell supported by this helper cell (265). Using the principle of feedback regulation, the suppressor factor (possibly TsF 120) released from the T8$^+$ suppressor-effector cell also restrains the activity of the T4$^+$ suppressor-inducer cell (*see* Fig. 3 and ref. 265).

Both helper T cell and the suppressor-inducer cell express, in addition to the T4$^+$ marker, a receptor capable of interacting with the Fc portion of IgM (Tμ^+). The T8$^+$ suppressor-effector cell (but not the T8$^+$ suppressor-precursor cell) expresses a receptor interacting with the Fc portion of IgG (Tγ^+). It was found, however, that Tμ^+ Tγ^+ classification for helper and suppressor cells does not correlate with the T4$^+$ T8$^+$ classification (275).

A further complication is that, under certain conditions, activation of the T4$^+$ cells may induce the appearance of another T4$^+$ subset that directly inhibits T4$^+$ helper cell function (266), these cells being designated as T4$^+$ suppressor-effector cells.

If the help provided by T4$^+$ helper effector-cells to B cells is not optimal, these helper cells are protected from being suppressed by the T8$^+$ suppressor-effector cells. The cells responsible for this protective effect are designated contrasuppressor cells, which are also a subset of the activated T8$^+$ cellular population

(*266,276*). Besides their role in antigen presentation, the presence of macrophages in relatively high levels may result in negative signals, causing suppression of various types of immunological activities (reviewed in *1*).

Any description of the immune system in humans is not complete without a discussion of the role of the NK cell. NK cells may be found in the peripheral blood of normal individuals, and their activity is not dependent on prior sensitization. They express cytotoxic activity against a variety of tumor cells, as well as against some microorganisms or microbially infected cells. The NK cells may thereby serve as first defense line against disease (*6*). Human NK cells appear as large lymphocytes with an indented nucleus and prominent azurophilic granules in the cytoplasm, and are often referred to as large granular lymphocytes (*23*). Virtually all NK cells react with the monoclonal antibody NKP-15 (or Leu 11a), which was originally raised against the LGL (*267*). Although the NK-cell activity may be developed by unstimulated cells, it may be considerably augmented by administration of INF or INF-inducing reagents.

2. Hodgkin's Disease

Hodgkin's disease (HD) is a lymphoproliferative disorder defined by the histologic appearance of giant cells (Reed-Sternberg cell) in the lymph nodes (*277,278*). The Reed-Sternberg cell is a neoplastic cell of uncertain descent, perhaps of macrophage lineage (*277*). Some reports are more specific in describing the antigen-presenting reticulum cell in thymus-dependent areas of lymphoid tissue as its antecedent (*279,280*). Various immunological disturbances are associated with the disease (reviewed in *277*), the most well-documented being the lack of a DTH response to tuberculin (*281*) and other natural antigens (e.g., mumps virus, *282*), impaired immunity after BCG vaccination (*283*), reduced cutaneous hypersensitivity after sensitization with DNCB (*284*), impaired skin graft rejection (*285*), impaired PHA (*286–289*), Con A, (*287,288*) and pokeweed mitogen (PWM, *288*) mitogenic responses, impaired in vitro proliferative response to purified protein derivative (PPD, *288*), impaired heterologous (*290*) or autologous (*277*) MLR, a reduced capacity to produce MIF (*291*) and leukocyte inhibitory factor (*292*), and a reduced capacity to generate cytotoxicity (293) or to form rosettes between patients' T cells and sheep erythrocytes (E-RFC, 294).

It was further found that the supernatants of some unstimulated HD mononuclear cells were able to suppress the lymphoproliferation of normal cells to PHA (292). According to one publication, the PHA mitogenic response defect was more pronounced in patients with more extensive disease (295), but another report suggests a poor correlation between this in vitro test and the disease intensity (296). The PHA mitogenic response was still at a very low level 2–8 yr after the termination of radiotherapy, when the patients were in continuous remission (295). Independent studies confirmed the existence of immunological defects in long-term disease free survivors (297–299), or indicated increased incidence of bacterial and viral infections in such individuals (300,301). In contrast to cellular immunity, primary and secondary antibody production is usually normal in HD patients (277). Thus, one may suggest that the disturbances of cellular immunity in HD patients are associated with serious infection episodes (277) and sometimes even with secondary neoplasms (302).

The impaired cellular immunity observed in HD could be associated with augmented suppressor-cell activity. Analysis of the suppressor and helper cell phenotypes and their relative representation may be an indicator of the patients' immunoregulatory balance. Tγ cells, which used to be classified as suppressor T cells (303), are present in the peripheral blood (303–309) and the lymph nodes (303) of treated and untreated HD patients at higher proportions than in normal individuals. Consequently, the ratio of Tμ (which used to be classified as helper T cells; 303) to Tγ is reduced in HD patients in comparison with normal individuals, possibly contributing to the impaired cellular immunity. For instance, one report (308) indicated that the Tμ:Tγ ratio found in the blood of normal individuals (n = 30) was 4.8, whereas that found in the blood of HD patients (n = 18) was 1.2. Similar low levels of Tμ:Tγ ratios were also found in the blood of non-Hodgkin's lymphoma patients and patients with solid tumors. It should be emphasized, however, that in contrast to the low Tμ:Tγ ratios in the patients' peripheral blood and lymph nodes, the ratio of Tμ:Tγ cells in the patients' spleen is relatively high (306,307).

More recent studies have assessed relative levels of helper cells and suppressor cells using monoclonal antibodies of the CD4 (T4, Leu3) and CD8 (T8, T5, Leu2) clusters, respectively

(*267,271,310,311*). Using these reagents for analyzing the ratios of helper cells to suppressor cells in the peripheral blood of HD untreated (*312–314*) or splenectomized (*314*) patients did not reveal a higher proportion of suppressor cells in comparison with normal individuals (*312,313*). It was, however, indicated (*314*) that the T4:T8 ratios of long survivors were low (0.78) in comparison with the normal ratio (2.00; *see* also ref. *315*) probably because of the treatment effects of irradiation and chemotherapy. Although Romagnani et al. (*316*) claimed a significant reduction of helper/inducer cells in the periperal blood of HD patients, the T4:T8 cellular ratios of the patients (1.61) were actually very close to those of normal individuals (1.84).

The percentage of helper/inducer cells and cytotoxic/suppressor cells in involved and uninvolved spleens of HD untreated patients is not markedly different from that of normal individuals (*312,313,317*). The percentage of helper/inducer cells and the cytotoxic/suppressor cells in the lymph nodes of HD patients is often quite variable (*279,318,319*), a fact that complicates the analysis of the T4:T8 cell ratios in these organs. Bearing this latter fact in mind, the general data indicate high helper:inducer to cytotoxic:suppressor cell ratios (about 5) in the lymph nodes of HD patients (*279,318,319*), in comparison with that of normal individuals' peripheral blood (from 2 to 3; *see* ref. *310*) or even with that of non-Hodgkin's hyperplastic lymph nodes (*279,319*), these ratios being independent of the treatment, if any (*279*). Another study found no differences in the helper/inducer to cytotoxic/suppressor ratios in the lymph nodes of HD patients and normal individuals (*313*). Furthermore, to the opposite extreme, Martin et al. (*320*) claimed that lymph nodes of HD patients exhibit a higher proportion of suppressor cells than hyperplastic lymph nodes of control individuals (helper/inducer to cytotoxic/suppressor ratios of 3.5 and 5.4; $p < 0.025$, respectively). These conflicting results could be explained in part by the variability of cellular subpopulation found in the lymph nodes of HD patients (*279,318,319*), and in part by the observation that OKT4 and Leu 3 monoclonal antibodies may also react with macrophages (*321*).

In general, these findings do not agree with the conclusion, based on analysis of Tμ:Tγ ratios, that suppressor cells are represented in the blood of HD patients in higher proportions than in normal individuals (*303,309*). However, Tμ and Tγ cellular populations do not correlate either phenotypically or functionally with the cellular subpopulations marked by T4/Leu3 and T8/T5/Leu2 antibodies, respectively. Both T4 and T5/T8 cell subsets contain Tμ and Tγ cells (275), making direct comparison between the two types of cellular population impossible. Furthermore, it has been found that T4$^+$ cells activate in vitro both helper and suppressor functions (265,322), and that suppressor-effector cells may bear a T4$^+$ marker, but not T8$^+$ marker (266), thus high helper/inducer: cytotoxic/suppressor ratio is not necessarily indicative of reduced suppressor cell function. It should further be borne in mind that organ-localized T8$^+$ cells could be cytotoxic rather than suppressive.

Although phenotypic characterization of cellular subpopulations has failed to establish any firm conclusions about the contribution of suppressor T cells to HD immune deficiency, more conclusive results may be obtained by functional studies. Several authors have found that the mononuclear cellular population of HD patients' peripheral blood contains a higher percentage of monocytes than normal individuals (309,323–325); the respective percentage values in three different studies are the following: 38.5 $\pm$ 4.3 vs 12.6 $\pm$ 3 (323), about 40 vs less than 25 (324), and 21 $\pm$ 2.4 vs 14.5 $\pm$ 1.2 (325). These differences were more pronounced in active disease (323,325), and were less significant (323) or absent (325) in inactive states. Other authors have not found differences between the levels of peripheral blood monocytes in normal individuals and patients (305,326). It should be borne in mind that, even if the absolute number of monocytes is not elevated in the peripheral blood of HD patients, there relative expression might be higher than normal because of a decrease in the level of the PBL. For instance, Sibbitt et al. (305) found similar percentages of monocytes in the blood of HD patients and normal individuals (13.2 $\pm$ 8.7% and 10.0 $\pm$ 1.0%, respectively), but the ratio of lymphocytes to monocytes was markedly lower in the patients (2.7) than in controls (6.6), the result of a substantial reduction of peripheral blood lymphocytes. A considerable reduction of lymphocytes in the blood of HD patients was also found by Schechter and colleagues (323,327), the lymphocyte:monocyte ratio of normals was 4.4 and that of HD patients 0.6.

As previously discussed (1), raised concentrations of monocytes may cause a substantial nonspecific suppression of the immune response. The notion that suppressor monocytes are associated with the immune deficiency found in HD is supported by several experimental approaches.

If an excess of monocytes in the peripheral blood of HD patients is responsible for the depressed in vitro immunological activities of the lymphocytes, removal of the monocytes from the blood sample should restore the immunological function. Sibbitt and associates (305) and Twomey and colleagues (324) applied peripheral blood MNC of HD patients to glass wool columns. The glass nonadherent cells exhibited stronger proliferative responses to PHA than the original cellular population. When the adherent cells were added back to the nonadherent cells, the PHA proliferative response was once again suppressed (305). Therapy did not affect the results (305), since the same pattern was found in both treated and untreated patients. In addition, Twomey et al. (324) demonstrated that the glass wool nonadherent cells exhibited augmented Ig synthesis after in vitro stimulation with PWM. This Ig synthesis almost reached the levels obtained from healthy individuals' MNC responding to the PWM stimulus. It was further demonstrated that mononuclear cells of HD patients suppressed the PWM-induced Ig synthesis of normal MNC when both cellular populations were cultured together. The degree of suppression of both the PHA proliferative response and Ig synthesis correlated with the number of monocytes in the peripheral blood of the patients, the more monocytes counted the more severe was the suppression observed, suggesting that glass-wool-adherent monocytes are responsible for the suppressive effect. In addition, the levels of PHA proliferative response and Ig synthesis suppressions correlated with each other, suggesting that the same mechanism inhibits both types of immunological activities. As we shall see later, Twomey et al. (324,328) found that, whereas some HD patients present suppressor monocytes, others present suppressor lymphocytes.

Schechter, Soehnlen, and colleagues (323,327,329) removed the monocytes from HD patients' MNC population by feeding them with carbonyl iron followed by their differential centrifugation over a Ficoll-Hypaque density gradient. The monocyte-depleted cellular population generated an augmented proliferative response after stimulation with PHA, PWM, and streptococcal antigen (streptolysin 0), an observation that was confirmed by the manifestation of intensive blastogenesis seen by light microscopy. The enhancing effect of monoctye removal (showing their inhibitory effect) was not, however, always consistent during periods of relapse in advanced disease. In certain cases, removal of monocytes enhanced the mitogen-induced proliferative response, whereas in others, it failed to do so. Because in all instances the patients were treated with radiotherapy and/or chemotherapy, it would appear that the suppressive effects were not treatment-related. The removal of monocytes did not, however, affect the mitogenic responses in remission or in localized diseases. In addition, the monocyte inhibitory effect did not correlate with the monocyte concentration in the blood, but did correlate with low lymphocyte:monocyte ratios, caused by a profound decrease of lymphocytes in the peripheral blood of HD patients. Adding back autologous plastic-adherent cells to monocyte-depleted MNC populations of HD patients inhibited the PHA mitogenic response. The same monocytes failed to inhibit the PHA mitogenic response of allogeneic normal MNC, but the relevance of this observation is uncertain since suppression of the PHA response, under these specific experimental conditions, may require HLA-identity. Since the same number of monocytes required to inhibit the autologous PHA responses of HD patients' MNC failed to inhibit the autologous PHA response of normal MNC, the authors suggest that the disease activates the monocytes (*see* also ref. *330*), which subsequently express a more efficient suppressive activity. In contrast, Twomey et al. (*324*) found that monocytes of HD patients exhibit a simple quantitative inhibition similar to that demonstrated by normal monocytes.

Hillinger and Herzig (*326*) found that MNC population of HD patients contain suppressor cells that inhibit the ability of autologous lymphocytes to proliferate after stimulation with allogeneic cells in MLC. Suppressor cells were found in treated or untreated patients with active disease, as well as in treated patients in remission. The suppressive activity of some patients' MNC was lost after removal of cells that ingested carbonyl iron or removal of nylon-wool-adherent cells. Mononuclear cells of the same or other patients retained their suppressive activity after depletion of cells forming rosettes with sheep erythrocytes (E^+ cells), suggesting that in all these cases the suppressor cells were monocytes. Nevertheless, we shall see later that suppressor T cells were found by the same authors in other patients (*326*).

Han (*331*) isolated T cells from HD patients' MNC by separating cells forming rosettes with sheep erythrocytes (E rosettes) from a Ficoll-Hypaque gradient. T cells of some patients (especially those with systemic symptoms) responded less efficiently to PHA than those of healthy subjects, suggesting an intrinsic defect of the T cells. Patients' cells depleted of E rosettes were exposed to iron particles and then were applied to a Ficoll-Hypaque gradient. Two cellular populations were separated from the gradient, a monocyte-enriched fraction, and a monocyte-depleted fraction (B cells were included in this second fraction). Monocyte-enriched cellular fractions from patients with active disease suppressed the autologous PHA mitogenic response of T cells. No suppressor T-cell activity was observed in both active and remission patients. In addition, suppressor macrophages were not found in the spleens of patients with active disease. In contrast, a different study (332) reported the detection of suppressor cells, inhibiting Ig synthesis after PWM stimulation, in the spleens of such patients.

The suppressive mechanism mediated by HD patients' monocytes has been the object of intensive research. Schechter et al. (327) found that MNC of HD patients failed to produce IL-1 after stimulation with LPS, PPD, or PHA, and the production of this monokine was completely restored after removal of monocytes ingesting carbonyl iron. It is possible that residual monocytes released from arrest following elimination of suppressor monocytes express their ability to produce IL-1 essential for initiating proliferative immunological activities.

In trying to answer how the suppression is mediated, Goodwin and colleagues (333) demonstrated that addition of indomethacin, an inhibitor of PG synthetase, to MNC of HD patients completely restored their ability to proliferate after PHA stimulation, suggesting that PG are responsible for the inhibitory effect. Indeed, PHA-stimulated MNC of HD patients produced approximately fourfold more PG than did normal MNC. Removal of glass-adherent cells substantially decreased both the enhancing effect of indomethacin upon the PHA proliferative response and the production of PG. In the separate study, Goodwin et al. (334) demonstrated that exogenous PG inhibits mitogen-induced proliferation of human lymphocytes. These experiments as well as others (335,336) indicate that PGs produced by monocytes of HD patients are responsible for the depressed mitogenic response observed in the stimulated MNC of these patients. Similar mechanisms have been observed for normal MNC (334), but as indicated before, they produced less PG than the MNC of HD patients. The observation that indomethacin augments mitogenic responses of HD patients' MNC has been confirmed by other studies (305,324,325,337–340). In addition, Bockman (341,342) demon-

demonstrated that indomethacin and flurbiprofen (another PG synthetase inhibitor) enhanced T-cell colony formation in HD patients' blood and spleen cell culture, suggesting that PGs control this function. Indeed, it was further found that adherent monocytes of HD patients synthesize more PG than adherent cells of normal individuals (342), and that PGs inhibit the clonal expansion of precursor T cells, which give rise to colonies (343). The authors recorded a progressive reduction of colony formation with more advancing stages of the disease, but they do not think that this phenomenon is solely related to increased production of PG, since PG synthetase inhibitors do not restore completely the T-cell lymphocyte colony formation. Schechter et al. (327) reported, however, that the indomethacin did not always augment the PHA proliferative response of HD patients' MNC (*see* also refs. 289 and 326), whereas the augmenting effect of monocyte-depletion exhibited more consistent results. In most cases where an enhancing effect of indomethacin was noted, the effect of monocyte depletion was more pronounced. It was concluded, therefore, that monocytes of HD patients use, in addition to PG production, other mechanisms that cause inhibition of mitogenic responses.

In contrast to Goodwin et al. (333), Fisher and Bostick-Bruton (336) indicated that neither monocyte depletion nor addition of indomethacin restored the PHA-induced mitogenic proliferation of the patients' MNC to the normal level, although they significantly augmented their response. These authors stimulated the MNC with suboptimal doses of PHA, which maximizes the differences between the mitogenic responses of lymphocytes from patients and normal individuals, whereas Goodwin et al. (333) used optimal doses of PHA. These different experimental protocols may explain the contradictory results. The fact that indomethacin or macrophage depletion, in some instances, only partially restored the PHA mitogenic responses of patients' MNC, suggests that a significant factor of HD immunodepression is either a different suppression mechanism or else an intrinsic defect in the T cells themselves. It should be indicated that long-term disease-free survivors of HD display depressed T-cell mitogenic proliferation, but they do not present significant augmentation of this response after addition of indomethacin (336), again suggesting an intrinsic defect of the T cells. This latter abnormality may be either a permanent defect acquired with the disease or a genetically determined predisposing factor with a possible etiological significance.

The finding that MNC (327,333) or adherent cells (341,342) of HD patients, both newly diagnosed and those in remission, produce greater amounts of PG than MNC of normal subjects has been confirmed by a later study (325). Again, no direct correlation was found between the activity of suppressor monocytes and the level of PG (*see* also ref. 327). Furthermore, the amount of PG secreted into the medium of cultures of MNC of HD patients, while in excess of those seen in normal MNC cultures, was still 100-fold less than the amount of exogenous PG required to induce a suppression comparable to the suppression observed in the patients' MNC (325). These results confirm that PG excessive production is not the sole mechanism of lymphoproliferation inhibition by monocytes. Even more importantly, whereas the PG level of HD patients' MNC inversely correlated in this particular study (325) with their in vitro PHA response, it did not correlate with the anergy of the patients (for supportive data, *see* ref. 344) nor with their clinical stage.

DeShazo (337) administered indomethacin orally to four HD patients (750 mg over 8 d). The MNC of two patients exhibited an enhanced PHA mitogenic response, compared with the response of the MNC of the same patients before the administration of the drug. The indomethacin treatment did not alter, however, the DTH skin test of these patients.

Activated macrophages produce highly reactive oxygen metabolites, such as hydrogen peroxide (H_2O_2). Such a product has been implicated as a mediator of macrophage-mediated suppression of lymphocyte proliferation (345). The suppressive mechanism mediated by activated monocytes of HD patients may also be associated, at least in part, with oxygen metabolites. In order to test this possibility, DeShazo and colleagues (339) tested the ability of antioxidant compounds to augment the PHA mitogenic response of HD patients' MNC. Catalase, an enzyme promoting the degradation of hydrogen peroxide, and vitamin E, a free radical scavenger, were employed for this purpose. Whereas addition of the antioxidants alone slightly and insignificantly augmented the PHA proliferative response of the patients' MNC, it significantly increased the enhancement effect of indomethacin. This observation was confirmed by independent study (336). This latter study indicates, however, that the net proliferative response of the patients' cultures, containing catalase plus indomethacin, remained significantly lower than the proliferative response of comparable cultures obtained from normal individuals. Removal of nylon-adherent cells abolished the enhancing effect of indomethacin or the combination of indomethacin and antioxidants (339). This finding suggests that adherent cells producing toxic oxygen metabolites as well as PG may be responsible, at least partially, for the lymphoproliferation inhibition found in HD patients. The synergistic effect of indomethacin plus catalase may be explained by the fact that PG exerts negative feedback on the production of oxygen radicals by macrophages (346). Thus, suppression mediated by hydrogen peroxide may be enhanced by the presence of indomethacin. On the other hand, oxygen radicals may augment PG synthesis (345). In contrast to the majority of the other investigators, Han (331) failed to find SFs associated with the suppressor monocytes.

Arresting cellular division by irradiation (323,331) or MMC treatment (326) did not affect the suppressive capacity of HD patients' monocytes, indicating that their suppressive function is proliferation independent. Whereas suppressor monocytes were detected in some HD patients, suppressor lymphocytes or more specifically suppressor T cells have been found in other patients. Twomey et al. (324) demonstrated that glass-wool-nonadherent lymphocytes from 5 of 11 untreated patients suppressed the ability of autologous cells (but not allogeneic cells) to proliferate after stimulation with allogeneic cells (MLC). A previous work of Twomey et al. (328) demonstrated that MNC of some patients failed to stimulate effectively the proliferation of allogeneic cells (in MLC), but the stimulation was improved if glass-adherent cells were removed from the stimulator cellular population. It was suggested, however, that the stimulator cellular population contains suppressor lymphocytes, since removal of phagocytic cells (by magnetic separation of cells that have engulfed carbonyl iron) did not affect the suppressive activity.

As indicated before, Hillinger and Herzig (326) found suppressor monocytes in some treated and untreated HD patients, whereas in others they found suppressor T cells. Both types of suppressor cells were detected by their ability to inhibit the capacity of autologous cells to proliferate after stimulation with allogeneic cells (MLC). The suppressor T cells were identified by their inability to adhere to nylon wool, the elimination of suppressor cell function after the removal of E^+ cells, and the presence of suppressor cells in the E^+ cellular population.

The suppressor cells found in the patients of Hillinger and Herzig (326) exhibited genetic restriction, they inhibited the MLC of autologous cells, but not that of allogeneic cells. Furthermore, one of the patients in this study had a sister with identical HLA. The patient's suppressor cells inhibited its own MLC and that of his sister to the same extent, but they failed to inhibit the MLC of an unrelated subject.

These results were confirmed by Engleman and colleagues in an independent study (347,348). They prepared cellular preparations enriched for T cells (95%) and non-T cells (mostly Ig positive cells and few monocytes) by an E-rosetting separation technique. The T and the non-T cells of HD patients were tested for their ability to suppress an MLC in which the responder cells were autologous to the tested suppressor cells. These authors found, like Hillinger and Herzig (326), that cells derived from both treated and untreated patients exhibited suppressive activity. Some patients presented suppressor T cells (which were possibly genetically restricted; 347), whereas others presented non-T suppressor cells, or even both types of cells. Hillinger and Herzig (326) found suppressor cells among 80% of their active patients and in 60% of their inactive patients, and Engleman and associates (348) found such cells in two-thirds of both treated and untreated patients. It should be noted, however, that the former group used an 8:1 suppressor to responder ratio in their studies, whereas the latter group used a 1:1 ratio, which probably was not sufficient to detect suppressor cells with weak activity. Engleman et al. (348) found a lack of correlation between activity of suppressor cells and age, sex, duration of disease, histological classification, clinical stage, or HLA. They also noticed that suppressor T cells were more common in treated patients. This is not surprising since it is well known that total lymphoid irradiation, widely used in therapy of HD, induces the appearance of suppressor T cells (349). Lack of correlation between activity of suppressor cells and histological classification or clinical stage of the disease was indicated also in ref. 289. Both Hillinger and Herzig (326) and Engleman et al. (348) did not detect SFs (like PG) in their systems. The suppressor T cells were effective after irradiation (324,348) and MMC treatment (326), indicating that their activity was proliferation independent.

Zarling and colleagues (*350*) applied MNC of HD patients to columns of Sepharose beads conjugated with histamine coupled to rabbit serum albumin. Patients' MNC with weak capacity of generating cytotoxic cells after in vitro stimulation with allogeneic cells, acquired an efficient capacity to generate such cells after passage over the column, suggesting that at least some HD patients express suppressor cells with histamine receptors. The authors presented evidence that these cells were not monocytes, but their classification as T cells requires experimental support.

The function of Con A induced suppressor cells in HD patients has been investigated by several workers. Schulof and colleagues (*351*) found a reduction in the activity of Con A-induced peripheral blood suppressor cells, especially among patients with advanced disease. No correlation between absolute lymphocyte count, absolute T-cell number, or mitogenic response to PHA and Con A-induced suppressor-cell activity was found (*351*). Akbar et al. (*352*) found that the activities of Con A-induced suppressor cells derived from the blood or the spleen of HD patients were no different from the corresponding cells of normal subjects (the suppressor cells were tested for their ability to inhibit Ig expression by PWM-induced autologous cells). Those individuals (both normals and patients) who exhibited a high level of Con A-induced suppressor cells demonstrated a lower level of spontaneous suppressor cells and vice versa, suggesting that both types of cells derived from the same cellular pool.

Although Vanhaelen and Fisher (*353*) also found no difference in the activities of Con A-induced suppressor cells of normal subjects and untreated HD patients, they did demonstrate that the untreated HD patients' MNC were more sensitive to allogeneic Con A-induced suppressor cells than MNC of normal subjects (i.e., when incubated with such cells, the patients' MNC demonstrated significantly lower proliferative response after Con A stimulation). MNC of patients with advanced disease were more sensitive in this respect than MNC of patients with early disease. The Con A-induced suppressor cells must be alive in order to express their activity, but arresting their division capacity by irradiation or MMC treatments did not change their function. A suppressor factor was not found in the supernatants of the suppressor cells, nor was PG involved in the suppressive mechanism. In a different study Fisher and colleagues (*354*) found that MNC of untreated HD patients were also more sensitive to monocyte suppressor cells (derived from normal subjects) than MNC of normal individuals. A profound sensitivity to Con A-induced suppressor cells and monocyte suppressor cells was demonstrated also by MNC of treated long-term HD survivors (*355*). The authors think that this sensitivity is associated with the disease, or perhaps even with the etiology of the disease, and not with the treatment, because MNC of similarly treated long-term survivors with diffuse histiocytic lymphoma demonstrated the same low sensitivity to suppressor monocytes as MNC of normal individuals (*355*). This study suggests that the low mitogen-induced proliferative response of HD patients' MNC is associated with increased sensitivity of these cells to direct cell-associated suppressive signals.

In summary, HD patients express considerable depression of cellular immunity, and at least some of their reduced in vitro tested immunological activities correlate with the activity of suppressor cells. The suppressor-cell activity does not correlate, however, with the in vivo manifestations of the HD immunodeficiency expressed by weak DTH to standard tested antigens. Similarly, the suppressor-cell function does not correlate with the disease activity. These facts cast doubts upon the association between the suppressor cells and the in vivo immunodeficiency in HD and, consequently, between the suppressor cells and the primary or the secondary (e.g., infections) pathological manifestations of the disease. However, because the suppressor cells were detected by in vitro tests, one cannot exclude the possibility that another suppressive mechanism, which may include a different subpopulation of suppressor cells, refractory to in vitro detection, may be responsible for the immunodeficiency and its consequences in HD.

It may be further suggested that the immunosuppression observed in HD is at least partially mediated by the hormone 1,25 dihydroxyvitamin D_3, which may be secreted by the HD cells themselves. This hormone, as well as causing hypercalcaemia (*356,357*), may induce the differentiation of monocytes from marrow precursors. In addition, the hormone may induce the activation of these monocytes (*358,359*) and, consequently, the expression of their suppressive function. This vitamin D metabolite also has a profound inhibitory effect upon helper T cells (*360*), possibly by blocking the release of IL-2 (*361*).

A second possibility could be the suppression resulting from the efforts of an immune system to overcome the enhancement of immune responses by the Reed-Sternberg cells themselves. The

Table 1
Suppressor Cells in Hodgkin's Disease[a,b]

Type of suppressor cells (S:R)	Effect of suppressor cells	Properties of suppressor cells	SF	Comments	Ref.
Monocytes (1:1)	Inhibition of PHA mitogenic response	Adhere to glass; bear C3 receptor (?)	Yes PG	Treated and untreated patients	305
Unknown (2:1 to 1:1)	Inhibition of PHA mitogenic response	Con A-induced suppressor cells	Yes PG	Untreated patients; decrease of suppressor cells in patients	309
Monocytes (1:2 to 1:5)	Inhibition of PHA, PWM and SLO mitogenic responses, and IL-1 production	Engulf carbonyl iron; adhere to plastic and glass; resist 3000 rad	Yes PG	Treated patients	323, 327, 329
Monocytes (1:1)	Inhibition of PHA mitogenic response and PWM induced-Ig synthesis	Adhere to glass	Yes PG	Untreated patients	324
T cells	Inhibition of MLR	Glass nonadherent; resist 2500 rad; genetically restricted			
Monocytes	Inhibition of PHA mitogenic response	Adhere to plastic	Yes PG	Untreated patients	325

Cell type	Function/assay	Characteristics	PG/oxygen metabolites	Patient status	Reference
Monocytes (8:1)	Inhibition of MLC	Engulf carbonyl iron; adhere to NW; resist MMC	No	Treated and untreated patients	326
T cells (8:1)		E$^+$; resist MMC; genetically restricted			
Monocytes (1:2 to 1:5)	Inhibition of PHA mitogenic response	Engulf carbonyl iron; resist 6000 rad	No	Treated and untreated patients	331
Monocytes	Inhibition of PHA mitogenic response	Adhere to plastic	Yes PG hydrogen peroxide	Untreated patients	336
Monocytes	Inhibition of PHA mitogenic response	Adhere to NW	Yes PG and Toxic ox. metab.	Treated and untreated patients	337, 339
Monocytes	Inhibition of T cell colony formation	Adhere to plastic	Yes PG	Untreated patients	341–343
Non-T cells (1:1)	Inhibition of MLC	E$^-$; resist 1000 rad	No	Treated and untreated patients	348
T cells (1:1)		E$^+$; resist 1000 rad; genetically restricted			
Undefined, perhaps T cells	Inhibition of cytotoxic cells generated in MLC	Bear histamine (H$_2$) receptor		Treated patients	350

[a]The suppressor cells recorded in this table are nonspecific.

[b]New abbreviations used in this table: NW, nylon wool; SLO, streptolysin O; S:R, suppressor:responder ratio; Tox. Ox. Metab., toxic oxygen metabolites.

Reed-Sternberg cells are genetically restricted efficient antigen-presenting cells (280), and are effective stimulator and accessory cells in MLC and responses to mitogens, respectively (362,363). The increased load of active immune accessory cells in the lymphoma could then result in a poorly regulated suppression.

For both suggestions, a rule may be envisaged for suppressor cells of different types, and their heterogeneity could then reflect both the heterogeneity of the lymphoma itself, by no means uniform (364), and the relative integrity of the immune system during the malignant state. In any event, the relevance of the suppressor cells to the HD malignancy is unclear, and attempts at potentiation of apparently depressed immune function would have at present no rational basis, and may even exacerbate the malignancy. The properties of HD suppressor cells are summarized in Table 1.

3. Non-Hodgkin's Lymphomas, Leukemias, and Multiple Myelomas

3.1. Introduction

The hematologic neoplasms encompass two classes of malignant lymphoproliferative disorders distinguished by their apparent site of origin or location, these being the lymphomas arising from lymph nodes and lymphoid components of other tissues, and the leukemias characterized by abnormal maturation in the marrow and accumulation of the abnormal cells in the peripheral blood (365). Both morphological and surface marker analysis suggest that each hematologic malignancy has been arrested at a distinct maturational stage, probably representing the initial malignant event (366). As a result, the hematologic neoplasms offer a means of dissecting hematopoietic development. For example, cells of unclassified acute lymphoblastic leukemia (ALL) are negative for both T and B cell markers, but positive for terminal deoxynucleotidyl tranferase, a marker for pre-T cells, and possibly other immature hemopoietic cells. The leukemic cells of common ALL (c-ALL) have the characteristics of pre-B cells, and those of Burkitt's lymphoma appear similar to early B cells. Both B cell chronic lymphocytic leukemia (B-CLL) and prolymphocytic leukemia (B-PLL) have the characteristics of an intermediate stage of B cell differentiation, whereas leukemic cells of nodular lymphoma or diffuse poorly differentiated lymphoma appear to be arrested at a mature B cell stage. The cells of multiple myeloma (MM) are functionally equivalent to a mature immunoglobulin-secreting plasma cell, the final stage of B cell differentiation (366). Similarly, lymphomas and leukemias may also carry markers characteristic of different levels of T cell differentiation. The T cell lymphoblastic lymphomas (T-LL) and T cell acute lymphoblastic leukemias (T-ALL) may be arranged in an early putative differentiation sequence for T cells based on the selective expression of a large panel of surface markers (366), whereas cells of T cell chronic lymphocytic leukemia (T-CLL) may express either helper (T4, Leu3) or suppressor (T8, Leu2) T cell markers (366), suggesting the malignant event occurs at the point of commitment to either the suppressor or helper pathway. Meanwhile, cells of Sézary Syndrome or adult T cell leukemia (ATL) are invariably T4-positive, suggesting transformation after commitment to the helper/inducer T cell line (366,367).

Chronic mylogenous leukemia (CML) is a clonal myloproliferative malignancy arising from transformation at the level of the pluripotent stem cell and characterized clinically by an overproduction of granulocytes. In most cases, the malignant cells of the patients are characterized by a specific chromosome abnormality, the Philadelphia (Ph[1]) chromosome (366,368). Although the above theoretical aspects of the malignant transformations may be still a matter of debate, the association of particular surface markers with stages of differentiation or maturation is rapidly gaining acceptance as a means of diagnosis complementary to histopathology of the neoplasm.

Since the lymphoid and the myeloid tissues provide the cellular structure for the immune system, the disturbance of their functions by malignancy must cause severe damage to the normal immunological activity. For example, malignant lymphoid or myeloid cells that do not mature to express their normal biological program will not express their immunological functions as well. Furthermore, their early differentiation antigens may even induce the appearance of suppressor cells, which subsequently may restrain any immunological activity against the tumor. On the other hand, dominant expression of malignant mature cells, such as helper or suppressor T cells, may cause a collapse of the normal immunoregulation because of the imbalance of T cell subsets.

In the following sections, such surface markers will be used to dissect and analyze the possible role of suppressor cells, either normal endogenous cells or malignant in origin, in complications of malignancy (e.g., opportunistic infections) or else in enabling the tumor to progress unabated by immunological efforts at rejection.

3.2. Non-Hodgkin's Lymphoma

The lymphomas may be conveniently divided into Hodgkin's Disease and the non-Hodgkin's lymphomas (NHL). This latter group may be divided further into the lymphomas of a nodular nature and those of a diffuse nature. Within each group, differentiation of subtypes is usually determined by histology, but more recently, surface-marker analysis has been used to enhance this classification. The majority of non-Hodgkin's lymphomas appear to derive from B cells and, to a lesser extent, from T cells or histiocytes (369,370). Progressive improvement of immunological detection techniques may increase the frequency of diagnosed T cell lymphomas. In agreement with this notion, a recent study proposed that 53% of lymphomas were of B cell origin and 42% were of T cell origin, most of them carrying the helper T cell phenotype (371). Non-Hodgkin's lymphomas with a suppressor T cell phenotype (T8$^+$) have also been characterized (371,372,373). The last report (373) describes NHL associated with long-standing hypogammaglobulinemia. A linkage between suppressor cell function of the OKT8 cells and the hypogammaglobulinemia was suggested with no attempt to prove this by functional studies. It should be finally emphasized that the development of lymphomas in different compartments of the lymph nodes leads to malignant cells expressing varying degrees of differentiation (369,370).

During the late course of the diseases, bacterial, fungal, and viral infections may occur. A leukopenia may be present, resulting from treatment and may be associated with early bacterial infections (369). The infectious complications are presumably associated with immunodepression caused by the disease, the disease treatment, or both. Evidence that the immunodepression is associated with the lymphoma itself was presented by Jones (374), who demonstrated that more than half of the untreated patients injected with recall antigens exhibited marked impairment of DTH. This observation was confirmed by a later study (375). However, marked heterogeneity in this response was observed; patients with diffuse histology and constitutional symptoms displayed more severe immunodepression than those with nodular histology and who had lacked symptoms (*374*). The majority of NHL patients manifest a defect of primary antibody synthesis (*376*). Furthermore, a marked decrease in the number of T cells was found in the lymph nodes of patients with NHL (*319,377*). Whereas the overall helper T cell:suppressor T cell ($T_H:T_S$) ratios (defined with Leu-3 and OKT8 antibodies, respectively) of the patients' blood was no different to that of normal individuals (2.18 and 2.12, respectively), patients with unfavorable clinical course demonstrated significantly lower $T_H:T_S$ ratios (1.76) than patients with favorable clinical course (2.82), suggesting that the higher relative helper T cell representation correlates with better prognosis. In contrast, neither treatment nor tumor stage had a clear-cut influence on the extent of the relative T cell representation in the lymph nodes (*377*). A T cell zone was found around the neoplastic follicles of patients with centroblastic-centrocytic lymphoma. Suppressor T cells were present more frequently within neoplastic follicles than within normal follicles, and the ratio of helper to suppressor cells (T4:T8) demonstrated a shift toward an excess of $T8^+$ cells (*367*). Yet, in another study, the malignant cells in the lymph nodes presented the $T8^+$ phenotype solely (*378*).

The possibility that suppressor cells are associated with the low in vitro immunological activity of lymphocytes obtained from the blood of untreated lymphoma patients was explored by Whisler and colleagues (*379,380*). These authors found that fresh MNC of NHL patients responded poorly to Con A, but they gained partial ability to respond to this mitogen after an in vitro incubation for 3 d. Fresh MNC of more than half of the patients suppressed, most of them incompletely, the ability of the cultured MNC to respond to Con A. Suppressor activity was detected mainly in patients with diffuse histology or constitutional symptoms (*379,380*). Mononuclear cells from NHL patients, depleted of monocytes by carbonyl iron engulfment and magnetic removal, exhibited an augmented mitogenic response to Con A. This response was abolished by addition of fresh (but not cultured) plastic adherent cells to the monocyte-depleted MNC (*379*), indicating that monocytes mediate the suppressive effect. Careful analysis of the overall data further reveals that the effect of the suppressor monocytes was incomplete, suggesting that other mechanisms besides suppressor-cell function inhibit the mitogenic responses of the patients' MNC. Furthermore, the patients' lymphocytes also expressed an intrinsic defect, since their mitogenic activity, even after culture in vitro, never returned to the response generated by normal cells. In contrast to untreated patients, successfully treated patients demonstrated either normal responses to Con A, or profound irreversible impairment of this immunological activity (*380*). The possibility that MNC of NHL patients contain suppressor monocytes that mediate their effect by PG was suggested by Han (*335*) and Han and Winnicki (*338*). The patients' MNC proliferative response to PHA, Con A, and PWM was slightly enhanced after addition of indomethacin, a PG synthetase inhibitor, but this effect occurred only if monocytes were present in the culture.

Suppressor cells, detected by their ability to inhibit local xenogeneic GVHR were found in the bone marrow and the mediastinal mass of a patient with poorly differentiated diffuse malignant lymphoma (*381*). The authors suggest that the suppressor cells are T cells, although direct evidence for this statement was not provided.

The presence of suppressor cells bearing histamine receptors in treated NHL patients was suggested by the augmentation of the allogeneic cytotoxic response of the patients' MNC after their passage over histamine-coated columns (*350*). A different study indicates that cells bearing the T3$^+$, 4$^+$, 8$^-$ phenotype of a patient with cutaneous T cell lymphoma suppressed the PWM-induced Ig synthesis of cocultivated normal cells (*382*). The lymph node malignant cells of another patient (T8$^+$ phenotype) helped the in vitro IgM immunoglobulin synthesis, but suppressed the in vitro IgG immunoglobulin production (*378*).

Mangan and associates (*383*) explored the suppressor T cell function during the treatment course of a patient with diffuse well-differentiated lymphocytic lymphoma. A life-threatening pancytopenia-aplasia developed almost immediately after treatment with human α-INF. During this time, marrow progenitor cells, CFU-E (erythroid colony-forming unit), and BFU-E (erythroid burst-forming unit) were undetectable. In contrast, the proportions of marrow T8$^+$ (cytotoxic/suppressor) lymphocytes and/or Leu7$^+$ NK cells and Tγ cells were markedly elevated. In addition to the possible direct effect of INF on the cell proliferation (*384*), it may also activate T8$^+$ and NK cells (*384,385*), both of which may be implicated in the inhibition of erythroid progenitor cells (*383,386*). Furthermore, the α-INF activated suppressor cells may release γ-INF (*387,388*), which may further activate immuno-suppression.

In agreement with this notion, Mangan et al. (*383*) found that removal of T cells by E-rosetting, as well as OKT3 or OKT8 monoclonal antibodies and C, markedly increased the CFU-E in the bone marrow cells of the α-INF-treated patient, and readdition of autologous T cells (but not heterologous normal cells) to the T-depleted cells completely inhibited the CFU-E. Corticosteriod-androgen treatment did not improve the hematologic state of the patient, but a dramatic change occurred after subsequent treatment with antilymphocytic globulin (ATG). The patient exhibited a rise in blood neutrophils, reticulocytosis, loss of the in vitro activity of suppressor cells on erythroid progenitor cells, and a remarkable reversal of the blood and the marrow T4:T8 ratios. Because of the direct effect of INF on marrow progenitor cells and its ability to affect the immunoregulation balance, the authors suggest cautious employment of the drug.

Thus, the immunosuppression of NHL patients could be mediated at least in part by suppressor monocytes or suppressor T cells. Nevertheless, the association between this immunosuppression and the disease is a matter of speculation.

One such speculation proposes that activation of suppressor cells causes immunosuppression, which is associated with the creation of an environment encouraging either the initial malignant transformation or else its progression. This concept, however, cannot be general, since Burkitt's lymphoma may provide an example of the reverse situation: failure of suppressor cell function committed to control B cell expansion may cause uncontrolled proliferation of Epstein-Barr virus (EBV)-infected B cells and their subsequent malignant transformation. In agreement with this notion, Whittle and colleagues (*389*) found that the T cell control of EBV-infected B cells is lost during *P. falciparum* malaria. The geographical coincidence of Burkitt's lymphoma and malaria may therefore provide the etiological basis for the lymphoma. On the other hand, the success of T cells to control the proliferation of EBV-infected B cells in infectious mononucleosis (*390,391*) may explain why this disease is not malignant. The question as to whether the T cell function controlling the B cell expansion is synonymous with suppressor T cell function is mostly dependent on the flexibility of the suppressor cell function definition; in this instance, T cells controlling Ig production by myeloma cells have also been considered as suppressor T cells (1). In a separate study, it was found that an excess of EBV antigen induced the appearance of specific suppressor T cells (T8$^+$) in cultures of MNC of EBV seropositive individuals (392). Similar suppressor cells induced in vivo may control the EBV-infected B cell proliferation (as documented in infectious mononucleosis; (390,391) or inhibit the immune response against the virus-induced tumor or the virus itself (possibly exemplified by EBV-associated nasopharyngeal carcinoma).

The suppressor cells may therefore exert a dual effect, and the balance between the two forces may determine the prognosis of the disease. As indicated before, environmental factors such as malarial infection, may have a considerable influence on the immunoregulatory balance and therefore on the disposition to malignancy. The properties of NHL suppressor cells are summarized in Table 2.

3.3. Acute Lymphoblastic Leukemia

Acute lymphoblastic leukemias tend to be leukemias of childhood and adolescence, characterized by a progressive malignant infiltration of the bone marrow and lymphatic organs by immature cells resembling lymphoblasts (393,394). The leukemic cells of the different ALL may express considerable variation in surface phenotypes, and this presumably represents the point in maturation pathway at which the final malignant event occurred. As a result, ALL may be associated with a lymphoid stem cell (c-ALL), with B cells (pre-B-ALL;B-ALL, which presumably represent Burkitt's lymphoma in a leukemic phase; 394), with T cells (pre-T-ALL;T-ALL), or with immature null cells. It has been recently suggested that the majority of the null cells may be pre-B cells (394–396).

Using anti-H$_2$ serum (directed against histamine receptors), it has been found that tumor cells of 80 percent of T-ALL patients express the TH$_2^-$ phenotype, whereas the rest of these patients exhibit the TH$_2^+$ phenotype (397). The TH$_2^-$ cellular subset accounts also for 80% of the PBL of normal individuals, and it provides a helper function. In contrast, the TH$_2^+$ subset comprises 20% of the normal PBL, and it contains both the cytotoxic and the suppressor cell populations (398,399). Using monoclonal antibodies with other specificities reveals that the majority of the T-ALL patients express either prothymocyte phenotypes, $T10^+$ or $T9^+$, $T10^+$, or the common thymocyte phenotype, $T10^+$, $T6^+$, $T4^+$, $T8^+$, and very few express the medullary mature phenotype $T10^+$, $T3^+$, $T4^+$, $T8^-$ or $T10^+$, $T3^+$, $T4^-$, $T8^+$ (400,401), i.e. either helper cells or cytotoxic/suppressor cells, respectively.

Patients with ALL exhibit a reduced NK activity, which does not appear to be mediated by suppressor cells (402). However, such patients do exhibit enhanced activity of short-lived suppressor cells that control T-lymphocyte colony formation in vitro. The suppressor cells were found in remission, but not during the acute phase of the disease (403).

Precursors of suppressor-effector cells may exist in T-ALL patients, although their function may not be detected because of the absence of suppressor-inducer cells [the suppressor-inducer cell ($T4^+$) activates the differentiation of the suppressor-precursor cells into mature suppressor-effector cells that can be either $T8^+$ or $T4^+$ cells; 265,266,404–406; Fig 3]. In line with this concept, Broder and colleagues (407) found that the leukemic cells of a boy with T-ALL contain precursors of suppressor-effector cells but not suppressor-inducer cells. Pokeweed mitogen-stimulated normal B cells supported by irradiated normal helper T cells exhibited an efficient Ig synthesis. ALL cells added to this cellular mixture did not inhibit the Ig production, unless normal T cells were also introduced into the cellular mixture. These results suggest that radiosensitive normal suppressor-inducer cells permit the differentiation of ALL suppressor-precursor cells into mature effector cells as detected by their ability to suppress the PWM-induced Ig production. ALL cells failed, however, to support differentiation of normal suppressor-precursor cells into mature suppressor-effector cells, indicating that they do not contain inducer-suppressor cells. ALL cells preincubated with normal T cells for 48 h, and then freed of them by killing the normal T cells with specific antiserum and C, were still capable of suppressing the Ig synthesis in the indicator cellular mixture. This experiment indicates first that the normal T cells contain the suppressor-inducer cell function and the ALL cells contain the suppressor-precursor cells, and second that the already differentiated ALL suppressor cells do not require the presence of suppressor-inducer cells in order to express their function. A factor released from the normal suppressor-inducer cells also stimulated the differentiation of the ALL suppressor-precursor cells into mature suppressor-effector

Table 2
Suppressor Cells in NHL, B-CLL, CML, and Myelomas[a,b]

Disease	Type of suppressor cells (S:R)	Effect of suppressor cells	Properties of suppressor cells	Comments	Ref.
NHL	Monocytes (1:1)	Inhibition of Con A mitogenic response	Engulf carbonyl iron; adhere to plastic; lose activity after in vitro incubation	Untreated patients	379, 380
NHL	T cells (?) (1:20)	Inhibition of local xenogeneic GVHR	E^+(?); EAC^+(?)	A treated patient; THF reverses the suppressor cell activity	381
NHL	Marrow $T3^+$ $T8^+$ cells	Inhibition of erythropoiesis	Induced with INF; sensitive to ATG given in vivo	An INF-treated patient	383
B-CLL	$T\gamma^+$ cells (3:1)	Inhibition of PWM-induced proliferative response	E^+	No treatment within 3 wk of study	424
B-CLL	$T\gamma^+$ cells (1:1)	Inhibtion of erythropoiesis	E^+	No treatment within at least 1 mo of study; reversion of the suppressive effect after drug induced remission	431, 435

B-CLL with Richter Syndrome	T3$^+$ T4$^+$ T8$^+$ cells	Inhibition of PHA and PWM mitogenic responses and MLC	E$^+$; adhere to plastic; ingest latex (?)	A treated patient	434
B-CLL	T cells (1:1)	Inhibition of PWM-induced Ig synthesis	E$^+$	Treated and untreated patients; no evidence for in vivo suppression of Ig synthesis	438
B-CLL	B and T cells (1:4)	Inhibition of PHA mitogenic response	E$^+$ and E$^-$ cells	No treatment within 3 wk of study; no SF	439
CML	Unknown (1:1)	Inhibition of PHA mitogenic response	Con A-induced and spontaneous suppressor cells	Suppressor-cell activity does not correlate with the disease	506
MM	Tγ^+ cells (1:1)	Inhibition of PWM-induced mitogenic response and PWM-induced Ig synthesis to the same extent as normal Ts	Radiosensitive to 2000 rad	No treatment at the time of study or untreated patients; B cells do not secrete Ig; normal function of Th and Ts (Tγ); lack of suppressor function in T non γ cell population	517

Table 2 (*Cont.*)

Disease	Type of suppressor cells (S:R)	Effect of suppressor cells	Properties of suppressor cells	Comments	Ref.
MM	Tγ⁺ cells (1:20)	Inhibition of PWM-induced B cell differentiation		Untreated patients	523
MM	T8⁺ cells (1:2)	Inhibition of PWM-induced B cell differentiation		Untreated patients; normal function of helper T cells	526
MM	Monocytes (1:1)	Inhibition of PWM-induced Ig synthesis or B cell differentiation	Engulf carbonyl iron; adhere to plastic and glass; resist 2000 rad	Treated and untreated patients; myeloma marrow cells do not exhibit suppressive activity	533–535

MM	EA-RFC, EAC-RFC, E-RFC and monocytes (1:1)	Inhibition of PWM, TT, and SKSD mitogenic responses and PWM, TT, and PP-induced Ig synthesis; inhibition of MLC	Resist MMC but cells must be viable; enhancement of suppressor-cell activity after Con A incubation	No treatment at the time of the study; suppressor cells release SF	536, 537
MM	Tγ⁺ cells (1:1)	Inhibition of PWM mitogenic response		Normal function of T_h; Ts of MM more effective than Ts of normal; MM B cells are more sensitive to suppression than normal B cells	539

[a]The suppressor cells recorded in this table are nonspecific.

[b]New abbreviations used in this table: PP, pneumococcal polysaccharide; SKSD, Streptokinase-streptodornase; Th, helper T cells; Ts, suppressor T cells; THF, thymus humoral factor; T nonγ, T cells that lack Fc receptor to IgG; TT, tetanus toxoid.

cells, as indicated by their function and the expression of new membrane antigens (IL-2 receptor designated Tac and to a certain extent T8$^+$). ALL cells incubated alone for 48 h gained the T3$^+$ marker, but this change was not accompanied by acquisition of a suppressive function.

3.4. Chronic Lymphocytic Leukemia

Chronic lymphocytic leukemia (CLL) is a disease associated with aging (median age of 60 yr). It is characterized by lymphadenopathy, peripheral lymphocytosis, bone marrow infiltration, and eventual interference with normal hematopoiesis (408). According to Dameshek (409), accumulation of immunologically incompetent lymphocytes throughout the body is the important pathological feature of the disease. The CLL may be subclassified by surface markers into B and T cell CLL, the vast majority being B-CLL (366,394,408,410). The classification of chronic lymphocytic leukemia may also include lymphosarcoma, B and T cell prolymphocytic leukemia, and hairy cell leukemia (408). Other T cell proliferative diseases such as cutaneous T cell lymphoma (mycosis fungoides/Sézary syndrome; 370,411,412), chronic T cell lymphocytosis with neutropenia (or Tγ -lymphoproliferative disease, Tγ -LPD; 394,413,414), and ATL (394,415) will be included in this section as well. It should be pointed out that ATL may appear in either subacute or chronic manifestations (reviewed in 394,415).

Patients with CLL exhibit an impaired immune system, especially immunoglobulin production (408,416), but also cell-mediated immunity, which may be detected by in vitro proliferation assays (290,293). Consequently, the risk of fungal, bacterial, and viral infections is markedly increased during the progression of the disease (408,416).

B Cell Chronic Lymphocytic Leukemia

B cell chronic lymphocytic leukemia is usually characterized by uncontrolled lymphocytosis of small, mature lymphocytes that infiltrate the peripheral blood, bone marrow, and other organs. The patients usually have benign indolent clinical courses and relatively long survival. B cell prolymphocytic leukemia (B-PLL) is characterized by marked lymphocytosis, massive splenomegaly, moderate hepatomegaly, minimal peripheral lymphadenopathy, and elderly male predominance (reviewed in 366,394).

An increased number of cells bearing receptors to IgG Fc (Tγ cells) were found in B-CLL or B-PLL patients, and consequently low ratios of Tμ:Tγ cells were recorded (e.g., 1.46 in B-CLL patients vs 4.18 in normal individuals; *417*). The Tμ:Tγ ratios of normal individuals are in the range of 2 (*418,419*) to 6 (*420*). B-CLL and B-PLL patients with relatively low Tμ:Tγ ratios have been described by other authors as well (*418–426*). If it is accepted (*303*) that Tμ is a marker of helper T cells and Tγ is a marker of suppressor T cells (a statement that has been, however, criticized; *275,427*), then the low Tμ:Tγ ratio reflects an immunoregulatory imbalance that favors suppressor cells. The ratio between helper cells and suppressor cells in B-CLL patients is reduced according to another criteria: the relative representation of helper T4$^+$ cells and cytotoxic-suppressor T8$^+$ cells in the circulating cellular pool. Whereas the ratio of these two cellular populations is from 1.8 to 2.2 in normal individuals, this ratio is around 1 or less in B-CLL patients (*426,428–436*). The increase of T8$^+$ cells was found in both treated and untreated patients (*432*), and it tends (although statistically insignificant) to be more profound in the advanced stages of the disease. The activity of the enzyme 5-nucleotidase is considerably reduced in T8 cells of B-CLL patients (*437*), indicating the abnormality of these cells.

Hersey and associates (*438*) demonstrated excessive suppressor T cell function in the MNC of most B-CLL patients compared with normal individuals. T cells of the patients inhibited the ability of cocultivated normal helper T cells to support the PWM-induced Ig production by normal B cells. In addition, the T cells from five of eight patients failed to directly support the Ig production of normal B cells, indicating defective function of helper T cells. Also, the patients' B cells could not gain support from normal helper T cells in order to produce Ig, implying that the B cell function of the patients was also defective. These observations were indicated in both treated and untreated patients.

Although functional suppressor T cells were found in the blood of B-CLL patients (*438,439*), in a few instances (*440*), the potential of such cells was not expressed because of the absence of collaborating cells in the suppressor cell circuit (*see below*). In addition to functional suppressor T cells, Faguet (*439*) detected functional suppressor B cells in B-CLL patients, and both inhibited upon cocultivation the mitogenic responses of normal cells stimulated with PHA. Suppressor factors were not found in the patients' sera or supernatants of the leukemic cells.

Lahat and colleagues (*434*) found that MMC-inactivated plastic adherent T cells of a B-CLL patient with a large lymphoma

(Richter's syndrome) suppressed the PHA mitogenic response of cocultivated autologous blood MNC, or the PWM and the MLC responses of normal cells. Because adherent T cells could not be recovered from normal individuals' MNC, it was impossible to appropriately control this experiment. Kay (424) demonstrated that T cells of B-CLL patients inhibited the PWM-induced proliferative response of cocultivated normal B cells mixed with normal T non-γ cells (T cells depleted of Tγ cells containing the helper T cell function). The suppressor cells demonstrated an excessively effective suppressor function in comparison with that of normal individuals. Furthermore, the irradiated T non-γ cells of B-CLL patients failed to support the PWM-induced proliferation of cocultivated normal B cells efficiently, indicating defective helper-cell function in B-CLL patients. This notion received further support from the observation of decreased IL-2 production and sensitivity to its effects in T cells of patients with B-CLL (441). Defective helper T cell function in B-CLL patients was described in a few other independent papers (438,442,443).

The above-described findings conflict however with other reports indicating lack of a suppressor cell effect (440,444,445), or normal functions of suppressor (425,442,446) and helper (420,425,440,446,447) cells in B-CLL patients, sometimes despite low Tμ/Tγ ratios (420). The inability of B cells from such patients to differentiate Ig-producing cells (425) may be related to an intrinsic defect or to the replacement of the normal B cells by a neoplastic clone.

The defect in the suppressor cell pathway of B-CLL patients was elegantly explored by Bloem and colleagues (440). Under normal conditions, suppressor-precursor cells (Leu-2$^+$, T8$^+$, Tγ$^-$), are activated by antigen-stimulated suppressor-inducer cells (Leu-3$^+$, T4$^+$), and consequently, they differentiate into suppressor-effector cells (Leu-2$^+$, T8$^+$, Tγ$^+$), which may release an SF (265,404; Fig 3). The SF is detected by its ability to inhibit the antigen-specific in vitro antibody response of normal MNC. Lymphocytes of B-CLL patients expressed the suppressor-inducer cell function after their incubation with the antigen—these cells being detected by their ability to activate, in the presence of specific antigen, the differentiation of suppressor-precursor cells of normal individuals to suppressor-effector cells. In contrast, antigen-stimulated suppressor-inducer cells derived from normal individuals failed to activate, in the presence of specific antigen, the differentiation of B-CLL cells to suppressor-effector cells. This experiment indicates that functional suppressor-precursor cells are absent from the MNC of B-CLL patients, despite Leu2$^+$ cells being present in this cellular population. Interestingly, just the opposite situation was found in the leukemic cells of a T-ALL patient. They contain suppressor-precursor cells, but not suppressor inducer cells (407).

The fact that some patients were subjected to treatments whereas others were not and the employment of different assays for measuring the cellular activities of the patients may explain the contradictory functions of B-CLL cells (*see* Table 3). Focusing on the use of different assays, one may remember that the cells' proliferation does not necessarily correlate with the ability to produce Ig (448); therefore, a comparison between these two sets of tests (e.g., the assays described in refs 424 and 447, Table 3) is not constructive. The patients' average age, which may differ from one set of experiments to another, may be an additional important factor contributing to the conflicting results, since aging considerably affects the immunological functions (449).

Anemia is a common complication of B-CLL. Assuming that the anemia is not entirely the result of occupation of haemopoietic areas by malignant cells, some investigators have postulated that the observed suppressor cells may inhibit red-cell production. This association between anemia and suppressor cells in B-CLL patients was investigated by Mangan and colleagues (431,435,450,451). They found that marrow T cells or Tγ cells (but not B cells) of the patients suppressed erythroid colony growth (CFU-E, BFU-E) of cocultivated autologous or allogeneic B-depleted and T-depleted marrow cells (null cells), which were cultured in the presence of erythropoietin. The suppressive effect of Tγ cells was more profound than that of unseparated T cells (431,435). It appears also that suppressor T cells taken from patients with more advanced disease (435) developed more intensive suppressive activity. The suppressive effect disappeared, however, when drug-induced remission had been achieved (431). The suppressor cells were found in both transfused and untransfused patients (435), and they inhibited the erythroid colony growth of a normal allogeneic cellular population, but not the proliferation of granulocytes in diffusion chambers (431), indicating their restricted activity. The authors suggested that the anemia occurring in the course of B-CLL is the result of a general accumulation in the marrow of Tγ lymphocytes, which suppress the erythroid progenitor cell growth (435). Suppressor cells inhibiting

Table 3
Variability in the Cellular Functions of B-CLL Patients[a]

Ref.	The status of immune cellular functions in B-CLL patients	Assay used to determine status of immune cellular functions[a]	Type of treatment of patients
420	Normal function of Th	PWM-induced B cell differentiation	No treatment
424	Excessive function of Ts; deffective function of Th	PWM-induced proliferative response	No treatment within 3–4 wk of study
425	Normal function of Ts and Th; defective function of B cells	PWM-induced B cell differentiation	No treatment or no treatment for at least 6 mo
434	Effective function of suppressor adherent T cells	PHA mitogenic response of autologous MNC; PWM and alloantigen-induced proliferative responses	Chemotherapy
438	Excessive function of Ts; defective function of Th; defective function of B cells	PWM-induced Ig synthesis	No treatment or treatment with chemotherapy or leucapheresis
439	Effective function of suppressor B and T cells	Mitogenic response	No treatment within 3 wk of study

440	Normal function of suppressor-inducer cells; defective function of suppressor-effector cells; normal function of Th	Antigen specific antibody response	No treatment at the time of the study
442	Normal function of Ts; defective function of Th	Spontaneous and Con A-induced suppressor cells were tested in PWM-induced proliferative response of autologous MNC; Th were tested in SRBC induced PFC response of normal tonsillar B cells	Splenectomy, chemotherapy
443	Defective function of Th	SRBC-induced antibody response	No treatment, splenectomy; steroid therapy
444	Lack of suppressor cell function	MLR	Not indicated
445	Lack of suppressor cell function	PHA mitogenic response	Not indicated
447	Normal functions of Ts and Th; defective function of B cells	PWM and antigen-induced B cell differentiation to PFC	No treatment

^aUnless otherwise indicated, the assay was performed in a mixture of B-CLL cells and cells of normal subjects.

erythroid colony growth have been found by other workers in
T-CLL patients (452,453), but not in B-CLL patients (452). In contrast to B-CLL, hairy cell leukemia (considered by most investigators as a B cell disorder as well, 454) does not exhibit immunepa-
resis (455) or abnormal Leu-3:Leu-2 ratios (456).

T Cell Chronic Lymphocytic Leukemia and T Cell Prolymphocytic Leukemia

T-cell chronic lymphocytic leukemia is characterized by massive splenomegaly, lymphocytosis, cutaneous infiltration, anemia, neutropenia and recurrent infections, aggressive clinical
courses, and relatively to B-CLL, short survival (reviewed in 394).
The features of T cell-prolymphocytic leukemia (T-PLL) include
hyperleukocytosis, splenomegaly, lymphadenopathy, cutaneous
infiltration, relatively aggressive clinical courses, and elderly male
predominancy (reviewed in 394,457).

The leukemic cells of patients with T-CLL or T-PLL may express a helper cell phenotype (T4$^+$,T8$^-$; 394,458–462), a cytotoxic-suppressor cell phenotype (T4$^-$,T8$^+$; 394,457–459,461–467) or
both phenotypes (394,458,459,468–470; the ratio of T4:T8 in the
case reported in ref. 468 was 0.33). When both phenotypes were
described, it is not always clear if they were coexpressed on the
T-CLL cells or they were distinctively expressed on T4 or T8
T-CLL subpopulations of the same patient. This fundamental difference must be illucidated in the future studies. Receptors for the
Fc portion of the IgG were identified on T-CLL leukemic cells either independently (screening for T4, T8 phenotypes was not performed) or in conjunction with the T4$^-$,T8$^+$ cytotoxic-suppressor
phenotype (458,463,464). Several studies have examined resident
immunological functions in patients carrying the cytotoxic-
suppressor cell phenotype. Their peripheral blood MNC failed to
express an efficient NK cell activity (453,463,464,468,471).
Antibody-dependent cellular cytotoxicity could be developed by
cells of some patients (453,458,464,471), but not by others
(463,468). A reduced ability to respond by proliferation to PHA
(453,468,472) or release IL-2 on such stimulation (461) has been
reported (*see also* Ref. 466). Interestingly, the cells that failed to
respond to PHA could proliferate in response to Con A according
to one report (453), but not another (472). This last report (472)
describes the absence of a PWM mitogenic response and MLC in
T-CLL patients. The cells of T-CLL patients with suppressor cell
phenotype (T8$^+$) formed colonies in agar after PHA stimulation,

but only in the presence of IL-2, whereas the cells of T-CLL patients with helper cell phenotype (T4$^+$) could form colonies independent of IL-2 (*461*).

According to one study (*468*), the function of helper cells, supporting the PWM-induced Ig synthesis, was normal in T-CLL patients. This study (*468*) indicates also that the function of Con A-induced suppressor cells was low, but it returned to normal level after chemotherapy. Although cells of some T-CLL patients expressed cytotoxic-suppressor phenotype, in at least two reports this phenotype was not associated with functional suppressor activity (*464,473*). Another report (*470*) described T-CLL cells (T4$^+$T8$^+$) with normal helper (support of Ig secretion) and suppressor (inhibition of mitogenic response) functions.

In contrast to the above reports, other groups have found that cells from T-CLL patients do suppress various immunological functions of normal cells (*452,453,463,466,468,471,472*). For instance, the T-CLL cells suppressed the ability of cocultivated normal cells to produce Ig or to differentiate into mature B cells after PWM stimulation (*453,458,463,468* but for a contradictory finding, *see* ref. *466*). Such suppression may be associated with the hypogammaglobulinemia found in T-CLL patients (*453,463*), but it is difficult to separate hypogammaglobulinemia caused by active suppression of B cell function from that caused by passive inhibition of B cell maturation because of infiltration of the marrow by malignant cells. In a different study (*468*), however, correlation between the function of suppressor cells inhibiting PWM-induced Ig synthesis and hypogammaglobulinemia was not found. According to this last report (*468*), the augmented suppressor-cell activity disappeared after chemotherapy. The ability of T-CLL cells to suppress the mitogenic responses of cocultivated normal MNC to PHA, Con A, and PWM (*471,472*), or MLC (*466,472*) and generation of cytotoxic cells after allogeneic stimulation (*466*) was reported in different studies. Although the suppressor T-CLL cells described in ref. *466* were allogeneic to both the stimulator and the responder cells, it appears that the inhibition was not associated with nonspecific allogeneic effect, because third-party allogeneic cells failed to abolish the MLC.

The T-CLL cells (obtained before or after blood transfusion) also suppressed the ability of cocultivated normal bone marrow cells to form erythroid colonies in the presence of erythropoietin (*452,453*). Suppressor cells inhibiting such erythroid progenitor cells were also found in B-CLL (*431,435,450*) and pure red cell aplasia associated with thymoma and panhypogammaglobuline-mia (474). The last report (474) speculated an association between the suppressor cells (OKT11$^+$, OKT3$^+$, OKT8$^+$) and pure red-cell aplasia. As with the hypogammaglobulinemia, the proposal that anemia in T-CLL is associated with the in vivo activity of the suppressor cells (452,453) needs to be supported by considerably more solid experimental evidence. Thus, there exists the possibility, at present not well supported, that the dominant representation of leukemic cells with suppressor cell function in some T-CLL patients may cause a change in the immunoregulatory balance and, consequently, complications of the disease may result.

Sézary Syndrome

Sézary syndrome is considered as the leukemic phase of cutaneous T cell lymphoma, mycosis fungoides. The clinical spectrum of the disease commonly observed in individual patients proceeds from multiple cutaneous lymphoid tumors with accompanying exfoliative erythroderma to infiltration of regional lymph nodes and beyond with eventual leukemic and visceral involvement (475). The malignant cells of Sézary patients are very heterogenous (476). Some reports show that lymphocytes of Sézary patients express T4$^+$,8$^-$ helper phenotype (367,477,478) or possess helper activity (479,480). Other reports show that the Sézary cells express T4$^-$,T8$^+$ cytotoxic/suppressor phenotype (462) or that they do not develop helper activity (481), but rather suppressed the PWM-induced Ig production by normal cells or the differentiation of normal B cells after PWM stimulation (478,481,482). The ability of normal cells to proliferate after PHA stimulation can also be suppressed by Sézary cells (478). Although malignant cells from Sézary patients suppressed PWM-induced Ig synthesis in vitro, there is no evidence of hypogammaglobulinemia in those patients (467,471).

The cells of one of the above-described Sézary patients (478,483), which expressed a T4$^+$,T8$^-$ phenotype (normally characterizing helper T cells, and perhaps suppressor-inducer cells; 265; Fig. 3), suppressed the PHA-induced proliferative response of cocultivated normal cells even after the elimination of T8$^+$ suppressor-precursor cells (with OKT8 antibody and C) from both the normal and patient cell populations (467), indicating a presence of suppressor-effector cells associated with the T4$^+$ Sézary cells. T4$^+$ suppressor-effector cells have also been demonstrated before among normal peripheral blood cell population (266,405,406).

The suppressor cells of the T4$^+$ Sézary patient were effective only when administered at the initiation of the culture (the first 24 h). These suppressor cells were effective even in the presence of excess of exogenous IL-2, indicating that their suppressive mechanism is not mediated by their ability to absorb IL-2. The growth of an IL-2-dependent murine line (a human line was not tested) was unaffected by the presence of the Sézary patient suppressor cells. Furthermore, the suppressor cells inhibited also the IL-2-independent calcium ionophore A23187-induced T cell proliferation of cocultivated normal MNC. The authors suggest that the target of the suppressor cell activity is, perhaps, an important intracellular event controlling DNA replication, which is common to both IL-2-dependent and independent T cell activation processes (483).

Adult T Cell Leukemia

Adult T cell leukemia appears mostly in an endemic form clustering geographically in Southwestern Japan (415), the Caribbean basin (484), and in certain areas of the southeastern USA (485). The disease, which was first described in Japan, is associated with the following characteristics: adult onset, subacute or chronic leukemia with rapidly progressive terminal course, hypercalcemia, frequent skin involvement, common lymphadenopathy and hepatosplenomegaly, and leukemic cells with T cell phenotype (394,415). A retrovirus, human T cell leukemia/lymphoma virus (HTLV), has been isolated recently and found to be associated with ATL. Almost all patients have serum antibody to the viral antigens (486). The cells of ATL, like those of most Sézary patients, exhibit the helper-inducer phenotype (T4$^+$,T8$^-$ or Leu2$^-$,Leu3$^+$; 487–495), or T4$^+$,T8$^+$ phenotype (495), but they do not express helper activity (487,490–493). The only exception is the Japanese T-cell lymphoma, which is perhaps a variant of ATL, also associated with HTLV. We shall see below that patients with this disease do display helper cell function (494).

ATL cells failed to proliferate after mitogenic or allogeneic stimulation (496) and were not able to express NK-cell activity (493). The cells of most but not all (e.g., ref. 495) ATL patients displayed, however, suppressive activity, as indicated by their ability to inhibit PWM-induced Ig synthesis or B cell differentiation by cocultivated normal cells (*487,490–495,497,498*). The patients' cells were also able to suppress the proliferative responses of normal cells stimulated with PHA or allogeneic cells (MLC; *496*). In a few instances, an SF was found in the supernatants of the leukemic suppressor cells (*496,497*). Although the suppressor cells inhibited the in vitro Ig synthesis, hypogammaglobulinemia was not observed in ATL patients (*490,497*).

An ATL cellular population that suppressed the PWM-induced Ig synthesis by cocultured normal cells expressed high proportions of $T4^+,T17^+$ phenotypes (*495*). Similar high proportions of $T4^+,T17^+$ phenotype were found among suppressor leukemic cells of Caribbean ATL patients (*491*) and in a patient with Sézary syndrome (*478*). Further, $T17^+$ cells of an ATL patient separated by fluorescence-activated cell sorter (FACS) expressed the suppressor-cell activity, whereas the $T17^-$ cells did not (*495*). It seems, therefore, that leukemic cells with $T4^+,T17^+$ phenotype express suppressor-cell activity.

Lymph-node cells ($Leu2^-,3^+$, helper phenotype) of different patients with HTLV-associated T cell lymphoma contained either helper cells or suppressor cells that could respectively support or inhibit the PWM-induced B cell differentiation of cocultivated normal cells (*494*). Lymph-node cells from one patient displayed both helper and suppressor functions. These lymph-node cells inhibited the PWM-induced B cell differentiation of cocultivated normal B and T cells. However, after exposure to 1000 rad X-irradiation, the lymph-node cells of this patient could display an efficient helper activity for the normal B cell differentiation induced by PWM (*494*), suggesting that radioresistant helper cells coexisted with radiosensitive suppressor cells in the lymph nodes of the patient. The radiosensitivity of ATL suppressor cells (including the $T4^+$ suppressor-inducer cells) has also been demonstrated in other studies (*490,493*).

Conflicting results are available as to whether the $T4^+,8^-$ ATL cells are suppressor-inducer (*265,404*) or suppressor-effector (*405,406*) cells. Morimoto and associates (*493*) demonstrated that ATL cells suppressed the ability of a mixture of normal B and normal $T4^+$ cells to produce PWM-induced Ig only in the presence of normal $T8^+$ cells (suppressor-effector cells), suggesting that the ATL cells exert a suppressor-inducer function. In contrast, Waldmann and colleagues (*492*) demonstrated that ATL cells suppressed the PWM-induced Ig synthesis by a mixture of normal B cells and normal T cells, even after removal of $T8^+$ cells by anti-T8 serum and C. A T cell line derived from the ATL leukemic cells (T4$^+$,T8$^-$) was shown to produce an SF, inhibiting the PWM-induced Ig synthesis by B cells in the presence of normal irradiated helper T cells. These experiments suggest that the ATL cells manifest a suppressor-effector function, rather than a suppressor-inductive activity. The different geographical locations of the patients described in these two studies (Japan vs USA) may explain in part the conflicting results.

Despite both cells of Sézary syndrome and cells of ATL in general sharing the T4$^+$,T8$^-$ phenotype, cells of former have been found to express, in different studies, either helper (479,480,492) or suppressor activity (478,481,482,492), whereas most ATL cells expressed a suppressive activity only (487,490–498). A further difference is found in expression of the IL-2 receptor (detected by anti-Tac antibodies), ATL cells, and a few Sézary cells expressing this receptor, whereas, most of the Sézary cells did not (492). Sézary cells with characteristics similar to ATL cells (suppressive activity and expression of IL-2 receptor) were derived from patients carrying HTLV antibodies, whereas Sézary cells with characteristics unlike ATL cells (lacking suppressive activity and IL-2 receptors) were isolated from patients who were HTLV negative. All the ATL patients (nine patients) were HTLV positive (*see also* ref. 494), and their cells bore IL-2 receptors. The cells of five of the nine ATL patients could also express suppressive activity (492). Thus, the suppressive activity of the leukemic cells and the expression of IL-2 receptors on their surface is associated in most, but not all, cases with the presence of antibodies to HTLV in the sera of the patients. Any conception about the association between the virus, the IL-2 receptor, the suppressor-cell function, and the malignant process, although very attractive, must wait until more experimental data has been accumulated.

Chronic T-Cell Lymphocytosis with Neutropenia (or Tγ-Lymphoproliferative Disease; Tγ LPD)

T cell lymphocytosis with neutropenia appears to be an independent entity of lymphoproliferative disorder. The disease is characterized by frequent infections resulting from severe granulocytopenia, severe anemia, bone-marrow infiltration, and lymphocytosis composed of predominantly Tγ cells with the cytomorphological features of the LGL. The course of the disease is often chronic, indolent, and nonprogressive, and karyotypic studies showed no abnormalities (394). As a result, the neoplastic nature of the disease is sometimes questioned (499–501). In most cases, the cells of the patients with lymphocytosis and neutropenia exhibit a cytotoxic-suppressor cell phenotype (T4$^-$,T8$^+$; 382,413,500,502,503) and a receptor for the Fc portion of IgG (382,413,499–504). A patient with helper-cell phenotype (T4$^+$,T8$^-$) was also identified (499). Although the cells of the patients bear cytotoxic-suppressor-cell phenotype markers, most of them failed to exhibit a suppressive activity, as indicated by various in vitro tests (413,500,503,504). Exceptions are reports by Rümke et al. (382) and Callard and colleagues (503) describing the ability of a patient's cells to suppress the PWM-induced Ig synthesis by normal cells, as well as the proliferative response of normal cells stimulated with PHA, respectively. Whereas the patients's cells demonstrated ability to mount an ADCC (413,500,502,503), they failed to exhibit NK-cell activity (413,500,502).

These results presented above lend support to the notion that the surface phenotype of a cell (e.g., T4$^-$,T8$^+$) does not necessarily indicate that the cell expresses the expected immunological function (e.g., suppressive activity). We may assume that, in the case of T cell lymphocytosis with neutropenia, the disease process itself restrains the function of the suppressor cells.

3.5. Chronic Myelogenous Leukemia

Chronic myelogenous leukemia is a myeloproliferative disease characterized by intense expansion of the myeloid population in the bone marrow, liver, and spleen. In most cases, a specific chromosome abnormality (Philadelphia chromosome, Ph^1) characterizes the leukemic cells (505).

Incubation in vitro of CML MNC in the absence or presence of Con A resulted, respectively, in the generation of spontaneous (or fetal calf serum induced; 195) or Con A-induced suppressor cells, which inhibited the PHA-induced proliferative response of cocultivated autologous responder cells (506). Con A-induced suppressor cells from first, second, and third remission stages of CML patients were more potent than the corresponding suppressor cells obtained from normal individuals. Mitogen-induced suppressor cells have also been described in CLL patients (507). Spontaneous suppressor cells from the first and the second remissions of CML patients were also more potent than the corresponding normal suppressor cells, but those of the third remission were not, indicating that the suppressor-cell activity does not necessarily correlate with the progression of the disease (506).

3.6. Human T Cell Lines with Suppressor-Cell Characteristics

Phenotypic and functional characteristics of suppressor cells have also been determined in T cell lines derived from leukemic patients. The leukemic T cell line HSB-2 released a factor that induced in lymphoid cells of C3H/He mice radiosensitive suppressor T (Thy-1$^+$) or non-T cells that produced an SF. The cells suppressed the generation of antitrinitrophenyl (TNP) cytotoxicity by normal C3H/He splenocytes stimulated with syngeneic trinitrophenylated spleen cells (508), a suppression that did not cross the species barrier. A T cell line derived from a patient with mycosis fungoides released an SF that inhibited the Ig biosynthesis induced in normal mononuclear cells by polyclonal activators (509). Another leukemic T cell line (designated 8402) expressing a precursor thymocyte phenotype responded to TPA by differentiating into a mature cell line. In the presence of a stimulus provided by conditioned medium from lymphocyte culture, the line further differentiated and a fraction of the cells displayed the T8$^+$,T4$^-$ phenotype of cytotoxic-suppressor cells (510). The leukemia T cell line PF-382 derived from the pleural effusion of a child with T-ALL exhibits a suppressor function along with markers of early thymocytes (OKT6, Leu-1, and Leu-9) and more mature OKT8 antigen of suppressor/cytotoxic phenotype. The line and factor released from it suppressed the PWM-induced differentiation of normal B cells supported by normal helper T cells. Interestingly, a chromosomal translocation between chromosome X and chromosome 15 is present in most of the line cells (511).

3.7. Multiple Myeloma

Multiple myeloma is characterized by a malignant transformation of a plasma cell resulting in the establishment of a cellular clone that grows progressively and produces immunoglobulin or a subunit of it; the majority of myelomas secrete their Ig product, but a small proportion are incapable of extracellular secretion. In addition to MM, Waldenstrom's macroglobulinemia and heavy chain disease are also considered to be plasma-cell neoplasms (512). Bone marrow replacement with malignant plasma cells, osteolytic bone lesions, and paraprotein production are typical features of the disease. Despite the increased synthesis of paraprotein, there is considerable impairment of normal polyclonal Ig synthesis, expressed functionally by a reduced capacity to form specific antibody and clinically by an increased susceptibility to certain bacterial infections (513–515). Whereas leukemic B cells of B-CLL patients did not proliferate after mitogenic stimulation even in the presence of normal T lymphocytes (516), the peripheral B cells of myeloma patients proliferate after stimulation with PWM in the presence of autologous T cells. However, these B cells subsequently fail to differentiate and secrete Ig (517).

Several hypotheses have been put forward to explain the impaired-host polyclonal Ig synthesis. These include the presence of mitotic inhibitors or chalones that block polyclonal B cell differentiation (518), the alteration of antigen-binding cells by infective RNA subunits derived from the malignant plasma cells (519), or the influence of circulating immunosuppressive factors released by the plasmacytoma cells (520). The possibility that suppressor-cell activity is responsible for the impaired Ig synthesis in MM patients has obviously attracted much attention, followed by several experimental approaches aimed at investigating the role of suppressor cells in MM.

The ratio of helper cell: suppressor cell represented either by $T\mu:T\gamma$ (521–523) or T4:T8 (524–527) criteria was reduced in MM patients, indicating a relative increase of the suppressor-cell phenotype. The low ratio was found in both treated and untreated patients (523,525,526), as well as in patients diagnosed at different clinical stages (525,526). However, a low helper:suppressor ratio that was limited to the treated group was also reported (524). Interestingly, it was also reported that patients with indolent or well-controlled disease and not those with progressive disease displayed an elevated proportion of $T\gamma$ cells (522).

Massaia and colleagues (527,528) indicated that the T8$^+$ cells of MM patients were deficient in activity of the enzyme Ecto-5′ nucleotidase and severely compromised in their clonogenic potential (529). A cytochemical assay proved a decreased number of enzyme-positive cells rather than a decreased enzyme activity per cell (527). The decreased number of enzyme-positive cells was linearly correlated with the increased number of OKM1$^+$ granular cells in purified CD8$^+$ subpopulation of MM patients (527). If the OKM1 monoclonal antibodies can faithfully discriminate between

CD8$^+$ cytotoxic cells (OKM1$^-$) and CD8$^+$ suppressor cells (OKM1$^+$) (275,530,531), then these results suggest that, in at least some MM patients, the proportion of CD8$^+$ suppressor cells is increased on the account of CD8$^+$ cytotoxic cells (the total number of CD8$^+$ cells is kept normal in MM patients; 527). Since the above-mentioned change is correlated with a decreased number of enzyme-positive cells, it may be concluded that the CD8$^+$ OKM1$^+$ suppressor cells are deficient with Ecto-5' nucleotidase, and this deficiency may be used as a marker of suppressor-cell expansion in MM patients. A similar enzyme defect was observed in CD8$^+$ cells of B-CLL patients (437). It should be emphasized, however, that the existence of enzyme-deficient suppressor cells (CD8$^+$ OKM1$^+$) in MM patients has not been proven by functional tests, at least as far as indicated in the above report (527).

Different reports described, however, functional suppressor cells in the peripheral blood of MM patients (532–534). The suppressor cells inhibited the PWM-induced Ig synthesis of cocultured normal cells. Bone marrow cells of the patients consisting mainly of malignant plasma cells did not exert a suppressive effect, indicating that tumor cells themselves are not involved in the immunodepression. The suppressor cells were identified as radioresistant phagocytic monocytes, since they could be removed by a carbonyl-iron and magnet procedure, and they were effective even after exposure to 2000 rad. Furthermore, glass-adherent cells of MM patients could also mediate the suppressive effect.

Pokeweed mitogen could induce a significant proportion of multiple myeloma MNC to develop into Ig-positive cells, if plastic-adherent cells were partially removed, whereas the total cell population developed only a low proportion of Ig-positive cells under similar conditions. The enhancing effect of monocyte removal upon MNC of normal individuals, subsequently stimulated with PWM, was relatively less efficient than the corresponding effect on patients' MNC (535).

Monocytes were not the only suppressor cells found in MM patients. Multiple types of suppressor cells were detected in MM patients by Paglieroni and MacKenzie (536,537). The suppressor cells were represented within several cell types, including EA-RFC (cells forming rosettes with human type O Rh positive erythrocytes coated with human anti-D immunoglobulin), EAC-RFC (cells forming rosettes with sheep erythrocytes coated with IgM anti-sheep erythrocyte antibody and C3 from human serum), monocytes (plastic-adherent cells), and E-RFC (cells forming rosettes with sheep erythrocytes). In a later study (538), the EA-RFC were identified as B cells (CD5[+], CD19[+], CD20[+], CD21[+], HLA-DR[+]). According to one report (537), suppressor cells were found in both treated and untreated patients, but the earlier communication (536) claimed that most of the treated patients did not express abnormal suppressor-cell function. Such suppressor cells were found neither in normal individuals nor in individuals with benign monoclonal gammopathy. The suppressor cells were detected by their ability to inhibit the proliferative response of cocultured normal cells stimulated with PWM, tetanus toxoid, streptokinase-streptodornase, or allogeneic cells (MLC). A further assay of suppressor-cell function was provided by the ability to inhibit the PWM, tetanus toxoid, and pneumococcal polysaccharide III-induced Ig synthesis of cocultured normal cells (536,537). Using this latter assay, EA-RFC (detecting cells bearing Fc receptors) expressed the most profound suppression (537), but their effect was detected at the initiation of the culture only (538). The suppressor cells must be viable; otherwise, they could not express their function. In addition, the suppressor-cell function was resistant to MMC indicating that their function was replication independent (536). At least the EA-RFC suppressor cells released an SF (mol wt of 10,000–20,000; 538).

The ability of Tγ[+] (517,523,539) or T8[+] (526) cells of MM patients to suppress the PWM-induced proliferation (517,539), Ig synthesis, or B cell differentiation (517,523,526) of cocultured normal (517,523,526,539) or autologous (517,539) cells has been reported by other groups. Some investigators reported that the suppressor T cells of MM patients were more potent than those of normal individuals (523,539), whereas others did not find any such difference in the suppressive activities (517,526). Radiosensitive spontaneous and Con A-induced suppressor cells were found in non-γ T cell fraction of MNC of normal individuals, but not in the corresponding cellular population of MM patients (517).

The function of helper cells of MM patients was normal as indicated either by the PWM-induced Ig synthesis and B cell differentiation assays (517,526) or the PWM-induced proliferation assay (539). In addition, the PWM-induced proliferation assay (539) implied that the myeloma B cells were more sensitive than normal B cells to the suppressive effect of normal Tγ cells. Suppressor cells inhibiting Ig secretion by myeloma cells have also been implicated in animal experimental modes (540,541).

The hypogammaglobulinemia of the MM patients could be the result of the in vivo effect of the suppressor cells characterized by the in vitro assays. The following observations do not agree, however, with such a proposal. Although helper cells of MM patients express normal function indicated by their ability to support the PWM-induced Ig synthesis of normal B cells, such cells cannot support PWM-driven Ig synthesis of autologous B cells (517). This experiment implies that the defect of B cells is intrinsic and independent of the suppressor-cell activity. The suppressor cells, however, may yet serve an important function. Lauria and colleagues (526) found that the absolute number of the T8$^+$ cytotoxic-suppressor cells was high only during the developmental early stages of MM. This fact may suggest an unsuccessful attempt on the part of suppressor cells to restrain the expansion of the myeloma clone. Interestingly, other papers (542,543) reported that patients with stable disease presented a much lower helper cell:suppressor cell (T4:T8) ratio than normal individuals or patients with active disease, indicating a more pronounced representation of suppressor cells at the time during which the disease is under control.

In conclusion, if the suppressor cells of MM patients (and perhaps of B cell lymphoma and B-CLL patients as well) are committed to control the proliferation of the malignant cells, we may explore how to increase the effectiveness of the suppression together with intermittent chemotherapy to reduce the tumor load, the interval between treatments allowing for recovery of white cell counts and expression of suppressive function. Such an immune regulatory mechanism has already been described in experimental animal models of myeloma (544 and discussed in our previous review, 1). The properties of B-CLL, CML, and MM suppressor cells are summarized in Table 2. The properties of T-ALL, T-CLL, Sézary syndrome, ATL, and Tγ LPD suppressor cells are described in Table 4.

4. Cancer of the Head and Neck

Most of the head and neck malignancies arise from the surface epithelium, and are therefore squamous-cell carcinoma or one of its variants, including lymphoepithelioma, spindle-cell car-

Table 4
Suppressor Cells in T-ALL, T-CLL, and Related Diseases[a]

Disease	Type of patient cells (S:R)	Effect of patient cells	Properties of patient cells	Comments	Ref.
T-ALL	$T3^+$, $T10^+$, $T8^+$, Tac^+ cells (after activation with inducing factor) (1:1)	Inhibition of PWM-induced Ig synthesis	Ts: Function of suppressor-precursors but not suppressor-inducer cells		407
T-CLL	Suppressor T cell (1:1)	Inhibition of erythropoiesis	Ts: sensitive to ATG	A treated patient	452
T-CLL	$T\gamma^+$ suppressor T cells (1:2 to 1:10)	Inhibition of PWM-induced B cell differentiation and erythropoiesis	General: No PHA mitogenic response; negative NK; positive ADCC. Ts: sensitive to ALS and resist freezing and thawing	A treated patient; no SF	453
T-CLL	$T\gamma^+$, $T3^+$ $T4^-$, $T8^+$ suppressor T cells (1:1)	Inhibition of PWM-induced B cell differentiation	General: Negative NK; negative ADCC. Ts: radiosensitive to 3000 rad	A treated patient	463

Disease	Cells	Inhibition	General/Ts characteristics	Comments	Ref
T-CLL	T4$^+$, T8$^+$ suppressor T cells (1:1)	Inhibition of PWM-induced Ig synthesis (before but not after therapy)	General: Reduced PHA mitogenic response and Con A-induced suppression; reduced NK and ADCC; normal function of Th	A treated patient	468
T-CLL	Suppressor T cells (1:2)	Inhibition of PHA, Con A and PWM mitogenic responses and MLC	General: No PHA, Con A and PWM mitogenic responses; no MLC; do not provide a stimulating effect. Ts: resist 3000 rad; radiosensitive to 6000 rad; resist MMC; genetically unrestricted		472
Sézary Syndrome	T3$^+$, T4$^+$, T8$^-$, T17$^+$ suppressor T cells (1:1 to 1:10)	Inhibition of PHA mitogenic response and PWM-induced B cell differentiation	General: Weak PHA, Con A and PWM mitogenic responses. Ts: resist 2000 rad	A treated patient; no evidence for in vivo suppression of Ig synthesis	478

(Continued)

Table 4 (*Cont.*)

Disease	Type of patient cells (S:R)	Effect of patient cells	Properties of patient cells	Comments	Ref.
Sézary Syndrome	Suppressor T cells (5:1)	Inhibition of PWM-induced Ig synthesis	General: Defective function of Th; normal function of B cells	A treated patient; suppressive effect is uncertain due to the high S:R ratio	481
Sézary Syndrome	Suppressor T cells (1:4 to 1:100)	Inhibition of PWM-induced Ig synthesis		A treated patient; no evidence for in vivo suppression of Ig synthesis	482
ATL Japan	$T3^+$, $T4^+$, $T5^-$, $T8^-$ suppressor T cells (1:1)	Inhibition of PWM-induced B cell differentiation	General: No function of Th. Ts: Tac^+	Two of three patients with Ts	487
ATL Japan	$Leu1^+$, $Leu2^-$, $Leu3^+$ suppressor T cells (1:3)	Inhibition of PWM-induced B cell differentiation	General: No function of Th. Ts: radiosensitive to 1000 rad; resist MMC	10 of 16 patients with Ts; no evidence for in vivo suppression of Ig synthesis	490
ATL (Caribbean)	$T1^+$, $T4^+$, $T8^-$, $T17^+$ suppressor T cells (1:1)	Inhibition of PWM-induced Ig synthesis	General: No function of Th. Ts: radiosensitive to 4000 rad	HTLV positive; three of five patients with Ts	491

ATL (USA)	T3$^+$, T4$^+$, T8$^-$, suppressor T cells (1:1)	Inhibition of PWM-induced Ig synthesis	General: No function of Th. Ts: function of suppressor-effector cells and not suppressor-inducer cells	HTLV positive and Tac positive	492
Sézary Syndrome (USA)	T3$^+$, T4$^+$, T8$^-$ helper or suppressor T cells (1:2)	HTLV$^+$ (but not HTLV$^-$) patients: inhibition of PWM-induced Ig synthesis	General: HTLV$^-$ patients: effective function of Th; HTLV$^+$ patients: no function of Th	HTLV negative and Tac negative or HTLV positive and Tac positive	493
ATL (Japan)	T4$^+$ T8$^-$ suppressor T cells (1:2)	Inhibition of PWM-induced Ig synthesis	General: Negative NK; no function of Th. Ts: function of suppressor-inducer cells but not suppressor-effector cells; radiosensitive to 1500 rad		
T cell lymphoma associated with HTLV (Japan)	Leu2$^-$, Leu3$^+$ helper or suppressor T cells (1:1)	Activation (helper cells) or inhibition (suppressor cells) or both activation and inhibition of PWM-induced B cell differentiation	Ts: Radiosensitive to 1000 rad	HTLV positive; the cells were obtained from the lymph node; the helper function of one patient was detected by removal of radiosensitive Ts	494

(Continued)

Table 4 (*Cont.*)

Disease	Type of patient cells (S:R)	Effect of patient cells	Properties of patient cells	Comments	Ref.
ATL (Japan)	T3$^+$, T4$^+$ T17$^+$ suppressor T cells (1:1)	Inhibition of PWM-induced Ig synthesis	General: No function of Th. Ts: radiosensitive to 2000 rad	Untreated patients	495
ATL (Japan)	Leu2$^-$, Leu3$^+$ suppressor T Cells (1:1)	Inhibition of PHA mitogenic response and MLC	General: No PHA mitogenic response and MLC. Ts: resist MMC	SF in two of three patients	496
ATL (Japan)	T4$^+$, T8$^-$ suppressor T cells (1:1)	Inhibition of PWM-induced B cell differentiation		Three of six patients with Ts; SF was found in one patient; no evidence for in vivo suppression of Ig synthesis	497
ATL (Japan)	T4$^+$, T8$^-$ suppressor T cells (1:5)	Inhibition of PWM-induced B cell differentiation		HBLA positive	498
Lymphocytosis with neutropenia (Tγ LPD)	Tγ$^+$, T3$^+$ T4$^-$, T5$^+$ T8$^+$ T cells	No inhibition of PHA mitogenic response and PWM-induced B-cell differentiation	General: negative NK; positive ADCC	A treated patient	413

Disease	Cells	Function	General	Patient	Ref.
Lymphocytosis with neutropenia (Tγ LPD)	Tγ$^+$, T3$^+$ T4$^-$, T8$^+$ T cells	No inhibition (test was not indicated)	General: negative NK; positive ADCC	A treated patient	500
Lymphocytosis with neutropenia (Tγ LPD)	Tγ$^+$, T3$^+$ T4$^-$, T5$^+$, T8$^+$ T cells		General: negative NK; positive ADCC	A treated patient	502
Lymphocytosis with neutropenia (Tγ LPD)	Tγ$^+$, T3$^+$ T4$^-$, T8$^+$ T cells (1:2)	Inhibition of PHA mitogenic response; no inhibition of Con A mitogenic response and PWM-induced Ig synthesis			503
Lymphocytosis with neutropenia (Tγ LPD)	Tγ$^+$ T cells	No inhibition of PWM-induced Ig synthesis	General: positive ADCC	Treated patients	504

^{a}New abbreviations used in this table: ALS, Anti lymphocyte serum; HBLA, human-B cell lymphocyte antigen.

cinoma, verrucous carcinoma, or an undifferentiated carcinoma (545). Patients with a head or neck carcinoma frequently exhibit a hyporeactivity or anergy in the DTH response to DNCB (546–549), and their lymphocytes may express decreased proliferative responses after stimulation with mitogens (549–551) or alloantigens (MLC, 552).

The T4:T8 ratios of head and neck cancer patients were either normal (553,554) or above the normal values (555; Lipscomb et al. reported in the 11th Midwest Autumn Immunology Conference, Chicago, 1982, that elevated T4:T8 ratios were found also in patients with uterine cervical cancer). These ratios decreased, however, below the normal levels after radiotherapy (553,554), or surgery and radiotherapy (553). The decreased T4:T8 ratios were not associated with surgery, since patients subjected to surgery alone displayed normal T4:T8 ratios (553). It is possible that radiotherapy may cause a relative decrease in the helper-cell presentation, and a subsequent immunodepression perhaps followed by opportunistic infection may result.

The possibility that suppressor monocytes are responsible for the depressed mitogenic response was supported by the observation of enhanced PHA-induced proliferative response of patients' mononuclear cells depleted of glass-adherent cells (556,557). In line with these results, Zighelboim et al. (549) and Berlinger et al. (552) found that elimination of monocytes either by magnetic removal of iron-ingesting cells (549) or by filtering the cells on Sephadex G-10 column (552) resulted in an increase of the mitogen- or alloantigen-induced proliferative responses, respectively. In an earlier report, Berlinger and associates had described a similar enhancement effect after monocyte removal on testing the MLC of patients with assorted malignancies (558).

Readdition of the adherent cells to an MLC mounted by autologous monocyte-depleted MNC resulted in a reexpression of the suppressive effect (552), indicating that suppressor monocytes downregulate the proliferative activity. Of 54 patients described in this study (552), 67% developed a low MLC, and the MNC of 56% of these generated a significantly increased proliferative response after removal of monocytes. These facts imply that immunodepression is not a general phenomenon among head and neck cancer patients, and even where it exists, it is not necessarily mediated by suppressor monocytes. Furthermore, the level of the MNC responsiveness to the external stimuli, which may reflect the intensity of the suppressor monocyte activity did not

correlate with the stage of the disease (549,552) or with the absolute number of circulating lymphocytes or T cells (549).

While Berlinger and colleagues (552) did not describe the
therapy protocols of their patients, Zighelboim and associates
(549) indicated that their patients were treated with weekly infu-
sions of C. parvum in conjunction with chemotherapy (e.g.,
dexamethasone and methotrexate) after conventional surgery and
radiotherapy had failed. Surgery (559) and C. parvum treatment
(*see* chapter entitled Induction of Suppressor Cells by Immunostimulants in this book) are potential inducers of a suppressor-cell
function; hence, it is not easy to evaluate the interrelationships
between the disease and the immunodepression, independently
of the therapy protocols.

The reduced mitogenic responses of head and neck cancer
patients' MNC were augmented or even restored to the normal
level by addition to the assay of indomethacin (551,557,560–563)
or RO-205720 (551), both PG synthetase inhibitors. The highly depressed mitogenic responses of head and neck cancer patients exposed to radiotherapy also recovered after indomethacin treatment (563). The notion that PG produced by patients' monocytes
is responsible for the suppressed proliferative responses is supported by the following observations:

(1) patients' MNC produced significantly more PG than normal
     individuals' MNC (551)
(2) the isolated monocytes but not the lymphocytes of the pa-
     tients produce the PG (551) and
(3) their MNC depleted of adherent cells failed to produce an
     augmented mitogenic response after addition of indometha-
     cin (560).

Nevertheless, the augmenting effect of indomethacin was not associated with the primary tumor site, disease stage, type of treatment (surgery, radiotherapy, or chemotherapy), or the patient's
age or race (551). One study (561) reported that inactivation of
monocytes by their ingestion of CAR or silica augmented the
PHA mitogenic response of the patients' MNC to the same extent
as removing the monocytes by plastic adherence or indomethacin
administration, also implying that monocytes producing PG mediate the suppressive effect.

As an endpiece, the depressed function of Con A-induced
suppressor cells has been observed in the blood of a patient with
head and neck cancer (556). In another study, however, normal

activity of suppressor cells inhibiting NK-cell activity was found in the peripheral blood of patients with larynx and lyngual adenocarcinomas (564). In summary, it seems likely that the immunodepression observed in some head and neck patients might be associated with the disease therapy or the patient's age, rather than with the disease itself, whereas the role of the immunodepression in the initiation or the progression of the disease remains speculative.

5. Lung Cancer

The majority (90–95%) of lung cancers arise from the bronchial or bronchiolalveolar surface epithelium and from bronchial mucous glands. Among these, the most frequently observed types of lung cancer include squamous-cell carcinoma, small-cell carcinoma, adenocarcinoma, and large-cell carcinoma (565).

The immunological responses of lung cancer patients are frequently markedly depressed. The patients exhibit low T lymphocyte levels, defective ability to respond to DNCB, and a low antibody response to bacterial antigens (566–569). Impaired DTH to standard recall antigens (566,570,571) and weak in vitro proliferative responses after stimulation with mitogens have also been reported (344,570–574), although proliferation within the normal range was recorded for some of the patients (344,572,573,575). An improvement of the DTH and the in vitro mitogenic responses could be generated after treatment with the streptococcal preparation OK432 (571). An increased frequency of infectious complications observed in lung cancer patients (576) might be attributed at least in part to the patients' immunodeficiency.

The ratio of T cells bearing receptors to IgM and T cells bearing receptors to IgG (Tμ :Tγ) in the peripheral blood of lung cancer patients (577) is lower (1.1) than that found in normal individuals (2.5). If Tμ cells and Tγ cells truly represent helper and suppressor T cells, respectively (303,578), these ratios imply a relative increase in suppressor cells. Screening for T4 and T8 markers on T cells, other authors (579) found considerably lower levels for the helper to cytotoxic-suppressor cell ratio (T4:T8) in patients with lung metastases, but not in patients with primary squamous carcinoma, primary adenocarcinoma (579), or advanced non-small-cell lung cancer (580). Interestingly, the T4:T8 ratios of heavy smokers was also found to be low (579,581). The possible association between the immmunodepression observed in lung cancer patients and the suppressor cell function has been the object of extensive investigations, suppressor-cell activity being found in the blood and pleural effusions of some (*see* following sections) but not all (*582,583*) lung cancer patients.

Uchida and colleagues (*584–591*) have provided many reports describing the function of suppressor cells in lung cancer, but in some of them (*584–586*), they fail to distinguish between different malignancies, grouping together patients with lung, stomach, and breast cancer. We must assume, therefore, that similar suppressor-cell activity was found in all the above-mentioned malignancies.

Uchida and Hoshino (*584*) found that unfractionated blood MNC from patients developed lower than normal proliferative responses to PHA and Con A. This activity was considerably augmented after removal of Sephadex G10-adherent cells, suggesting that the adherent cells may have a suppressor function. These results are supported by independent studies (*344,556,557,574,592,593*), demonstrating either directly (mixture experiments, *592,593*) or indirectly [removal of plastic- (*344*) or glass-adherent (*556,557*) cells] that monocytes of untreated lung cancer patients suppressed the PHA (*344,556,557,592,593*) and the PWM (*592*) mitogenic responses of cocultivated autologous cells.

Han and Takita (*574*) found that the suppressive effect of the monocytes was abolished by addition of the PG synthetase inhibitor, indomethacin (*574*), implying the suppression was mediated by monocyte-producing PGs (*see also* refs. *344* and *557*). Han and Takita (*592,593*) further found that peripheral blood monocytes from normal individuals (*592,593*) or from patients with benign lung lesions (*593*) failed to suppress the mitogenic responses. In the absence of suppressor monocytes, T cells of lung cancer patients were fully capable of proliferating in response to PHA, demonstrating that the cells were intrinsically functional (*593*). The suppression exerted by the monocytes correlated fairly well with the severity of the disease and with the tumor histology (small-cell lung cancer being the most severe). In addition, the suppression mediated by monocytes significantly diminished during remission (*593*). The same authors (*593*) found that, in addition to suppressor monocytes, lung cancer patients also developed another type of suppressor cell found in the cellular population depleted of monocytes and E^+ cells.

The peripheral-blood plastic-adherent cells (monocytes) of patients with non-small-cell carcinoma of the lung subjected to complete resection of the tumor and to subsequent intrapleural administration of BCG suppressed the proliferative responses of cocultivated autologous lymphocytes stimulated with PPD. Monocytes of normal subjects did not demonstrate this effect (594). Nevertheless, the radiosensitive suppressor cells of these patients could be equally associated with the postoperative BCG treatment as with the malignant state. Suppressive activity was also found in the pulmonary alveolar macrophages of some but not all lung cancer patients. These cells suppressed the mitogenic responses of autologous and normal allogeneic lymphocytes to Con A (583).

The carcinomatous pleural effusions of patients with primary or secondary lung cancer contained little or no NK activity, in contrast to the nonmalignant effusions of patients with congestive heart failure that had significant NK-cell activity (595). Low NK-cell activity was also found in the peripheral blood of the patients (595–597), although it was higher than that of the effusion cells from the same patient (595). Large granular lymphocytes isolated from the patients' blood or effusion by discontinuous Percoll gradient centrifugation displayed, however, an appreciable natural killing activity not only against NK-sensitive target cells (K562 cells), but also against the autologous fresh tumor (596).

The possibility that suppressor cells inhibit the NK-cell activity in the pleural effusion of lung cancer patients was explored by Uchida and colleagues (587–591). Mononuclear cells isolated from the carcinomatous pleural effusion of lung cancer patients (untreated at the time of the study) suppressed the NK-cell activity of autologous or normal allogeneic blood lymphocytes if incubated with them 24 h prior to the cytotoxic assay (587,588). The augmented NK-cell activity induced by the addition of INF to the cultivated mixture of NK cells and target cells was also inhibited by the addition of pleural effusion suppressor cells (588,590).

The suppressor cells were, however, ineffective if added directly into the cytotoxicity assay (blood MNC incubated 4 h with K562 erythroleukemic target cells, 587,588). The suppression was not an artifact resulting from changes in NK activity during the preincubation with putative suppressor cells, since NK cells incubated alone for 20 h developed the same level of cytotoxic activity as uncultured NK cells (591). Contaminating tumor cells were not responsible for the suppression, since malignant cells incubated with the blood lymphocytes failed to suppress the NK-cell activity (*587*). Effusion cells of patients with congestive heart failure also failed to suppress the NK-cell activity (*587*).

The pleural effusion suppressor cells were characterized as macrophages, since Sephadex G-10 and plastic-adherent cells mediated the suppression (*587,591*). In the pleural effusions of some patients, the suppressor cells could have been T cells, since they adhered neither to nylon wool nor Sephadex G-10 (*587*). Suppressor cells with anti-NK-cell activity have not been found, however, in the blood of lung cancer patients (*597*).

Although pleural effusion suppressor macrophages needed to be incubated with the NK cells for 24 h before assay to exert their suppression, they could then be removed by Sephadex G-10 adherence before assay, while the NK cells still remained suppressed (*587*). If, however, the suppressor macrophages were removed from the effusion MNC by adherence to Sephadex G-10 column and the residual cells were incubated alone for additional 24 h, they could then express an appreciable NK-cell activity, indicating that such suppression was reversible (*587,588*). The recovery of viable blood lymphocytes after preculture with suppressor cells was comparable to that without suppressor cells (*587*), indicating that the suppressive effect was not mediated by killing the NK cells, but rather by affecting their function.

Suppressive factors were not found in the supernatants of effusion cells incubated either alone or with blood MNC (*587*), suggesting that the suppressive effect is mediated by cell-to-cell contact. Addition of indomethacin to the preculture of blood lymphocytes and effusion macrophages did not abolish the suppressive activity (*587*); thus PG was probably not involved in the suppressive mechanism.

In a subsequent study (*591*), the suppressor-cell mechanism was explored in more depth. Adherent cells were isolated from the malignant pleural effusions of lung cancer patients by centrifugation on discontinuous Ficoll-Hypaque gradients and adherence to serum-coated plastic dishes. These cells suppressed the NK-cell activity of LGL purified from the peripheral blood of normal individuals by centrifugation on discontinuous Percoll gradients and further depletion of high-affinity E-RFC. A 24-h preincubation of the suppressor cells with the LGL was required in order to detect an appreciable suppressive activity in the cytotoxic assay. The suppressor cells also inhibited the ability of the LGL to bind and, subsequently, kill target cells in a single-cell assay. These results conflict with the previous report (587) from the same authors, showing that the effusion suppressor cells of lung cancer patients failed to inhibit the binding of K562 target cells to the NK blood lymphocytes. The fact that in the former study unseparated MNC were used as targets for suppression, whereas in the last study LGL were used for this purpose, may explain the conflicting results.

Preincubation of the adherent effusion cells of lung cancer patients with normal LGL impaired the polarization of LGL and their ability to migrate from agarose droplets to the surrounding medium (591). Since cytochalasin B inhibits both the motility and the binding capacity of NK cells, the authors speculated that the microfilaments of NK cells were disrupted by the suppressor cells during the preincubation period, and consequently, their polarization, motility, and ability to bind target cells and kill them were impaired (591).

Intrapleural administration of streptococcal preparation OK432 resulted in a partial or complete disappearance of either pleural effusion or its tumor cells content or both in lung cancer patients. This effect was accompanied by an increase in effusion NK-cell activity with a simultaneous decrease in its suppressor-cell activity. The peripheral-blood NK-cell activity was not enhanced by treatment with this preparation. The possibility that OK432 abolishes the anti-NK suppressor-cell function was supported by the observation that pretreatment in vitro of plastic-adherent cells derived from the pleural effusions of untreated patients with OK432 preparation restrained their ability to suppress the NK activity of cocultured normal donor PBL (589,590). The authors suggest that OK432 abolishes the anti-NK suppressor-cell function in the pleural effusion, and subsequently, the desuppressed NK cells are activated by INF produced by OK432-activated effusion macrophages and/or mesothelial cells (590). The possible consequence of these events is the disappearance or the reduction of tumor cells in the pleural effusion.

The peripheral blood of lung cancer patients contains not only suppressor monocytes, but also suppressor T cells. The weak mitogen-induced proliferative responses of lung cancer patients' blood lymphocytes were only partially restored after removal of Sephadex G-10 adherent cells. The Sephadex G-10 column nonadherent cells were further applied to a nylon-wool column, and the adherent fraction revealed the maximal capacity of proliferation after the mitogenic stimulation. This experiment suggests that another population of suppressor cells resides in the nonadherent fraction after passage through nylon-wool, probably being T cells. Direct evidence for the presence of suppressor cells in the nylon-wool nonadherent cell population was obtained by demonstrating that the nonadherent MMC-treated cells of patients suppressed the mitogenic responses of cocultivated autologous or normal allogeneic cells, whereas nylon-wool nonadherent cells of normal donors did not suppress the mitogenic responses. The suppressive effect of the patients' nylon-wool nonadherent cells was more pronounced if the autologous patient lymphocytes were cultivated alone for 7 d prior to their incubation with the suppressor cells. It is possible that during the preincubation period suppressor cells, sensitive to the culture conditions, were eradicated and the nonsuppressed cellular population revealed a strong sensitivity to the readministration of suppressor cells. Indeed, preincubation of nylon-wool nonadherent cells resulted in a loss of their suppressive activity. The nylon-wool nonadherent cells also lost their suppressive function after removal of E-RFC (584), indicating that they were T cells. The possible involvement of suppressor T cell activity in the immunodepression seen in lung cancer patients was supported by an independent study (598), which also demonstrated the correlation between suppressor-cell activity and the clinical stages of the disease.

Lymphocytes of lung cancer patients treated with the streptococcal preparation OK432 revealed augmented proliferative responses after PHA and Con A stimulation, suggesting that the preparation inhibits suppressor-cell function. This receives some support from the observation that the suppressive activity was not detected in the nylon-wool nonadherent cellular population of patients that were treated with OK432 (585).

The blood LGL of patients with malignant pleural effusions, which express NK-cell activity, also express a suppressor-cell function (599). The proliferative response of the patients' PBL stimulated with autologous tumor (isolated from the carcinomatous pleural effusion) is very low or virtually absent. In contrast, appreciable tumor-induced proliferative responses were found in most cellular populations of small T cells derived from the high density fractions of discontinuous Percoll gradient of these PBL. The low-density fractions containing the LGL failed to express any proliferative response after the tumor stimulation. The assumption that the LGL express suppressor-cell function was directly proved by demonstrating that the isolated T cells cocultured with LGL failed to proliferate and generate antitumor cytotoxic cells after stimulation with autologous tumor. The suppressive activity of the LGL was lost after treatment with monoclonal antibodies expressing anti-NK specificity (Leu-7, Leu-11b) and C, but not after treatment with a monoclonal antibody expressing pan-T-cell specificity (OKT3). The LGL failed to suppress the antitumor cytotoxicity when added into the cytotoxic assay system, and they also did not block the ability of the patients' T cells to proliferate after stimulation with allogeneic PBL or PHA. These findings indicate that the LGL suppressor cells express at least partial specificity and that the suppressive activity was restricted to the induction phase of the immune response. The LGL released an SF when encountered with the autologous neoplastic cells. The factor inhibited the tumor-induced proliferative responses, but it neither killed the autologous tumor nor the responder T cells. These results suggest that distinct mechanisms for the NK-cell activity and the suppressor-cell function both reside in the LGL cells. The former uses a cell-to-cell contact, whereas the latter employs a release of a blocking factor. It should, however, be remembered that the NK-cell activity was also under control of independent suppressor-cell functions mediated by monocytes and T cells (*584,585*).

Although usually the effusions of lung cancer patients do not contain spontaneous suppressor cells inhibiting mitogenic responses, such cells have been found, as indicated before, in the blood of most patients. Con A-induced suppressor cells are usually found in the pleural effusion of most (*586*), and in the peripheral blood of a few (*556,586*), lung cancer patients. The peripheral blood of most patients does not contain Con A-induced suppressor cells (*586*). Interestingly, the Con A-induced suppressor cells were found in the blood of some of those patients who failed to express spontaneous suppressor cells (*586*). The Con A-induced suppressor cells of the pleural effusion and the spontaneous suppressor cells of the peripheral blood of the lung cancer patients exhibit similar characteristics. Both types of cells suppress the mitogenic responses of autologous and allogeneic lymphocytes, both of which belong to a group of nylon-wool nonadherent cells (E$^+$ T cells) expressing sensitivity to culture conditions and the function of both survive treatment with MMC (*586*). These similarities suggest that the spontaneous and the Con A-induced suppressor cells belong to the same cellular pool, but the former have already been activated and are not available for further activation by Con A.

Mononuclear cells of patients with non-small-cell lung cancer who had undergone complete resection and received postoperative intrapleural BCG treatment developed an enhanced proliferative response against PPD after removal of $T\gamma^+$ cells. The PPD-induced Ig synthesis of this depleted cell population was also augmented, suggesting that $T\gamma^+$ cells suppress these immunological responses. The effect was more pronounced in patients with negative skin test to PPD than in patients reactive to this antigen. Incubation of $T\gamma^+$ cells with the $T\gamma^+$ depleted cellular population (designated $T\gamma^-$) inhibited the proliferation of $T\gamma^-$ cells after PPD stimulation, but not after stimulation with PHA. Similarly, the addition of $T\gamma^+$ cells to $T\gamma^-$ cells suppressed the ability of the latter to support the PPD-induced (but not the PWM-induced) Ig synthesis by autologous B cells. Whereas such $T\gamma^+$ suppressor T cells were detected in some of the patients, radiosensitive suppressor monocytes were found in other patients. Since one patient with a positive skin test to PPD did not undergo complete resection and did not receive intrapleural BCG but had a pattern of reactivity similar to that of the other patients, whereas normal individuals (PPD negative) did not develop this type of suppression, the authors suggested that the apparently specific suppressor-cell function was related to the malignancy rather than to the BCG administration (594). Obviously, such a conclusion is tentative until it can be shown with greater confidence that the presence of suppressor cells is not related to the treatment procedure.

Other investigators (600,601), however, presented evidence that BCG treatment induced or augmented the appearance of suppressor or cytostatic monocytes in lung cancer patients. In contrast, patients who were not receiving BCG demonstrated predominantly nonadherent (T cell?) suppressor-cell activity.

The ability to induce tumor-specific suppressor cells was also reported by Akiyama and associates (582) and Uchida and Klein (599). The former authors (582) found, although indirectly, such suppressor cells in some lung cancer patients, whereas nonspecific suppressor cells were found in other patients and, in others, suppressor cells could not be detected at all.

In contrast to one report mentioned above (594), it was found that MNC of untreated lung cancer patients generated a poor response in the PWM-driven Ig synthesis assay, whereas the PWM-induced proliferation response of these cells was no different than that of cells from normal individuals (575). Mixing of enriched B lymphocytes of some but not all patients with autologous irradiated (1250 rad) T lymphocytes produced, however, augmented levels of Ig after stimulation with PWM, suggesting that radiosensitive T cells suppressed this immunological response in a nonspecific manner. The conflicting results of these two reports (575,594) suggest that the suppressor cells observed in the BCG-treated patients were associated with the treatment rather than with the malignancy (*see also* a previous section describing suppressor cells induced with immunostimulants). Alternatively, the conflicting results might be attributed to the different histological stage classification of the cancer cells inducing the suppressor cells.

Vose and Moore (602) isolated tumor-infiltrating lymphocytes (TIL) from tumors of lung cancer patients by stepwise application of velocity and density sedimentations on discontinuous Ficoll-Triosil or bovine serum gradients. In comparison with the autologous blood lymphocytes, the TIL generated a reduced proliferative response after stimulation by PHA or autologous tumor cells, a lack of cytotoxicity against the autologous tumor cells and virtually no NK-cell activity. These defects might be attributed to the presence of suppressor cells in TIL, since MMC-treated TIL suppressed the ability of cocultivated autologous blood lymphocytes to proliferate after stimulation with PHA or autologous tumor (602,603). The nature and characteristics of these suppressor cells were not described.

In summary, although one study stresses that the suppressor-cell activity is fairly well correlated with the extent of lung cancer disease and it significantly diminished during remission (593), other studies describe the absence of immunosuppression (344,572,573,575) or suppressor cells (582,583) in at least some of the patients. When suppressor cells were documented in lung cancer patients, they revealed quite heterogeneous properties and in most cases they were nonspecific (*see* Table 5). Taking all these facts into account, it is very difficult to evaluate the significance of the suppressor cells to the disease etiology or to the disease modification. In order to determine if the disease activity is associated with suppressor-cell function, it is most important to perform more longitudinal studies, relating specific suppressor function to development of disease, and secondly to eliminate those alterations in suppressor activity related to treatment or other unrelated conditions. For example, the presence of suppressor cells might be associated with inability to respond to PPD and not with the tumor activity.

6. Alimentary-Tract Malignancies

Tumors of the alimentary viscera include those arising in the esophagous, stomach, colon-rectum, liver, and pancreas. In addition to the arbitrary regional classification, these are variations in the types of the tumors arising in each site.

More than 90% of malignant esophageal neoplasms are squamous-cell carcinomas developing from the squamous-cell ep- ithelium of the esophageal lumen. Of the remaining 10%, adenoid cystic carcinoma, oat-cell carcinoma, and leiomyosarcoma have been observed (*604*).

Ninety-five percent of the neoplasms of the stomach are adenocarcinomas, the remainder including adenoacanthoma, squamous-cell carcinoma, carcinoid tumors, and leiomyosarcoma. As a result, the term gastric cancer usually refers to adenocarcinoma (*605*). Of the colorectal cancers, over 98% are also adenocarcinomas (*606*). Two-thirds of the hepatomas are of the nodular form, 30% are of the massive form, and 5% are of the diffuse type (*607*). Finally, neoplasia of the exocrine portion of the pancreas accounts for 95% of pancreatic tumors, and the remainder are islet tumors (*608*).

As for all instances of a site-localized tumor, as opposed to a diffuse malignancy, such as leukemia, if any changes in immune function are to be observed, this would most likely be in the draining lymph node. As a result, the relevance of measurements taken using peripheral blood must be rigorously examined. Nevertheless, in several instances, alterations in immune function, apparently associated with the tumor, may be detected in the peripheral blood.

Some, but certainly not all, patients with gastric (*609*) or colorectal (*610*) carcinomas exhibit a depression of mitogen and alloantigen-induced proliferative responses, in comparison with normal individuals. These depressed responses, however, are not necessarily associated with circulating peripheral blood suppressor cells (*609*).

Zembala and colleagues (*611*) reported that 76 of 245 (31%) patients with gastric cancer presented increased suppressor-cell function, assessed by the ability of their MNC to inhibit the PHA mitogenic response of cocultivated lymphocytes derived from normal individuals. The suppressor cells were characterized as plastic-adherent cells (monocytes). The presence of similar suppressor monocytes (as well as suppressor T cells) in patients with stomach cancer was previously demonstrated by other authors (584). The suppressor-cell function in these gastric cancer patients (611) was more frequently detected with increasing severity of the disease, and may have been associated with decreased PHA mitogenic responses seen in these patients. Among those patients whose tumors were surgically resectable, the suppressor-cell activity was frequently reduced in comparison with the level before surgery. Interestingly, patients with advanced disease who presented increased suppressor-cell activity survived longer than similar patients with less suppressive activity (611).

Nonspecific suppressor cells have also been found in the blood (610,612) and the lymph nodes (561,603) of patients with colon cancer. One of these studies (612) indicated that the spontaneous suppressor-cell function, inhibiting the PHA mitogenic response of cocultivated normal MNC, did not correlate with the stage of the disease, the level of oncofetal antigens, or serum immune complexes.

Some evidence from the experiments of Balch and colleagues (610) implies that PG produced by monocytes of colorectal cancer patients suppressed the PHA and, to a lesser degree, the Con A mitogenic responses of the patients' lymphocytes. Addition of indomethacin, a PG synthetase inhibitor, restored the PHA mitogenic response of the patients' MNC. Furthermore, culture of the patients' MNC produced greater amounts of PGE_2 (10.1 ng/mL) than culture of the MNC of normal individuals (5.1 ng/mL), and the synthesis could be exclusively attributed to monocytes (610). Unfortunately, this report does not present evidence that the monocytes actually suppressed the mitogenic responses, since their activity was not demonstrated by cocultivation experiments.

These latter results are supported by previous studies (557, 561) presenting evidence that addition of indomethacin to blood MNC of colon patients enhanced their PHA mitogenic responses. In addition, it has been demonstrated that removal of monocytes by plastic (561) or glass (557) adherence or their inactivation with CAR or silica (561) augmented the mitogen-induced proliferative response of the patients' MNC.

Toge and colleagues (*613,614*) found that the blood of patients with advanced gastric cancer contains increased levels of precursors of suppressor cells that expressed suppressor-effector cell function after incubation with Con A. These suppressor-precursor cells populated the E rosette cellular fraction (i.e., they express a T cell phenotype) and after activation with Con A suppressed the PHA mitogenic response of cocultivated normal lymphocytes (*613*). A considerable reduction of the Con A-induced suppressor-cell function was noticed after tumor resection (*613*) and during the terminal stages of the disease (*614*). Nevertheless, this reduction during the terminal stages was associated with an increased spontaneous suppressor-cell function (meaning that Con A was not required for activation). The simplest interpretation would be that the precursor-suppressor pool is finite, and with increased tumor burden, there was an increased activation of suppressor cells, leaving less cells available for further activation by Con A. Perhaps supporting this notion, sera of patients with advanced gastric cancer induced the appearance of suppressor cells in a normal mononuclear cellular population (*615*). The ability of the sera to induce suppressor cell activity correlated with the activity of spontaneous suppressor cells derived from the sera donors. Furthermore, the ability of the sera to induce suppressor-cell function and the spontaneous suppressor-cell activity of the sera donors were markedly reduced after subjecting the patients to a few cycles of plasma exchange (*615*). Both tumor-serum-induced suppressor cells and Con A-induced suppressor populations contained increased levels of $T8^+$ cells (*615*). These findings all together support the notion that the tumor antigens or immune complexes of patients with advanced gastric cancer probably activate the same suppressor-precursor cell population that is activated by Con A.

Elevated Con A-induced suppressor-cell function was found also in thoracic esophageal cancer patients, which exhibited considerable depression of cell-mediated immunity (*616*).

As was noted before, there have been efforts to establish the levels of suppressor function not only in the peripheral blood, but also in the structured lymphoid organs. For example, suppressor T cells have been found in the E^+ cellular fraction derived from involved and uninvolved lymph nodes of colon cancer patients. These suppressor T cells inhibited the PHA and the Con A mitogenic responses of cocultured autologous PBL (*561*). The spleens of patients with advanced gastric cancer may contain spontaneous suppressor cells (*614,617*) and Con A-induced suppressor cells (*614*). Neither type of suppressor cell described in ref *614* adhered to glass, whereas both could be eliminated with T8 antibody and C, indicating their suppressor T cell phenotype. On separation of spontaneous and Con A-induced suppressor cells by velocity sedimentation over FCS, the spontaneous suppressor cells appeared to be larger than their Con A-induced counterparts (*614*). Since there were no normal controls in this study, the significance of the patients' splenic suppressor cells is uncertain.

Kanayama and colleagues (*618*) found that the supernatants of spleen cells (or splenic plastic nonadherent cells) and, to a lesser degree, of blood lymphocytes, both derived from advanced gastric cancer patients, contain an SF that inhibits the PHA proliferative response of normal lymphocytes. Interestingly, whereas the blood lymphocytes of advanced gastric patients did not develop PHA mitogenic responses as high as blood of individuals with benign diseases, spleen cells of these patients demonstrated normal responses, suggesting that they are refractory to the inhibitory effect of their own SF.

Koyama and colleagues (*619,620*) also claimed that the spleen and the peripheral blood of gastric cancer patients contain specific suppressor T cells. They found that nylon-wool-nonadherent cells of preoperative frozen PBL and spleen cells, both derived from resectable advanced cancer patients, inhibited the proliferative response of cocultivated autologous postoperative lymphocytes stimulated with a 3*M* KCl extract of the autologous tumor (*619*).

In separate studies, the above-mentioned group (*609,620*) demonstrated that blood MMC-treated IL-2-dependent cultured lymphocytes derived from all gastric cancer patients with nonresectable tumors suppressed the PHA and the alloantigen-induced proliferative responses of cocultivated autologous PBL. Similar cultured lymphocytes from patients bearing resectable tumors or from normal individuals as well as uncultured lymphocytes from patients with resectable and nonresectable tumors or from normal donors failed to exert these suppressive activities. The suppressor IL-2-dependent cultured lymphocytes of the patients carrying systemic metastases were characterized by appropriate antibodies as Leu-2$^+$, Leu-3$^-$ cells (*609*). The authors suggest that precursors of these cells may be activated in patients with large tumor burdens, and the consequential immunodepression may promote further tumor progression. Since the cells mediating the suppression were IL-2-dependent, the possibility that they block the alloantigen or mitogenic responses by absorbing IL-2 in the culture needs to be tested by adding exogenous IL-2 during the period of the suppression-cell function assay.

Gibson and colleagues (621) reported that MNC isolated from human intestinal mucosa of patients with colorectal carcinomas or other nonmalignant intestinal disease generated enhanced spontaneous cytotoxic cell activity after incubation in vitro for 24 h, whereas the uncultured cells expressed low or no activity. The depressed spontaneous cytotoxic cell activity of the intestinal MNC was attributed to toxic factors released during the collagenase digestion used to separate the cells from the mucosa. This conclusion was based on the fact that supernatants of the digested cells suppressed the spontaneous cytotoxic cell activity of peripheral blood MNC, but the inhibitory effect was reversed if the blood MNC were cultured for 24 h before the NK-cell assay. Nevertheless, the intestinal MNC slightly but significantly suppressed the spontaneous cytotoxic cell activity of cocultivated peripheral blood MNC, and this suppression was not reversed by a 24-h preincubation of the intestinal cells, indicating that toxic factors were not involved in this inhibition. In this instance, however, the suppressive activity of cancer patients' intestinal cells was no different than that of patients with nonmalignant diseases. As a result, artifactual causes of suppression, such as the ability to absorb IL-2 or the release of toxic factors, must be eliminated before drawing conclusions about suppression, which itself may be no greater than that developed by PBL from normal individuals, thus stressing the need for controls.

A tumor-derived acidic suppressogenic entity has been isolated from human colonic adenocarcinoma cell line extracts and a primary colon carcinoma supernatant, by pIEF. These human acidic soluble factors induced suppressor cells in murine splenocytes that inhibited, when injected into syngeneic mice, their DTH response to DNCB (245). The ability of isolated tumor fractions to induce suppressor-cell activity is discussed in the chapter entitled Antigenic Entities of the Tumor That Induces Suppressor Cells May Prevent the Functional Expression of Coexpressed Immunogenic Entities (p. 41).

Colon carcinoma has been shown to aggregate in families who demonstrate no evidence of preexisting precancerous conditions (622–626). Berlinger and associates (627) attempted to determine whether or not cancer-free individuals within family aggregates of apparently hereditary colon carcinoma exhibited an immundeficiency, as indicated by their ability to respond to alloantigen in MLC assay. Although the tested sample was limited in size, it suggests that the immunodeficiency aggregates in the families in which the colon carcinoma also aggregates. The relatively low MLC of the family members was restored, at least partially, by eliminating Sephadex G-10-column-adhering cells from the cellular cultures, suggesting that monocytes mediate the suppressive effect. The authors speculate that a genetically transmitted immunologic determinant may be contributory to the genesis of the colon carcinoma (627).

A recent report from the People's Republic of China indicates a marked reduction of $T\mu$:$T\gamma$ cell ratios in the blood of patients with malignant hepatoma (as well as in patients with gastric carcinoma, (628). In addition, low ratios of T4:T8 cell phenotypes have confirmed the increased expression of cells with suppressor phenotype in Chinese hepatoma patients (629). Finally, glass-adherent suppressor monocytes and Con A-induced suppressor cells have also been found in patients with cancer of the pancreas (556).

Analyzing the published data, firm conclusions about the association between suppressor-cell function and the above-mentioned malignant diseases cannot be formulated. Immunodepression is not always manifested in the cancer patients, and when it appears, it is not always mediated by suppressor cells (609). Furthermore, the suppressor-cell function, when apparent, is expressed in many cases during the advanced stages of the disease (611,613,614), but there are exceptions (612). This last fact stresses that the nonspecific suppressor cells (in most cases, only such suppressor cells were explored) are not associated with the permissive phases of the disease. In addition, since their function is not always expressed, it is doubtful whether they are involved in the promotion phases. The most provocative association is the observation that patients with advanced disease with an apparently suppressor-cell function survived longer than similar patients without such function (611). On the other hand, the finding of Berlinger et al. (627), showing the aggregation of immunodeficiency in family members of patients with colon carcinoma, does not oppose the notion that, in certain instances, suppressor-cell function is associated with one of the permissive phases of the disease. This interesting observation must, however, be confirmed by screening large number of families with a disposi-

tion to colon carcinoma and proving the association of immunodeficiency with a subsequent development of colon carcinoma.
Finally, it should be remembered that, in most cases (an exception is ref. *619*), the function of nonspecific suppressor cells was
explored, whereas the function of tumor-specific suppressor cells,
which might be more significant to the malignant process, has not
been investigated.

7. Genitourinary Malignancies

In this section, the suppressor-cell function observed in neoplasms of the kidney, bladder, and prostate will be discussed under the common title of genitourinary malignancies. Renal adenocarcinoma is the most common malignancy involving the kidney.
The tumors are of renal tubular epithelium origin (*630,631*).
Among the urothelial bladder tumors, 90% are of the transitional-
cell variety, 6–8% are squamous cell carcinomas, and 2% are adenocarcinomas (*632*). The most common tumor arising in the prostate is an adenocarcinoma, originating from the peripheral acinar
glands (*633*).

In patients with transitional-cell carcinoma of the bladder, a
deficiency in the DTH response to DNCB was observed, which
correlated with the stage of the disease, with the tumor burden,
and possibly with the disease prognosis (*634,635*). The in vitro
proliferative response to mitogens was often impaired in these
patients as well as in patients with other urological (kidney, prostate) cancers (*636,637*). In addition, in patients with advanced
prostatic cancer, a low helper:suppressor cell ratio (*638,639*) and a
relatively high proportion of monocytes (*639*) were found. These
observations were confirmed in rats bearing the Dunning prostate
adenocarcinoma (*640*).

The MNC proliferative response after allogeneic stimulation
of bladder cancer patients (MLC) was unaffected by the presence
of a malignancy, but the ability of the allostimulated cells to differentiate into cytotoxic cells was significantly reduced, an effect that
correlated with the stage of the disease, being more pronounced
in the invasive than in the superficial stage. Surgical removal of
the tumor improved the MLC-generated cytotoxicity of the patients, the improvement being greatest among those with
superficial-stage malignancies (*641*). The cytotoxic response of the
allostimulated MNC of patients with bladder tumors was restored

to the normal level after elimination of the monocytes by magnetic removal of carbonyl iron-ingesting cells (*641,642*), suggesting that monocytes mediated this suppression. The same effect of monocyte elimination was observed in postoperative patients with invasive tumors (*641*). Readdition of plastic-adherent monocytes to the MLC did not, however, completely regenerate the suppression observed before monocytic depletion (*641*). The authors suggest that the suppressive effect is partly mediated by a monocyte subpopulation that is not completely represented by the plastic-adherent cells used to reconstitute the suppression.

Catalona and colleagues (*637,643,644*) tested the activity of Con A-induced suppressor cells in patients with kidney, bladder, or prostatic malignancies, and found that it was no different than that of control individuals with benign urologic disorders (*637,643*). Con A-induced suppressor-cell function was found also in the regional tumor-draining lymph nodes of the patients (*643,644*), but the low number of control individuals tested in this study (*644*) precludes the drawing of any firm conclusions. Spontaneous suppressor cells, not requiring induction by Con A, could not be found in the peripheral blood or lymph nodes of the same patients (*644*).

Bean and colleagues (*645–647*) identified an unusual instance of a genetically restricted suppressor cell in the peripheral blood MNC of an untransfused patient with recurrent superficial bladder carcinoma. The suppressor cells inhibited the MLC response only of normal individuals expressing the HLA-B14 class I antigen, but not the MLC of those lacking this phenotype. The apparently restricted cells from the patient did not, however, cause lysis of the HLA-B14-positive cells, indicating a true suppressive effect (*646*). The suppressor lymphocytes were characterized as Ia positive, T3-positive, and T8-positive, but T4-negative, indicating that they were cytotox/suppressor T cells (*647*). The patients' suppressor and helper cells were isolated by incubating them with mouse OKT8 or OKT4 monoclonal antibodies, respectively, and subsequent absorption of these cells on petri dishes coated with goat antimouse IgG (panning technique). As few as 7800 of the positively selected OKT8$^+$ cells (suppressor:responder ratio of 1:16) suppressed the MLC of HLA-B14 donor by 75% (*647*).

In contrast to other reported cases (*648–652*), HLA-D compatibility between the patients' suppressor cells and the target cells to be suppressed was not required (*646*). The authors speculated that the patients' suppressor cells were activated in vivo by tumor-altered antigen, which coincidentally cross-reacts with HLA-B14 antigen. As a result, the suppressor cells could recognize and inhibit only allostimulated cells of HLA-B14 donors.

The effect of INF treatment on renal-cell carcinoma patients was explored by Braun and colleagues (653). The ability of the patients' MNC to proliferate after PHA stimulation was markedly impaired after the INF treatment, but this effect did not correlate with the clinical response to this immunomodulator. Addition of indomethacin during culture markedly enhanced the mitogenic response to PHA of the patients' MNC and, in certain cases, even restored this mitogenic activity to the pretreatment level. The suggestion that INF induced PG-producing suppressor cells was supported by an experiment demonstrating that INF could induce glass-adherent cells to suppress the PHA mitogenic response of autologous MNC on their subsequent coculture. This suppressive effect could be largely overcome by addition of indomethacin during the mitogen stimulation (653). The authors suggest that the INF treatment may be more successful if combined with indomethacin or other drugs that inhibit PG synthesis (653), thereby overcoming PG-mediated suppression, which may antagonize the antineoplastic effects of INF.

8. Gynecologic Malignancies

The function of suppressor cells in gynecologic malignancies will be discussed in this section. More than 80% of ovarian malignancies are epithelial carcinomas arising from the serosal mesothelial layer of the ovary (654), and 95% of uterine-cervical cancers are squamous-cell carcinomas (655), originating from the squamous-columnar junction of the endocervical canal or the portio of the cervix (656). Five percent of the uterine-cervix carcinomas are adenocarcinomas (655).

Macrophages isolated from ascites or collagenase-dispersed solid tumors of patients with ovarian carcinoma were able, in some but not all instances, to suppress the PHA mitogenic response of cocultured autologous blood lymphocytes. Monocytes isolated from the peripheral blood of some patients were also able to exert a similar suppressive effect. Suppressor activity was also detected in the purified tumor-cell fraction of some patients, yet tumor-cell contamination was insufficient to account for the suppression mediated by the macrophages (657).

Tumor-infiltrating lymphocytes isolated from the carcinomatous ascites of ovarian carcinoma patients by density separation on a Ficoll-Hypaque gradient followed by velocity sedimentation in fetal bovine serum developed a reduced NK-cell activity in comparison with the NK-cell activities of PBL from the same patients or normal donors (658,659). The suppression of the NK-cell activity of normal (658,659) or autologous (659) PBL by cocultivated TIL was noted in only a few of the patients, whereas in most cases, suppressive activity was not detected or was not convincingly demonstrated (the authors did not take into account the dilution effect in the mixed cellular population; hence, an inhibition of only 14% is at the limit of acceptance; 658,659). Both nylon-adherent and nonadherent cells, derived from the ascites of one patient, expressed anti-NK suppressor-cell function (659), suggesting that both T and non-T cells are involved in this activity.

Glass-adherent suppressor monocytes were found in the blood of an untreated patient with cervical cancer (657). In another study, the activity of the peripheral blood Con A-induced suppressor cells in uterine cancer was found to decline after the patients underwent a hysterectomy (660). This effect was accompanied by decreased mitogenic responses to PHA and Con A, indicating the influence of the operative trauma on these proliferative responses.

9. Cancer of the Breast

The most common breast cancer, accounting for almost 70% of the cases, is infiltrating duct carcinoma, in which no special type of histologic structure is recognized. This tumor commonly metastasizes to axillary lymph nodes, and its prognosis, relative to other breast carcinomas, is poor. Other invasive carcinomas that arise from the large ducts are medullary carcinoma, tubular carcinoma, mucinous carcinoma, and infiltrating papillary carcinoma. Lobular carcinoma arises from the small end ducts of the breast. It appears in both invasive and noninvasive forms (the noninvasive form accounts for 50% of all the mammary carcinomas, which themselves comprise almost 5% of all neoplastic lesions of the female breast; (661).

Petrini and colleagues (*662*) found relatively high levels of Tγ cells in the peripheral blood of breast cancer patients, whereas the levels of Tμ cells were normal. After radiotherapy, the proportion of Tγ cells falls with a consequent elevation in the Tμ :Tγ ratio (*662–664*). However, as mentioned before, the representation of helper and suppressor cells by Tμ and Tγ cells (*303*) has been questioned (*275*), for instance, by demonstrating that antibodies against antigens of monocytes react with Tγ cells (*275*). Furthermore, only 20–30% overlap has been reported between Tγ cells and suppressor/cytotoxic cells expressing the Leu-2$^+$ phenotype (*662*). The proportions of helper (Leu-3$^+$) and suppressor/cytotoxic (Leu-2$^+$) cells of breast cancer patients have not been shown to be any different than those found in normal individuals (*662,665*).

In contrast to their own previous report (*662,664*) and another group report (*666*), Petrini's group (*667,668*) as well as others (*663*) claimed that preoperative or postoperative radiotherapy reduced the helper:suppressor T cell ratios, indicated by expression of Leu-3 and Leu-2 phenotypes, respectively. The effect was observed one year (*667*) and even ten years (*667,668*) after treatment.

The same authors (*665*) also reported that the proportions of both helper (Leu-3$^+$) and suppressor (Leu-2$^+$) cells were markedly reduced during postoperative cyclic therapy with cyclophosphamide, methotrexate, and 5-fluorouracil. There was a greater reductive effect upon the helper cells with a resultant fall in the helper:suppressor cell ratio (*665,667*), which remained low two or even three years after completion of the chemotherapy (*665*). Patients subjected to surgery with no other treatments did not develop such changes in their helper:suppressor T lymphocyte ratios (*667,668*). In contrast to patients with acquired immunodeficiency syndrome (AIDS), who also present low helper:suppressor cell ratios (*670*), the treated breast cancer patients did not develop signs of serious infections (*667*). However, the helper:suppressor cell ratio in AIDS patients is markedly lower than that of posttherapy breast cancer patients (compare ref. *670* to ref. *667*).

The possible function of suppressor monocytes in the blood of breast cancer patients was demonstrated by the enhanced proliferative response of MNC depleted of glass-adherent cells and stimulated with PHA (*556,557*). Prostaglandins released from the monocytes possibly mediates the suppressive activity, since indo-

methacin added to the patients' MNC enhanced their proliferative activity (557). In addition to monocytes, Con A-induced suppressor cells were also detected in the blood of breast cancer
patients (556). The patients described in this experiment were not
subjected to surgical resection, and received neither radiation nor
chemotherapy for at least six months before assay.

Uchida and associates (671) explored the suppressor-cell
function in breast cancer patients who had undergone modified
radical mastectomy, including prophylactic lymph node dissection but were otherwise untreated. Whereas the preoperative
blood MNC developed a normal NK-cell function, the natural-
killer-cell activity of the postoperative blood MNC was reduced.
In contrast, the PHA mitogenic response of the postoperative
cells was normal. The NK-cell activity of the postoperative MNC
could be increased if monocytes were removed from the responding cells by plastic adherence, a further round of adherence
to Sephadex G-10 and then a 24-h culture of the monocyte-
depleted cells before assay. Removal of the monocytes after 24 h
of in vitro cultivation of the MNC but immediately before assay
did not augment the NK-cell activity, suggesting that the peripheral blood of postoperative cancer patients contains potentially
cytotoxic cells that are suppressed by monocytes, but could re-
cover their lytic function if the suppressor monocytes were absent
during 24 h. This assumption was confirmed by demonstrating
that plastic-adherent cells of postoperative patients, but not of
preoperative patients or normal individuals, suppressed the subsequent NK-cell activity of normal blood lymphocytes preincubated for 24 h with the plastic adherent cells. The PHA response
of normal lymphocytes, however, was unaffected by the presence
of postoperative adherent cells. Suppressor factors were not detected in the supernatuant of postoperative monocytes incubated
alone or with normal lymphocytes (671), suggesting that cell-to-
cell contact is required in order to mount an efficient suppressive
effect. Similar results were described by these authors in a separate communication (204), but in this instance, the type of cancer
of the postoperative patients was not stated.

In contrast to the previous finding (671), Eremin (672,673)
found normal NK cell function in the blood and the axillary
lymph nodes of breast cancer patients undergoing a mastectomy
and axillary clearance. The conflict of results is perturbing, but
may be accounted for in part by differing times of assay, the normal NK function being found immediately postoperatively (673),

whereas the suppression of NK activity was found 1–2 wk after surgery (*671*).

Tumor-infiltrating lymphocytes isolated by mechanical dis-aggregation, collagenase digestion, and passage through a Sephadex G-50 column failed to develop appreciable levels of NK-cell activity, but were able to suppress the NK cells of cocultivated autologous PBL (*673*). The possibility was not formally excluded that contaminating tumor cells in the TIL were responsible for the suppressive activity, although it was demonstrated that lymph nodes invaded by metastases contained a significant level of NK-cell function (*673*), suggesting that the tumor cells do not inhibit the NK-cell activity.

In agreement with the above-mentioned findings, Vose and Moore (*602*) reported that TIL from a breast malignancy isolated by stepwise application of velocity and density sedimentations on discontinuous Ficoll-Triosil or bovine serum gradients, failed to develop cytotoxicity against K562 cells or the autologous tumor. In addition, the proliferative responses of the TIL to PHA or autologous tumor cells were poor. In contrast, the proliferative responses of the patient's PBL to PHA or autologous tumor were relatively high, but were depressed when cocultured with TIL. The suppressive activity was subsequently located within the nylon-wool-nonadherent fraction of the TIL, presumably being T cells (*602*). If NK cells do restrain the local development of the tumor and its spread to other tissues (a prediction yet to be proven), blocking the *in situ* anti-NK-suppressor-cell function may en-hance the regression of the tumor and prevent the metastatic pro-cess.

10. Melanoma and Other Skin Malignancies

Melanoma is a neoplasm derived from melanocytes that spe-cialize in the biosynthesis and transport of melanin pigment (*674,675*). Basal and squamous cell carcinomas are nonmelanoma skin cancers arising from the epidermal cells (*676,677*). Both epi-demiological studies and animal experimental research have shown that the UV spectrum of sunlight is an important etiolog-ical factor in the development of skin malignancies (*678*). Kaposi's sarcoma has recently attracted much attention because of its asso-

ciation with AIDS (about one-third of all AIDS patients develop
Kaposi's sarcoma; *679*). The tumor is thought to arise from endo-
thelial cells and presents itself as raised pigmented lesions of the
skin (*680*).

Spontaneous regression of primary melanoma and late recurrence of the disease, sometimes 25 y after the removal of the initial primary tumor, suggests that the immune system can respond
to the melanoma antigens and sometimes even successfully control the disease. This notion is supported by the facts that both
cellular and humoral immunities against melanoma antigens are
detected in melanoma patients. Nevertheless, it has been found
that the melanoma patients are less easily sensitized to DNCB
than healthy individuals and their lymphocytes respond poorly to
PHA in comparison with normal individuals. Furthermore, patients with diffuse disease react less efficiently to recall antigens
than patients with local disease (*674*).

Considerable experimental research in animals, performed
by Kripke (*681–683*), Daynes (*681,685*), and their colleagues indicates that suppressor cells induced by UV irradiation may encour-
age the growth of UV-induced tumors. In fact, the UV irradiation
may provoke three dramatic events in the epidermis that may result in photocarcinogenesis. First, the UV light may cause
antigenic modification or production of neoantigen (*686*). Second,
it may cause depletion or functional failure of the epidermal
Langerhans cells (which may serve as APC, stimulating the
helper cells; *687,688*). Finally, the UV irradiation may cause malignant transformation in the skin cells (*689*). It is possible that the
neoantigen (or the altered antigen) activates suppressor cells, but
because of the altered function of the APC, no balancing helper
cells are induced. The skin UV-induced neoantigens could share
antigenic determinants with the UV-transformed cells; thus, the
uncontrolled suppressor cells induced by these skin antigens may
be further activated by the UV-transformed tumors. Consequently, these suppressor cells may restrain the immunological
rejection of UV-induced tumors, but not the rejection of other malignant cells. More experimental and theoretical details concerning the interrelationships between UV-induced suppressor cells
and UV-induced tumors are presented in our previous review paper (*1*).

The possibility that UV irradiation activates suppressor cells
in human beings was proposed by Hersey and colleagues
(*690,691*). The helper cell:suppressor cell (T4:T8) ratios were lower

in volunteers exposed to UV irradiation delivered by a commercial solarium (1.5 ± 0.8; *672*) or by sunlight (0.83 ± 0.2; *673*) than in normal individuals not exposed to these treatments (T4:T8 ratios of 2.0 ± 0.6 and 1.57 ± 0.32, respectively; the pretreatment values of the tested individuals were similar to those of the normal subjects), indicating better representation of T8 cytotoxic-suppressor cells after UV irradiation. Furthermore, irradiated (2000 rad) T cells of the UV-exposed volunteers provided more help for cocultivated B cells to produce Ig after PWM stimulation than T cells not subjected to X-irradiation. Such an enhancement effect was not expressed by X-irradiated T cells of normal individuals, (*690,691*). This finding suggests that the UV-exposed volunteers, but not the normal individuals, develop radiosensitive suppressor cells.

Impressed probably by the findings described in experimental animals, the authors speculated that the suppressor-cell function may be amplified by the melanoma antigens, and consequently, tumor progression may be enhanced in the patients (*691*). This specific speculation does not agree with the authors' own findings (*692*), implying that in many cases suppressor cells from melanoma patients and normal individuals provide the same degree of inhibition for PWM-induced Ig synthesis by cocultivated B cells. After surgical removal of the tumor, the levels of suppressor-cell activity were equivalent to the lowest level observed in the controls, implying that the tumor mass was maintaining a relatively high suppressor activity. This change was associated with a concomitant increase in the serum concentrations of IgM and IgG (*692*). The activity of Con A-induced suppressor cells of melanoma patients was no different than that of normal individuals, but this activity reached the upper level of the control after surgical removal of the tumor (the suppressor-cell function was measured by its ability to inhibit the mitogen-induced proliferation of cocultivated autologous lymphocytes). The reduced activity of Con A-induced suppressor cells of melanoma patients was associated, before the surgery, with elevated proportions of Tγ cells (*693*). Suppressor cells specific to the melanoma antigens were not, however, explored in these studies (*692,693*); therefore, any conclusion derived from the above-described nonspecific suppressor-cell function must be considered with caution.

Minassian and Kadagidze (*598*) found that the monocyte-depleted blood cellular population of melanoma patients contains suppressor cells inhibiting the PHA mitogenic response of

cocultured normal cells. The degree of the suppression was correlated with the clinical stage of the disease.

Several years earlier, Ninnemann (*694*) found that a selected
population of normal B cells was able to provide a suppressive
function for a cocultured selected population of normal T cells, if
they (the B cells) were previously incubated with serum from melanoma patients, whereas pooled serum from normal individuals
was not able to induce such function in the B cells. The suppressive activity was determined by testing the ability of the normal B
cells preincubated with melanoma patients' serum and normal T
cells to inhibit the proliferative response of cocultured autologous
lymphocytes stimulated with PHA (the responder lymphocytes).
The responder lymphocytes were separated from the regulatory
cells by taking peripheral blood MNC nonadherent to a cotton
column and applying them to a sodium metrizoate-Ficoll
(Lymphoprep) gradient. The responder lymphocytes were collected from the interface, whereas the regulatory cells were collected from the bottom of the tube. In order to obtain regulatory B
and T cellular populations, prior to the Lymphoprep separation,
the cells were separated into nylon-wool-adherent (B cells) and
nonadherent (T cell) fractions (*694*). The possibility that monocytes were involved in the suppressive mechanism was not excluded by direct experiments, although indirect observations
(*694*) suggest that they were not determinative in this process.
Finally, it should be noted that the immunosuppressive serum
was taken from patients who were treated with xenogeneic immune RNA. Obviously, this fact complicates the interpretation of
the results.

Mukherji and colleagues (*695–697*) recently described
regulatory circuits in melanoma patients mediated by specific
suppressor T cells, whose significance may far exceed the limits of
this specific experimental model. These authors found that lymph
node cells of melanoma patients sensitized in vitro with the
autologous melanoma cell line (PJ-M) and further stimulated with
IL-2 suppressed the ability of autologous cocultivated blood lymphocytes to generate anti-PJ-M cytotoxic cells after in vitro incubation with autologous PJ-M cells. Unsensitized lymph node cells
failed to display suppressive activity (*695*). Suppressor cells were
effective even when cocultured with the responder cells in excess
of IL-2, indicating that the suppressor-cell mechanism is not asso-

ciated with absorption of IL-2. An IL-2-dependent homogeneous lymphocyte line (I-10:1) bearing the T4$^+$ helper/inducer phenotype and a T4$^+$ clone (I-10.3) were derived from the tumor-sensitized lymph node cells, and both presented tumor-specific suppressive activities, indicated by their ability to block the generation of antitumor cytotoxicity in autologous PBL stimulated with the PJ-M cells (*696,697*). The specificity of the lymph-node-derived (*695*) and the cell-lines (*696,697*) suppressor cells was proved by their inability to suppress the cytotoxic responses induced in the autologous blood lymphocytes with allogeneic tumor cells.

T8$^+$ and T4$^+$ cells were separated from the tumor-sensitized lymph node cells by incubating the cells with OKT8 and OKT4 antibodies, respectively, and binding the coated cells to goat antimouse IgG attached to a plastic surface (panning technique). The T8$^+$ cells inhibited the antitumor cytotoxic response of the cocultivated blood lymphocytes relatively quickly, since the suppression was detected after 1 wk of cocultivation. In contrast, 3 wk of cocultivation were required for the T4$^+$ cells in order to exert a suppressive activity (*695*). This experiment suggests that the T4$^+$ cells express a suppressor-inducer function, i.e., they activate T8$^+$ suppressor-effector cells in the cellular population of cocultivated PBL (therefore, their effect is detected relatively late). This assumption was confirmed by demonstrating the ability of the suppressor cell line (I-10:1) to activate T8$^+$ suppressor-effector cells in autologous blood lymphocytes stimulated with the PJ-M tumor line. The isolated T8$^+$ cells of this cellular population suppressed, in a second culture, the antitumor cytotoxic response of autologous PBL (*696*). The existence of suppressor-cell precursors in the lymph nodes of melanoma patients was confirmed by a more recent study. Hoon and colleagues found that nodes closest to melanoma lesions contained higher activity of Con A-induced suppressor cells than those located further away. In contrast to the former group (*696*) Hoon et al. (*698*) failed to establish IL-2-supported suppressor-cell line.

Both experimental models (*695,698*) may explain why antitumor immunological activity is not detected in the lymph nodes of melanoma patients, whereas such activity, if it exists, may be critical for the eradication of tumor cells colonizing neighboring lymph nodes. Furthermore, the first model (*695,696*) elucidates the immunoregulatory circuits in these cancer patients and, subsequently, may enable the future planning of rational strategies of immunotherapy.

The majority of lymphocytes surrounding the skin tumors were shown to be T cells with helper cells outnumbering suppressor cells by ratios from 2:1 to 5:1. This extensive representation of helper cells is possibly of no benefit to the patients, because the Langerhans cells committed to activate helper cells by presenting the antigen to them are markedly depleted or absent in the tumor sites (699).

Suppressor cells may appear in melanoma patients as a consequence of treatment. Uchida and colleagues (700,701) found that melanoma patients treated with human α-INF exhibited, 12 h after treatment, a considerable impairment of NK-cell activity that returned to or exceeded the pretreatment level within the next 24 h. A similar initial reduction in the NK-cell activity after INF treatment was observed in independent studies exploring melanoma (702) and other cancer patients (703). Whereas in vitro exposure to INF augmented the NK-cell activity of PBL from untreated patients, this reagent failed to enhance the activity of PBL obtained 12 h post-INF injection. Blood monocytes obtained from patients treated 12 h (but not 24 h) earlier with INF suppressed, upon cocultivation, the ability of INF to enhance the NK-cell activity of nylon-wool-nonadherent PBL obtained from the same patients (701). The base line level of NK-cell activity of the PBL was not suppressed by the monocytes (but a different study indicates that the early INF-induced suppressor cells do suppress the base line level of NK-cell activity; 703). The ability of streptococcal preparation OK432 to augment in vitro the NK-cell activity of PBL was not prevented when suppressor monocytes (obtained from the INF-treated patients) were added to the culture, indicating that the suppressive activity of the monocytes was limited to the INF augmentation effect (701). The authors suggest (701) that the transient decline of the NK-cell activity observed 12 h after INF treatment is mediated by short-lived suppressor monocytes that inhibit the INF-induced transition of pre-NK cells to NK cells (pre-NK cells are marked by their ability to form nonlysable conjugates with the target cells, and this effect was not suppressed 12 h after INF treatment).

Karavodin and Golub (702) found that patients treated with INF displayed an augmented NK-cell activity that peaked 3–7 d after treatment and returned to the normal level 21 d after treatment. The augmentation of the NK-cell activity was associated with an increased proportion of Leu-3 helper cells and a decreased proportion of Leu-2 cytotoxic/suppressor cells, an effect that was more profoundly expressed by the helper cell: suppressor cell ratios. These ratios peaked on day seven (1.47) and returned to pretreatment values (0.67) by day 21, despite continuation of α-INF therapy. The correlation between the Leu-3:Leu-2 ratios and the NK-cell activity suggests that helper and suppressor cells regulate the NK-cell activity and that INF treatment may affect this regulation in the favor of helper cells. In a different study, Karavodin and associates (704) reported that INF-untreated melanoma patients displayed, at various disease stages, the same helper:suppressor cell ratios as normal subjects.

In contrast to Karavodin and Golub (702), Maluish et al. (705) and Ozer et al. (706) did not observe any change in the helper T cell or the suppressor T cell phenotypes after α-INF treatment. These conflicting findings may be explained by different treatment protocols. Indeed, other authors (707–709) found that different INF treatment protocols (the nature of the group of patients treated or the timing, route of administration, type and dose of INF used) resulted in different posttreatment representations of the helper:cytotoxic/suppressor cell ratios.

The ability of cimetidine to prevent the activation of H_2-receptor-bearing suppressor cells (*see* earlier chapter, Control of NK Cells by Suppressor Cells, p. 15, and refs. 214,215) was the rationale for using this drug in the treatment of melanoma patients. The clinical application of the concept was further encouraged by experiments demonstrating the rejection of tumors (710) or reducing the lung metastases (711) of animals administered cimetidine orally. Flodgren and associates (712) observed tumor regression in six out of 20 melanoma patients injected intramuscularly or intratumorally with α-INF and, subsequently, administered cimetidine orally. No objective antitumor responses were recorded when INF was administered alone. Histopathological examination of the responding patients' biopsy materials revealed marked lymphocyte infiltration and tumor-cell destruction. The combined therapy of α-INF and cimetidine affected patients with metastases confined to the skin and subcutaneous tissues, whereas patients with extensive and multiple-organ tumor involvement did not benefit from the treatment.

These findings may suggest that α-INF simultaneously activates NK cells and suppressor cells with H_2-receptors, some of them with anti-NK cell activity, as suggested by Uchida and colleagues (700,701). Blocking the suppressor cells with cimetidine may permit an uninterferable expression of the INF-activated NK cells.

Tilden and Balch (713,714) found that indomethacin, a PG synthetase inhibitor, enhanced the PHA and Con A mitogenic responses of blood MNC derived from melanoma patients. However, the conclusion that PG produced by monocytes displays the augmented suppressive effect in the melanoma patients could not be drawn from this finding, since the PGE_2 production by the patients' cultured MNC did not differ from that of cultured MNC derived from normal individuals, and both cellular populations revealed the same sensitivity to exogenous doses of PGE_2. Furthermore, another PG synthetase inhibitor (RO-205720) did not augment the mitogen responses of the melanoma patients' MNC (714). The authors suggest that indomethacin acts directly on the T cells, since preincubation of the drug with relatively purified populations of either T lymphocytes or monocytes and then recombining them revealed that the preincubation of the T cells, but not the monocytes, resulted in augmented mitogenic responses. These observations are most critical, since the indomethacin augmenting effect is usually interpreted as inhibition of the PG production, whereas in fact it may express other routes of function.

As far as UV-induced tumors of animals are concerned, solid evidence implies that immunodeficiency mediated by UV-induced suppressor cells supports the tumor progression (1). The evidence that a similar mechanism is involved in the progression of human skin tumors is fragmented and sometimes conflicting. In addition, caution must be exercised in extrapolating from immune responses in the peripheral blood to immune responses in and around the tumor. Until the number of variable factors is reduced and, consequently, more uniform results are obtained, it will be difficult to directly associate environmentally induced immunosuppression with skin carcinogenesis.

Patients with AIDS-associated Kaposi's sarcoma display markedly low helper:suppressor cell ratios. Modlin and colleagues (715) reported a helper:suppressor cell ratio of 0.6 ± 0.4 (controls 2.1 ± 0.3), Gottlieb et al. (716) reported a ratio of 0.55 (controls 1.72), Wallace and associates (670) found in his patients a ratio of 0.5 or less (controls 2–2.5), and finally, Lane and colleagues (717) observed a ratio of 0.2 (controls 2.2).

The low helper/suppressor cell ratio is a result of a decrease in the number of helper T cells (*718*), or a simultaneous increase in the number of suppressor T cells and a decrease in the numbers of helper T cells (*716*). The reduction of helper T cells is, however, more profound than the elevation of suppressor T cells (*716*). Interestingly, the helper:suppressor cell ratios of patients with Kaposi's sarcoma that is not associated with AIDS were significantly higher than normal controls because of a marked decrease in suppressor cells (*719*). In comparison with normal subjects, the reactive lymph nodes interfollicular T cell zones and mantle B cell regions of patients with AIDS associated Kaposi's sarcoma contained many more cells with suppressor phenotype (*715*).

Depletion of helper T cells that causes low helper:suppressor cell ratios is a hallmark of AIDS, including those disorders exhibiting opportunistic infections (*720*). The imbalance of T cell subpopulations of AIDS patients is associated with an inability to mount DTH responses and a deficiency of in vitro T cell functions such as responsiveness to soluble antigen (tetanus toxin), alloantigens (MLC), or mitogens (reviewed in *720*). The helper T cell function of AIDS patients (measured by the ability to provide help for B lymphocytes to produce Ig) is markedly deficient, but interestingly, the function of suppressor T cells was found normal (*717*). Another report (*721*) describes, however, an exclusive ability of supernatants from AIDS patients' MNC to suppress the differentiation of B cells into Ig-producing cells. T cell hybridomas obtained from these cells also produced such an SF (*722*).

The depletion of helper T cells in AIDS patients is caused by the retrovirus HIV, which is associated with AIDS (*723,724*) and displays a tropism for helper T cells (*725*). The massive depletion of helper T cells in the patients may cause severe immunodeficiency, and the subsequent opportunistic infections and malignancy. Therefore, AIDS is probably the best known human model supporting the existence of immunosurveillance of tumors.

11. Malignancies of the Central Nervous System

Gliomas, which comprise the majority of all primary neoplasms of the central nervous system (CNS), arise from tissue of neuro-ectodermal origin, and they constitute the bulk of the intrinsic intraparenchymal tumors of both brain and spinal cord (726). Interestingly, several primary malignancies of the CNS are associated with a broad impairment of the host immunocompetence (727–734). Perhaps this is surprising, because the blood–brain barrier would limit contact between the CNS tumor and the immune cells of the periphery. As a result, a general immunosuppression is likely to be a consequence of either a direct secretion of immunosuppressive entities by the tumor, or else secretion of a factor inducing suppressor cell function. Since the blood–brain barrier will limit exchange of large proteinaceous material between the cerebrospinal fluid and the plasma, it is likely that any material passing into the periphery will be small and lipophilic; of course, PG would be an ideal candidate.

Unfortunately, the limited scope of reports of immunosuppression in CNS malignancies are not particularly enlightening either with regard to the proposal above or with regard to mechanism in general. A depression of PHA mitogenic responses in cerebral malignancy has not been associated with an elevation in spontaneous, Con-A activated, or glass-adherent nonspecific suppressor cells (733), whereas in another study (557,732) glass-adherent suppressor cells possibly secreting PG were observed in patients with glioma but not in normal subjects. Meanwhile, a further report (735) proposed that a depressed ability to secrete Ig in response to PWM in patients with CNS malignancies was not the result of increased suppressor cell function, but the result of a combined defect of helper T cells and B cells. Table 5 describes the properties of suppressor cells in malignant diseases developing solid tumors.

12. Some Considerations of the Role of Immune Suppression in Human Malignancy

We have seen in previous sections that the mechanisms of suppression are quite heterogeneous not only in comparing one disease with another, but also when a suppressor function is compared in individuals presenting the same disease, as well as in comparison of results emanating from different laboratories. From Table 1, it is clear that in Hodgkin's disease monocytes/macrophages (e.g., refs. 326,331) or T lymphocytes (e.g., refs.

326,348) may mediate the suppressive activity. A similar hetero-geneity (*see* Table 5) in the mediation of suppression has been found in lung cancer (e.g., refs. *592,594*), as well as in stomach/gastric (*584,609,611*) and bladder malignances (*641,645*). The properties of the suppressor cells, even of the same cell type, may also vary; for instance, one study claims that the suppressor mon-ocytes of lung cancer patients are resistant to 6000 rad of X-irradiation (*592*), whereas, another study (*594*) finds that they are sensitive to 3000 rad.

Consequently, exploration of the mechanisms of immune suppression and the properties of the suppressor cells among dif-ferent subjects displaying the same malignant disease does not provide consistent trends, imposing a limitation on each individ-ual study. Despite this tremendous heterogeneity, several au-thors explored the immunosuppression in human malignancy in heterogenous populations of cancer patients, with no efforts to focus attention on specific diseases. Although this approach is limited by nature, we shall briefly discuss the major findings be-cause some of them support previously indicated observations, whereas others enlighten new aspects. Summing up this section, we shall call attention to few sources of artifacts that may appear if the experiments are not appropriately controlled.

In the previous chapters of this book, several reports were presented showing that monocytes of some patients with a vari-ety of malignant diseases inhibited the in vitro mitogenic re-sponses of cocultured normal cells, suggesting that suppressor monocytes are associated with the depressed immune responses. In agreement with this proposal, it has been found (*736*) that blood MNC of cancer patients with high proportions of mono-cytes (47%) generated significantly lower PHA-induced mitogenic responses than MNC of cancer patients with normal proportions of monocytes (27–29%). In a separate report, cancer patients with various solid tumors presented higher proportions of Tγ cells (presumably suppressor cells) and lower proportions of Tμ cells (Tμ:Tγ = 1.4) than normal individuals (Tμ:Tγ = 4.8; *308*). Similar low Tμ:Tγ ratios were found in HD (*308,737*) and NHL (*308*) pa-tients, and these ratios were further reduced in disease-free HD patients who were exposed to radiotherapy (*737*). Similarly, the T4:T8 ratios (1.3) of cancer patients with solid tumors were lower than those of normal donors (2.2; *738*), indicating a better repre-sentation of cells with cytotoxic-suppressor phenotype. A high concentration of monocytes/macrophages (*see* our previous re-

Table 5
Suppressor Cells in Malignant Diseases Developing Solid Tumors[a,b]

Disease	Type of suppressor cells (S:R)	Effect of suppressor cells	Properties of suppressor cells	SF	Comments	Ref.
Head and neck cancer	Monocytes (1:1)	Inhibition of the MLC	Adhere to plastic and G-10			552
Head and neck cancer	Monocytes	Inhibition of the PHA mitogenic response	Adhere to glass	Yes PG	An untreated patient	556, 557
Head and neck cancer (laryngeal cancer)	Monocytes	Inhibition of the PHA mitogenic response	Adhere to plastic; sensitive to CAR and silica	Yes PG	Untreated patients	561
Lung cancer	Monocytes	Inhibition of the PHA mitogenic response in 2 out of 14 patients	Adhere to plastic	Yes PG	Untreated patients; immunodepression in four out of 14 patients; suppressor cell activity does not correlate with skin tests	344

Lung cancer	Monocytes	Inhibition of PHA mitogenic response	Adhere to glass; sensitive to culture condition	Yes PG	Untreated patients; contain also Con A-induced suppressor cells	556, 557
Lung cancer	Monocytes; monocyte-depleted non-E cells (1:5)	Inhibition of the PHA and PWM mitogenic responses	Engulf carbonyl iron; adhere to plastic; resist 6000 rad.	Yes PG	Untreated patients; normal subjects do not contain suppressor cells	574, 592, 593
Lung cancer	T cells (2:1)	Inhibition of PWM-induced Ig synthesis in seven out of 18 patients	E^+; sensitive to 1250 rad		Untreated patients	575
Lung cancer	Alveolar macrophages (1:10)	Inhibition of Con A mitogenic response in five out of 20 patients				583

(Continued)

145

Table 5 (*Cont.*)

Disease	Type of suppressor cells (S:R)	Effect of suppressor cells	Properties of suppressor cells	SF	Comments	Ref.
Lung cancer	Blood monocytes	Inhibition of PHA and Con A mitogenic responses	Adhere to G-10		No treatment at the time of the study;	584, 585
	Blood T cells (10:1)	Inhibition of PHA and Con A mitogenic responses	E$^+$; NW nonadherent; sensitive to culture conditions and to OK-432; resist MMC		NW nonadherent cells of normal subjects did not inhibit the mitogenic responses	
Lung cancer	Pleural effusion Con A-induced suppressor cells (1:1)	Inhibition of PHA and Con A mitogenic responses	E$^+$; NW nonadherent; sensitive to culture conditions; resist MMC		No treatment at the time of the study; non-malignant pleural effusions do not contain suppressor cells	586

Lung cancer	Pleural effusion macrophages (1:10)	Inhibition of NK cell activity and the INF augmented NK cell activity; inhibition of binding of target cells to NK cells (LGL), and the migration of NK cells (LGL) from microdroplets	Adhere to plastic and G-10; express their activity when cultured 24 h with target cells; sensitive to OK-432	No	No treatment at the time of the study; non-malignant pleural effusions do not contain suppressor cells	587–591
	Pleural effusion T cells (few cases)	Inhibition of NK cell activity	NW nonadherent			
Lung cancer (non-small cell)	Monocytes and Tγ$^+$ cells (1:1 to 1:2)	Inhibition of PPD induced (but not PHA-induced)-proliferative response and PPD (but not PWM)-induced-Ig synthesis	Plastic adherent and Tγ$^+$ cells; sensitive to 3000 rad; PPD specific suppressor cells		Treated patients (surgery and BCG)	594

(Continued)

Table 5 (*Cont.*)

Disease	Type of suppressor cells (S:R)	Effect of suppressor cells	Properties of suppressor cells	SF	Comments	Ref.
Lung cancer	T cells (1:1)	Inhibition of the PHA mitogenic response	Monocyte-depleted fraction mediated the suppressive effect; resist MMC; indomethacin insensitive		Untreated patients	598
Lung cancer	LGL (1:5)	Inhibition of tumor-induced proliferative response of autologous cells and their ability to differentiate into cytotoxic cells	Leu 7$^+$; Leu 11b$^+$; resist MMC; specific suppressor cells	Yes	No treatment at the time of study; suppression of the induction phase	599

		response of autologous lymphocytes to PHA and autologous tumor cells				
Colon cancer	Monocytes in the blood	Inhibition of PHA mitogenic response	Adhere to plastic; sensitive to CAR and silica E^+	Yes PG	Untreated patients	561
	T cells in lymph nodes	Inhibition of Con A and PHA mitogenic responses of autologous cells				
Stomach cancer	Monocytes	Inhibition of PHA and Con A mitogenic responses	Adhere to G-10		No treatment at the time of the study	584
	T cells (10:1)	Inhibition of the PHA and Con A mitogenic responses	E^+; NW nonadherent; sensitive to culture conditions; resist MMC		NW nonadherent; cells of normal subjects did not inhibit the mitogenic responses	

(Continued)

Table 5 (*Cont.*)

Disease	Type of suppressor cells (S:R)	Effect of suppressor cells	Properties of suppressor cells	SF	Comments	Ref.
Gastric cancer	IL-2-dependent T cells (1:10)	Inhibition of PHA and alloantigen-induced proliferative responses	Leu-2$^+$, Leu-3$^-$; IL-2 dependent cell line; resist MMC		Untreated patients; Ts in nonresectable patients only	*609*
Colon cancer	Monocytes	Inhibition of PHA and Con A mitogenic responses	React with antimonocyte monoclonal antibody; produce PG	Yes PG	74% of patients exhibited suppression	*610*
Gastric cancer	Monocytes (1:20)	Inhibition of PHA mitogenic response	Adhere to plastic; esterase positive; resist MMC		Untreated patients	*611*
Colo-rectal cancer	Unknown cells (1:1)	Inhibition of PHA mitogenic response	Resist MMC		No evidence for PG involvement	*612*

150

Gastric cancer	Con A-induced and spontaneous suppressor T cells (1:1)	Inhibition of PHA mitogenic response	Populate the PBL and spleen; E$^+$, T3$^+$, T8$^+$; glass nonadherent; relatively fast on velocity sedimentation; resist MMC; serum factor induce Ts		Untreated patients	613–615
Gastric cancer	T cells	Factor derived from spleen cells and to a lesser degree from PBL of patients with advanced disease suppresses the PHA mitogenic response of normal lymphocytes	Plastic nonadherent	Yes		618

(Continued)

151

Table 5 (*Cont.*)

Disease	Type of suppressor cells (S:R)	Effect of suppressor cells	Properties of suppressor cells	SF	Comments	Ref.
Gastric cancer	T cells	Preoperative PBL and spleen cells from resectable advanced cancer patients suppress autologous postoperative proliferative response to the extracted tumor antigen	NW nonadherent; specific suppressor cells			619
Bladder cancer	Monocytes (1:3)	Inhibition of cytotoxic cells generation after allogeneic stimulation	Ingest carbonyl iron; adhere to plastic		Untreated patients	641

Tumor	Suppressor cell	Effect	Characteristics	Mediator	Comments	Ref.
Bladder cancer	T cells (1:1)	Inhibition of MLC of HLA-B14 subjects only	Ia$^+$, T3$^+$, T8$^+$; resist 2250 rad; HLA unrestricted	No		645–647
Renal cell cancer	Monocytes	Inhibition of PHA-induced mitogenic response	Adhere to glass; PG producing cells	PG	INF-treated patients; suppressor cells were possibly induced by INF	653
Ovarian cancer	Monocytes (1:1)	Inhibition of PHA mitogenic response; suppressive activity was observed in some but not all patients	FcR$^+$, esterase and acid phosphatase positive; slow in sedimentation velocity		Suppressor monocytes/macrophages have been isolated from the blood, ascitic or collagenase-dispersed tumors from patients undergoing surgery	657

(Continued)

Table 5 (Cont.)

Disease	Type of suppressor cells (S:R)	Effect of suppressor cells	Properties of suppressor cells	SF	Comments	Ref.
Ovarian cancer	TIL (1:1)	Inhibition of NK activity; suppressive activity was observed in some but not all patients	NW adherent and non-adherent cells			658, 659
Breast cancer	Monocytes	Inhibition of PHA mitogenic response	Adhere to glass	Yes PG	Untreated patients	556, 557
Breast cancer	TIL (T cells) (1:2)	Inhibition of proliferative response of autologous PBL after stimulation with PHA or autologous tumor	NW nonadherent; resist MMC			602

Breast cancer (postoperative)	Monocytes (1:5)	Inhibition of NK cell activity	Adhere to plastic; 24 h are required in order to exert the suppressive effect	No	No treatment at the time of the study	671
Breast cancer	TIL 1:1	Inhibition of NK-cell activity			Minimal NK activity in TIL	673
Melanoma	T cells (1:1)	Inhibition of PHA mitogenic response	Monocytes depleted cellular population mediate the suppressive effect; resist MMC		Untreated patients	598
Melanoma	Con A-induced suppressor cells (1:1)	Inhibition of Con A mitogenic response			Suppressor-cell activity was no different than that of normal subjects	693

(Continued)

Table 5 (*Cont.*)

Disease	Type of suppressor cells (S:R)	Effect of suppressor cells	Properties of suppressor cells	SF	Comments	Ref.
Melanoma	B cells cooperating with T cells (5:1)	Melanoma serum induced normal B cells to activate normal T cells to inhibit PHA mitogenic response	B cells: adhere to NW (>65% Ig^+ < 5% E^+); T cells: NW non-adherent (95% E^+)		The patients were treated with xenogeneic immune RNA	694
Melanoma	T4 suppressor-inducer and T8 suppressor–effector cells (1:10)	Inhibition of in vitro generation of antitumor cytotoxic cells	Tumor sensitized and IL-2-expanded patient LNC or IL-2 dependent line or clone ($T4^+$) derived from the patient LNC; the $T4^+$			695, 696

Melanoma	INF-induced monocytes (1:2)	Monocytes obtained 12 h after INF injection suppressed the INF (but not OK432)-induced NK cell activity	Adhere to plastic	suppressor-inducer cells activate T8$^+$ suppressor-effector cells; specific suppressor cells	No treatment at the time of the study	701
CNS	Monocytes	Inhibition of the PHA mitogenic response	Adhere to glass; sensitive to culture conditions	Yes PG	Treated and untreated patients	732

[a]Unless otherwise indicated, the suppressor cells in this table are nonspecific.
[b]New abbreviations used in this table: LNC, lymph node cells.

view paper, *1*) and/or a relatively high representation of cells with cytotoxic-suppressor phenotype, as observed in AIDS patients (*739*) may provide the cellular basis for the immunodepression frequently associated with malignancy.

The proportions of individuals with suppressor-cell activity detected by function (ability to suppress PHA or Con A mitogenic responses) were higher among cancer patients than among normal volunteers. The suppressor-cell activity was detected in 71% of the patients, in 75% of these, the suppressor cells were radiosensitive (4000–6000 rad), and in about 40%, they were thymic-hormone sensitive (*740*; but for contradicting results concerning the thymic hormone, *see* ref *741*). However, the intensity of the suppressor-cell activity varied markedly from case to case (*740*). These findings emphasize the heterogeneity of the suppressor cells, but perhaps this is not surprising, since the authors explored this suppressor-cell function in a variety of cancers of diverse origin (lung cancer, melanoma, testicular carcinoma, sarcoma, lymphoma, and leukemia).

Depressed cutaneous hypersensitivity reactions (*742*) and prolonged skin allograft (*743*) have been observed in cancer patients. These immunodeficiencies may be associated with defects in the mobilization capacity of the patients' MNC. Such defective cellular mobilization may also cause a reduced infiltration of MNC into the tumor site, thus reducing the effectiveness of any antitumor response. In fact, it has been claimed that the best prognosis exists for patients who display an increased infiltration of MNC at the tumor site (*744*).

In support, Hesse and colleagues (*745*) found that E^+ rosetting T lymphocytes of several cancer patients migrated less efficiently after stimulation with casein than T lymphocytes of normal individuals. Furthermore, T lymphocytes of cancer patients suppressed the ability of cocultivated normal T lymphocytes to migrate after stimulation with casein. The patients' lymphocytes lost their suppressive activity if preincubated for 24 h. However, an SF was not detected in the supernatants derived from cultures of these patients' cells. Since the patients' cells were contaminated with a small percentage of monocytes, their role in mediating or supporting the suppressive effect cannot be excluded.

In a separate study (*746*), the same group showed that T lymphocytes of some cancer patients did not produce appreciable amounts of chemotactic factor after stimulation with Con A, and this defect was not reversed by indomethacin. In addition, the patients' lymphocytes suppressed the ability of cocultured normal cells to produce a chemotactic factor after stimulation with Con A. The suppression could be localized to an erythrocyte-rosetting lymphocyte population that was Leu-2 positive.

In conclusion, at least some cancer patients display suppressor cells that inhibit MNC chemotactic locomotion as well as the ability of T cells to produce chemotactic factors. It is attractive, albeit unsupported, to associate these effects with a reduced antitumor response of cancer patients.

Of the types of human suppressor cells so far recognized, one is a thymus-derived cell bearing a histamine receptor (classified as H_2 type) and activated by histamine. The H_2-receptor-bearing suppressor cells produce an SF after stimulation with histamine, and cimetidine blocks this effect (214,215). If immunodepression in cancer patients is associated with H_2-receptor-bearing cells, the possibility exists that H_2-receptor antagonists may be of use in augmenting the antitumor responses of such patients. In this respect, it should be indicated that increased histamine levels were found in tissues of tumor-bearing animals (747).

Mavligit and colleagues (748) demonstrated that incubation of blood MNC from immunodeficient cancer patients with cimetidine improved their ability to mount a local GVHR in immunosuppressed rats in comparison with the inflammatory response generated by normal MNC injected intradermally in similar immunosuppressed animals. In a subsequent study (749), it was shown that administration of cimetidine to immunodeficient cancer patients also augmented the immunocompetence of their MNC as indicated by their ability to mount a local GVHR on transplantation to a xenogeneic host.

The cells of some cancer patients, however, are quite capable of generating a xenogeneic local GVHR even if not treated with cimetidine. Injection of cimetidine to one of these patients caused a detrimental effect: his cells lost the capacity to induce a GVHR inflammatory response. It should be further remembered that suppressor cells lacking histamine receptors would not be affected by H_2-receptor antagonists. This may explain why in vivo administration of cimetidine does not restore completely the immunocompetence of cells from immunodeficient patients.

Suppressor T cells cannot produce rosettes with sheep erythrocytes if the MNC are treated with theophylline (750); therefore, the isolated rosette-forming cells do not include suppressor cells under such conditions. Mavligit and Wong (751) demonstrated that T cells of some cancer patients, depleted of theophylline-sensitive suppressor cells mounted stronger local xenogeneic GVHR than the unfractionated cellular population. This experimental manipulation did not restore completely the immunocompetence of the patients' cells, suggesting the existence of other suppressor mechanisms or an intrinsic defect in the effector cells.

Prostaglandins and thromboxanes are synthesized by cyclooxygenation of arachidonic acid. They may develop inflammatory conditions, including local vasodilation, edema, and pain (reviewed in *161,162,171*). In addition, the PG directly inhibit several immunological functions mediated by lymphocytes, including responses to mitogen, cytolysis, and antibody or lymphokine production (reviewed in *161,162,171*). Prostaglandin exerts its direct inhibitory effect by activating adenylate cyclase and hence cyclic AMP levels, which in turn may inhibit phospholypase activity (752), thus leaving the cell refractory to further stimuli.

Among other cells, the macrophages are important producers of prostaglandins and thromboxanes. Their two major metabolites are PGE_2 and TxA_2, respectively. Various factors such as zymosan, *C. parvum*, bacterial endotoxin, antigen–antibody complexes, Con A, or colchicine induce the production of PG by macrophages (*170,171,753*). The tumors may also induce PG production by macrophages (*158*). Furthermore, the tumors themselves may produce PG, and consequently, high levels of PGs may be found in TBH (reviewed in *161,162*).

Prostaglandin E_2 at high concentrations may activate suppressor T cells, which may further inhibit the B cell differentiation and proliferative responses induced by PWM or alloantigens, respectively (754). In fact, antigen-stimulated lymphocytes release lymphokines that stimulate macrophages to produce PG. In turn, the PG inhibit the lymphocytes activity, thus forming a feedback loop that may regulate the lymphocyte function (reviewed in *171*).

The PG may also exert a direct inhibitory effect on the growth of the tumor (755), not only stressing the dual effect of this biological product, but partially explaining the inconsistency of results using indomethacin, which may be dependent upon the sensitivity of a particular tumor to PG. Furthermore, the proinflammatory effects of PGs may aid other antitumor activities mounted by the host. It should be further noted that many investigators, demonstrating the effect of PG on various in vitro immune responses, have employed nonphysiological concentrations of PG (10^{-4}–10^{-6}M), which may generate conditions quite unlike those found in vivo. In addition, it should also be remembered that, in many experiments, the involvement of PG is inferred from the results after addition of the PG-synthetase inhibitor indomethacin. However, besides its inhibition of PG production, indomethacin may exert other biological effects (reviewed in *161*); hence the involvement of PGs in suppression must be confirmed by use of other PG-synthetase inhibitors. Nevertheless, it is important to recognize that administration of indomethacin and other PG-synthetase inhibitors has resulted in the slowing of tumor growth or inhibiting the spread of metastases in animals, possibly by blocking of PG-mediated immunosuppression (*162*). It has also been claimed that indomethacin administration caused regression of head and neck cancer (*756*), skin cancer in xeroderma pigmentosum (*757*), and metastases in breast cancer (*758*). Each one of these studies must, however, be evaluated carefully, considering the effect of other drugs used before or during the indomethacin therapy, the presence of matched control patients, and the employment of objective tests measuring the levels of PG and the intensity of the immune responses prior, during, and after the therapy. In any event, as mentioned previously, the administration of indomethacin may directly affect tumor PG synthesis, and any increase in immunocompetence may reflect this aspect rather than a block of suppressor macrophage activity.

Enhancement of mitogenic responses after addition of indomethacin to the MNC of cancer patients (*759,760*) is not sufficient by itself to infer the presence of PG-producing suppressor cells. One must demonstrate that elimination of suppressor cells from the tested cellular population (e.g., removal of adherent monocytes) is associated with augmentation of the immune response to external stimuli; together with insensitivity of the suppressor's depleted stimulated cells to PG-synthetase inhibitors and with a decline of the PG levels in the culture supernatants (*334*).

Finally, one must remember that PG produced by cancer patients' monocytes may exert partial suppressive effects as indicated by in vitro mitogenic responses, whereas other factors such as the inability of cancer patients' monocytes to produce IL-1 may be the major cause of immunosuppression (*761*). Such immunodepression may be associated with decreased ability to generate suppressor cells after Con A stimulation (762), implying a generalized defect in the immune regulation of cancer patients.

Concluding this section, we must focus our attention on one source of possible misinterpretation that might be frequently observed using in vitro assays for assessing immune responses against tumors. The in vitro generation of cytotoxic cells against tumor cells may be inhibited by a simultaneous activation of suppressor cells. The interpretation that tumor-induced suppressor cells mediate this effect could be, however, mistaken. For instance, it has been shown that the generation of cytotoxic cells in human in vitro cultures stimulated by an allogeneic diffuse histiocytic lymphoma cell line was enhanced after removal of nylon-adherent cells (763). The suppressor nylon-adherent cells were not induced by the tumor cells, but by the in vitro culture conditions, possibly under the influence of the serum included in the culture medium (763). The mistaken interpretation was avoided by demonstrating that PBL incubated 4 d in the presence of autologous serum, human heterologous serum, or fetal bovine serum inhibited the generation of lymphocytes stimulated with the tumor (764). Thus, whenever suppressor cells are detected in tumor-stimulated in vitro cultures, one should determine which antigen is responsible for their induction. Finally, it must be proven that the observed suppression is not mediated by cytotoxic cells killing the responder or the stimulator cells, rather than by cells mediating a true suppression.

13. The Effect of Antineoplastic Chemotherapy on Human Suppressor-Cell Activity

Antineoplastic chemotherapy is aimed, in the first place, at eradicating the tumor cells themselves. However, various animal models reveal that several cytotoxic drugs employed in human cancer chemotherapy augment the immunological activities of the hosts injected with these drugs. In many cases, the augmentation of the immunological responses was associated with selective blocking of the suppressor cells that express a stronger sensitivity to these drugs than other cells of the immune system (for a review, *see* our previous review paper; 1). Similar effects were observed in cancer patients subjected to several differing chemotherapy protocols.

All melanoma and colorectal cancer patients tested developed an increased DTH response to keyhole limpet hemocyanin (KLH) after treatment with Cy, whereas without treatment with Cy, 7 of the 11 patients tested did not respond to KLH (765,766). Patients treated with Cy also revealed a decreased number of T cells (both helper and suppressor) and B cells. In addition, the proliferative responses of the patients' cells to PHA, Con A, and PWM declined 1–2 d after the drug treatment, returned to the pretreatment level 3 d after the treatment, and then declined again on the 14th d. The activity of Con A-induced suppressor cells also declined 1 d after the drug treatment, but it remained lower than the pretreatment suppressor-cell activity for at least 21 d (767,768). Thus, the impairment of the suppressor-cell activity was not a reflection of general impairment of T cell functions. The authors suggest that Cy selectively eliminates precursors of suppressor cells, or alternatively, such cells had a decreased capacity for repair of sublethal Cy-induced damage. This effect could account for the enhanced DTH observed after Cy treatment (765,766).

The effect of different drug treatment programs on the immune responses of cancer patients presenting various diseases was explored in a separate study (769,770). The patients received cytotoxic drugs as a single treatment or in combinations (e.g., phenylalanine mustard, 5-fluorouracil, Cy, adriamycin, methotrexate, MMC, methyl-chloroethyl-cyclohexyl nitrosourea, and Bis-chloroethyl-cyclohexyl nitrosourea). Of the 20 treated patients, 14 exhibited enhanced PHA mitogenic responses that reached or exceeded 150% of the pretreatment response. This effect was accompanied by a considerable reduction in the activities of glass-adherent and PG-producing suppressor cells assessed by the level of the PHA mitogenic responses after removal of the adherent cells or addition of indomethacin to cultures (769,770). These experiments suggest that suppressor monocytes are sensitive to the chemotherapy. However, the inclusion of a variety of solid tumors in one study and the variety of regimens do not aid interpretation of these results.

Further evidence that presuppressor cells are affected by chemotherapy is provided by the observation that Melphalan, an antiproliferative alkylating agent, prevented the induction of suppressor cells by Con A, but it did not affect already induced suppressor cells (771). Thymosin, a thymic hormone widely used as a biological response modifier (772,773), has been implicated in immunotherapy of cancer patients (774). Serrou and colleagues (775) found that this factor blocked the ability of cancer patients' suppressor cells to inhibit various mitogenic responses.

Interferon has also been used in cancer therapy because of its antiviral and antitumor effects, which are well established (776). In addition, this drug augments various immunological responses such as NK-cell activity or generation of cytotoxic cells, but it may inhibit other responses such as DTH (reviewed in 776). Cancer patients treated with INF exhibited a reduced T4:T8 ratio, indicating a relative elevation of the suppressor/cytotoxic cellular phenotype (777). OK-432, a streptococcal preparation, is an antitumor response modifier. Infusion of OK-432 into the peritoneum of patients with cancerous ascites caused infiltrations of neutrophils, lymphocytes, and monocytes followed by the disappearance of the tumor cells. In addition, a considerable reduction in Con A-induced suppressor cells was observed after this treatment (778).

In conclusion, the direct antitumor effects of the antineoplastic drugs may be enhanced by additional selective activities of the drugs against the suppressor cells. On the other hand, it is worth noting that at least some of these drugs may express activities against various immune functions, and consequently, they may diminish the drugs' net antitumor effects. Varying the dose of each drug, the time of its administration, or other parameters, optimal conditions may be established where the negative effects of the drug are eliminated, while its antitumor and antisuppressor cell effects are still preserved.

Suppressor Cells and Malignancy in Animal Experimental Models

A Brief Summary of Recent Findings

Since our previous review article was published (1), new information concerning suppressor cells in tumor-bearing animals has come our way, most of it published during the years 1985 to 1987. These papers may shed more light on some aspects described in this book and, hence, will be briefly reviewed.

1. Suppressor Macrophages and "Null" Cells

The role of macrophages in suppressing the immune responses of TBH has been the focus of much attention during the last decade, and previous review articles (1,2) dealt extensively with this issue. Jessup and associates (779) demonstrated, by adoptive transfer experiments, that macrophages are responsible for the depressed DTH of mice bearing chemical, virus, and spontaneously induced tumors. The immunodepression was not specific because it affected the DTH response to DNCB. The generation of the in vitro cytotoxic response to M109 spontaneous lung carcinoma by lymphocytes from mice bearing that tumor was also nonspecifically inhibited by macrophages. Removal of macrophages from the responder cell population enhanced the antitumor cytotoxic response (780). Nonspecific suppressor macrophages inhibiting mitogenic responses were also found in rats bearing chemically induced hepatoma (781).

One mechanism by which macrophages may exert their immunosuppressive effects is by the release of PG (1). Pelus and Bockman (782) demonstrated that splenic macrophages of

C57BL/6 mice bearing MCA fibrosarcoma synthesize significantly more PG than macrophages of their normal littermates. The elevated concentrations of the PG may be associated with the suppressive effect as shown by macrophages found in the spleen of C3H/Hen mice bearing plasmacytaema (783). Since indomethacin antagonized the suppressive effect of the macrophages, it was suggested that the effect is mediated mostly by PG. In support of this assumption, it was found that indomethacin and carrageenan (macrophages toxic substance) slowed the growth of the plasmacytoma in the syngeneic host. The role of PG in inducing immunosuppression in TBH was further demonstrated by immunizing mice bearing LLC against PG (784) or by passive administration of anti-PG antibodies to such TBH (785). The mitogenic responses of splenocytes derived from the treated mice were augmented in comparison with untreated TBH. Furthermore, the tumor progression was slowed in the passively immunized mice (785). In agreement with these findings, it was found (786) that the bone marrow of LLC-tumor-bearing mice exhibits increased hematopoiesis, increased in the proportions of monocytes and, as the tumor growth progressed, suppressor cell function was also elevated (nonadherent to nylon but Thy-1$^-$). The suppressor cells inhibited the Con A mitogenic responses of cocultured normal spleen cells, possibly by releasing PG. The authors suggest that LLC cells stimulate hematopoiesis, which results in the appearance of immature bone-marrow-derived suppressor cells, possibly of monocyte origin.

Another type of nonspecific immunodepression is mediated by leukemic splenocytes of mice infected with M-MuLV. The suppressor cell that inhibits the in vitro PFC immune response to SRBC is not, however, the leukemic cell itself, but a Thy-1 negative nylon-wool-nonadherent cell ("null" cell) that cooperates with T cells in executing this suppressive effect (787).

2. "Sneaking Through" of Low Doses of Tumor Cells Is Mediated by Suppressor Cells

Sneaking through is one of the most puzzling phenomena associated with the biological behavior of cancer cells: small inocula of tumor cells are not rejected by the host, unlike larger doses of the same tumor. Several explanations for this paradoxical observation have been proposed, and they were summarized in one of our previous reviews (2). The suggestion that a small inoculum of the tumor preferentially induces suppressor cells that hamper the immunological rejection of the tumor is supported by a study of Gatenby and colleagues (788). These authors demonstrated that a dose of 2.5 × 10^2 of Meth-A tumor cells was not rejected by most of the mice injected with this neoplasm, whereas a higher dose of 10^4 cells was rejected. Furthermore, about 50% of the mice preinjected with 2.5 × 10^2 irradiated Meth-A cells failed to reject a subsequent challenge of 10^4 viable Meth-A cells, which are normally rejected. The sneaking through of the tumor cells was abolished by injecting the recipient mice with Cy (100 mg/kg), suggesting that drug-sensitive suppressor cells mediate the effect.

McBride and Howie (789) demonstrated that small inocula (10^1–10^3 cells) of MCA-induced fibrosarcoma could induce an immunological tolerance to the tumor antigens. Moderately sized inocula (10^4–10^6 cells) were immunogenic, but larger cell doses again induced immunological tolerance. Whereas the low zone tolerance was mediated by tumor-specific suppressor T cells, the high zone tolerance was mediated by both specific suppressor T cells and nonspecific suppressor non-T cells. In support of the above observations, Kölsch and associates (790,791) demonstrated that injection of exponential increasing numbers of small doses of ADJ-PC-5 plasmacytoma cells induced specific suppressor T (Lyt-2$^+$) cells in syngeneic BALB/c mice.

3. Suppressor T Cells and Their Mechanism of Action

The above observations imply that sneaking of tumor cells through the barrier of the immunological surveillance is mediated by suppressor T cells. In general, suppressor T cells attracted much attention in many other tumor-host systems of experimental animals. Brodt and Lala (792) observed a considerable increase in the thymus and draining lymph node content of Lyt-2$^+$ cells 5 wk after the injection of a carcinogenic dose of 3-methylcholanthrene and prior to the appearance of histologically evident tumor cells. The number of Lyt-2$^+$ cells returned to a normal level a few weeks later, when the tumor cells were identified by histological examination. At that time, there was a moderate increase in the level of systemic Lyt-2$^+$ cells. The mixed lymphocyte response of the draining lymph node cells was suppressed, and the local growth and the metastatic spread of transplanted mammary tumor was enhanced during the period of an increased level of Lyt-2$^+$ cells in the thymus and the lymph node. High levels of Lyt-2$^+$ lymphocytes were also observed within the thymus, the draining lymph node, and the tumor site of retired breeder C3H/ Hef female mice bearing small, newly detected, spontaneous mammary carcinomas (793). These results suggest that localized immunodepression associated with the rise in Lyt-2$^+$ suppressor T cells may be of functional significance during the carcinogenetic process.

Yoshida and Tachibana (794) demonstrated that injection of 10^6 viable mammary tumor cells into the footpads of C3H mice induced the appearance of accessory T cells (Lyt-1$^+$) in the regional lymph nodes. These cells augmented the antitumor cytotoxic response of cocultivated immune cells derived from the peritoneum of mice immunized with irradiated homologous tumor cells. After 10 d, the accessory cells were replaced by suppressor cells (Lyt-1$^+$). If, however, the footpads were injected with irradiated tumor cells prior to the inoculation with the viable tumor, the regional lymph nodes were gradually populated with suppressor cells with no prior appearance of accessory cells. In both experimental protocols, the appearance of the suppressor cells was accompanied by the appearance of lymphatic metastases, and in such circumstances, it is tempting to suggest a role for suppressor cells in the establishment of lymphatic metastasis.

Mullen and colleagues (795) explored the effect of an already-growing progressor tumor on the growth of a subsequently transplanted regressor tumor in the same animal. Both types of tumors were induced either by UV irradiation of C3H mice or by injection of MCA into UV-irradiated C3H mice. The progressor tumors enhanced the growth of most of the regressor tumors, which are regularly rejected by normal mice. The regressor tumors gradually grew in the host and finally killed it, even after the removal of the original progressor tumor. In addition, regressor tumors isolated from mice bearing progressor tumors did not lose their original phenotype, indicated by their rejection when retransplanted into normal animals. The immunodepression state that permitted the growth of the regressor tumors in mice bearing progressor tumors was mediated by Thy-1$^+$, Lyt-2$^-$ suppressor T cells. The suppressor cells inhibited the immunological rejection of various syngeneic independently derived tumors induced by different carcinogens, but they did not induce a general immunodeficiency. Nevertheless, all the tumors used in this study, including the MCA tumors, were generated in UV-irradiated mice, which confers upon the tumors similar immunogenic properties (796). As a result, it is uncertain that suppressor cells express as wide a specificity as suggested by the authors (795); their activity may be restricted to antigens of tumors generated only in UV-irradiated mice.

On examination of the mechanism of action used by tumor-induced suppressor cells, it appears that cellular communication is required for mediating the suppressive effect. Ingenito and Calkins (797,798) found that spleen cells from DBA/2 mice bearing the MCA-induced lymphoma L5178Y suppressed the in vitro anti-SRBC PFC response of cocultivated normal spleen cells. The TBH suppressor cells expressing the phenotype of suppressor-inducer cells (Ala-1$^+$, Thy-1$^+$, Lyt-1$^+$, 2$^-$; 797,798) cooperated with precursors of suppressor-effector cells (Qa-1$^+$, Lyt-1$^-$, 2$^-$) residing among the normal splenocytes. This conclusion was inferred from the fact that Qa-1$^+$-depleted normal splenocytes could not be suppressed in the presence of TBH suppressor inducer cells (798). The number of suppressor-precursor cells in the TBH spleen is probably limited, since the in vitro anti-SRBC PFC response of the TBH splenocytes is not suppressed unless relatively high concentrations of cells are cultured (798).

These results were confirmed and further extended by Pope (799) and Almawi and Pope (800). Spleen cells from DBA/2J mice bearing the MCA-induced fibrosarcoma M-1 contained suppressor-inducer cells that activated suppressor-precursor cells (Thy-1$^+$, Lyt-1$^+$, 2$^+$) resident in the spleens of normal mice. The suppressor-effector cells of normal mice were induced by TBH suppressor-inducer cells when separated by a dialysis membrane, indicating release of a soluble SF. The normal activated suppressor-effector cells suppressed the in vitro anti-SRBC PFC response of cocultivated normal splenocytes either directly, or again when separated from the target population by dialysis membrane, indicating that they also released an SF. The suppressive effect of the activated suppressor-effector cells was reversed by the lymphokine IL-2, suggesting that IL-2 producing T cells are the target of the suppressor cells (799; and similar effect also seen in ref. 790). A continuous cell clone, releasing a protein SF, was established from the TBH suppressor cells by limiting dilution (800), and these cells maintained their original suppressor-inducer function although their surface markers altered (Thy-1$^-$, Ly-5$^+$, GM-1$^+$).

In another system, Halliday and colleagues (*801,802*) demonstrated that the serum of CBA mice bearing MCA-(*801,802*) or MSV-induced (*801*) tumors, contained a suppressor-factor (SF1) that blocked the ability of TBH antigen-stimulated Lyt-1$^+$ T cells to inhibit leukocyte adherence to a glass surface. The SF1 is specific for tumor antigens and exists in two forms of differing mol wt (>100,000 and 40,000–50,000 daltons; *801*). The smaller form has antigen-binding capacity and an I-J site on separate polypeptide chains (*803*). Lyt-2$^+$, I-J$^+$ T lymphocytes produced this factor only if accessory macrophages were also present (*804*). It has been found in a different tumor-host system that SF1 and the receptors of the cells that produce it share an idiotype with the antitumor effector cells of this system (*805*). On analyzing further the suppressor mechanism it was found that TSF1 does not affect directly the target population, but in the presence of specific antigen, it stimulates TBH Lyt-2$^+$, I-J$^+$ cells to produce a further suppressor factor (SF2) that blocked the leukocyte adherence inhibition (LAI). The SF2 appears also in two different molecular forms (>190,000 and 20,000–50,000), but in contrast to SF1, it suppresses the LAI in nonspecific manner (*802*).

The cooperation between suppressor T cells and accessory cells (probably macrophages) in the suppression mechanism was reported earlier by Moser and colleagues (*806*). These authors demonstrated that the MOPC-315 myeloma cells produced markedly less Ig if incubated across a cell-impermeable membrane with idiotype specific suppressor T cells, derived from mice injected with myeloma protein coupled to syngeneic spleen cells, demonstrating the release of an SF. However, the suppression could only be developed if accessory cells (macrophages?) were coincubated with the myeloma target cells. The authors suggest that the accessory cell function may involve processing of the SF or presentation of such factor to the myeloma cells.

Maier and colleagues (*264,807–809*) produced polyclonal (*264,807*) and monoclonal (*808,809*) antibodies against the SF extracted from suppressor T cells of DBA/2J mice injected with soluble membrane extracts of the syngeneic mastocytoma P815 (the antibodies were designated anti-SF). The polyclonal anti-SF blocked, in the presence of C, the ability of tumor-induced suppressor cells to inhibit the in vitro primary cytotoxic response against the tumor, but they did not affect the activity of the cytotoxic cells themselves (*264*). Regarding the effect of suppressor cells on cytotoxic cells, Haubeck and Kölsch (*790*) introduced an interesting point. They found that the cells in the induction phase (in contrast to effector-cytotoxic cells) are sensitive to the effect of the suppressor cells. Whereas the effector-cytotoxic cells are stable, the features of cytotoxic cell clones might be an object of various changes; therefore, it is preferable to transfer noncloned cytotoxic cells over cloned cytotoxic cells in an attempt to reject the tumor from the host (adoptive immunotherapy).

Injection of the polyclonal anti-SF into DBA/2 mice, early in the course of P815 tumor growth, slowed the progression of the tumor and prolonged the survival of the animals (*807*). Whereas the polyclonal anti-SF was effective only against the P815 mastocytoma (*807*), the monoclonal anti-SF conferred resistance against both the relevant P815 tumor and an unrelated syngeneic tumor. The ability of the monoclonal anti-SF to recognize public specificity on the SF or suppressor-cell receptor was further confirmed by demonstrating that splenocytes of mice injected with anti-SF monoclonal antibodies displayed stronger MLR than did equivalent controls (*808*). The mol wt of SF eluted from immunoadsorbent prepared with the anti-SF monoclonal antibody was analyzed and found to be a dimer composed of peptides of 40,000–46,000 daltons (*809*).

A separate aspect of immunoregulation was enlightened by the experiments of Strayer and Leibowitz (*810*), who injected rabbits with fibroma virus, inducing a progressive myxosarcoma. Seven days after the virus inoculation, considerable immunodepression was observed in the animals, but it disappeared four days later, even as the tumor progressed. The immunodepression was mediated by suppressor T cells or by an SF released from these cells. In keeping with the disappearance of suppressor cells at 11 d, a supernatant of rabbit spleen cells obtained 11 d after virus injection blocked the suppressive activity of spleen cell supernatant obtained 7 d after the virus inoculation. If the 11-d splenocytes were treated with goat antirabbit T cell serum, their supernatant no longer contained the contrasuppressive activity and, instead, developed a suppressive effect. The authors suggest that contrasuppressor cells that appear at d 11 after virus injection protect the immune cells from being affected by suppressor cells. This event occurs, however, too late for the immune response to prevent tumor growth.

Whereas IL-2 producing T cells may be target for suppressor-cell activity in some experimental models (790,799), in other models, IL-2 may enhance the activity of the suppressor cells themselves. Bruley-Rosset and Payelle (811) demonstrated that the spleens of old (18–24 m of age) C57BL/6 mice contain suppressor cells (Thy-1[+], CY resistant), which upon transfer into young mice interfered with their ability to be immunized against chemically induced fibrosarcoma. Injection of IL-2 into the old mice enhanced their suppressor-cell activity.

4. Suppressor T Cell Lines and Clones

Several groups have succeeded during the last year in establishing T cell lines or clones (791,800,812,813) as well as a T cell hybridoma (814) from tumor-induced suppressor cells. The availability of large amounts of pure material generated by these immortalized cells may allow isolation and characterization of SF and specific receptors mediating the suppression, as well as establishing the biomolecular basis for specific and apparently nonspecific suppression, using modern molecular biology techniques.

Koyama and colleagues (813) established from the spleen of mice bearing a S1509a MCA-induced fibrosarcoma an IL-2-dependent suppressor T cell line (Thy-1[+]). These cells suppressed the ability of tumor-induced cytotoxic cells to cytolyze the target tumor in an in vitro assay. In contrast to the suppressor cells obtained directly from the TBH (233), the established cell line also suppressed cytotoxic cells specific for irrelevant syngeneic tumor cells, indicating that long-term culture may change the properties of the cells. Kölsch and associates (791,812) established by a limiting dilution technique a suppressor T cell clone obtained from a draining lymph node of a BALB/c mouse bearing a plasmacytoma. The cells of the clone (Thy-1[+], Lyt-2[+]) specifically suppressed the in vitro primary cytotoxic response to the tumor, but did not show any cytotoxicity against the tumor cells themselves.

Steele and colleagues (814) produced a T cell hybridoma by fusing DBA/2 thymocytes from mice injected with P815 tumor membrane extract with a BW5147 thymoma (the thymocytes of the DBA/2-injected mice contained tumor-specific suppressor T cells). A factor released from this T cell hybridoma specifically enhanced the growth of P815 mastocytoma. Analysis of the SF with

SDS-PAGE under reducing conditions revealed a heterodimer with mol wt of 43,000 and 45,000 dalton.

Ultraviolet irradiation stimulates the appearance of suppressor cells, which enhance the growth of syngeneic UV-induced tumors, but not tumors induced by other carcinogens (reviewed in ref. 1). The induction of suppressor cells may be mediated by a soluble factor (1000–10,000 dalton) found in the serum of UV-exposed animals (*815*).

Palaszynski and Kripke (*816*) suggested that, after UV irradiation, the skin contains a UV-radiation-associated antigen that is also present in all UV-radiation-induced tumors; therefore, suppressor cells induced by such skin antigens can be activated by UV-induced tumors, but not by other tumors. Support for the prediction that all UV tumors express a common antigen that can be recognized by one clone of UV-induced suppressor T cells is provided by Roberts (*817*). This author cloned by limiting dilution an IL-2-dependent cell line derived from UV-induced suppressor cells. The cells of the clone (Thy-1$^+$, Lyt-2$^{+/-}$, I-J$^+$) enhanced the growth of a panel of UV-induced tumors, but they did not affect allograft rejection or contact hypersensitivity to 2,4-dinitrobenzene-1-sulfonic acid (DNBS). Although the cloned suppressor cells may slightly change their original surface markers (*817*), they preserved their restricted ability to recognize a common antigen on various UV-induced tumors.

5. Suppression of Concomitant Immunity

The ability of suppressor cells to downregulate concomitant immunity in TBH is another aspect on which several reports have appeared during recent years (*818–822*). Concomitant immunity describes the ability of an experimental animal with a progressing tumor to develop an immunological rejection against a small transplant of homologous tumor. North and colleagues have focused their efforts upon elucidation of mechanism in concomitant immunity, and their findings are summarized in a recent review paper (*820*). In one of their recent reports (*821*), evidence is presented that B6D2F1 mice bearing 9-d-old P815 mastocytoma contained immune cells that caused, on adoptive transfer, a rejection of a 4-d-old homologous tumor from irradiated (500 rad) recipients. The immune cells of the TBH were gradually replaced by suppressor T cells (Lyt-1$^+$) that abolished, when cotransferred with the immune cells, the rejection of the tumor from the irradiated recipient mice (the recipient mice were irradiated in order to remove their own suppressor cells). In another report, Bursuker and North (*818*) demonstrated that CB6F1 mice bearing a 9-d-old Meth A tumor failed to reject by concomitant immunity a smaller tumor if suppressor cells obtained from a host bearing a large tumor were previously transferred to them. If, however, the suppressor cells were removed from the TBH by 500 rad X-irradiation, the concomitant immunity could be effectively expressed, and consequently, the tumor would be rejected (*823*).

Dent and Finlay-Jones (*819*) reported that spleens of BALB/c mice bearing a small MCA-induced fibrosarcoma (MC-2) contained immune cells that inhibited the growth of homologous tumors in sublethally irradiated recipients (Winn assay). When the tumor increased in size, the immune cells disappeared, and instead, radiosensitive suppressor T cells appeared. This last event may be associated with the onset of metastases in the spleens of some TBH. The findings of North's group (*820*) were confirmed by Bear (*822*) in DBA/2 mice bearing a P815 mastocytoma. Spleen cells from hosts bearing a tumor early in growth generated specific cytotoxic cells when cocultivated with homologous tumors, whereas spleen cells from hosts bearing a tumor later in growth contained radiosensitive suppressor T cells (Thy-1$^+$). Interestingly, the immunocompetent cells of hosts bearing the early tumor were relatively resistant to the effect of the suppressor cells, but this resistance gradually disappeared as the tumor continued to grow. These findings illustrate the limited and insufficient ability of immune cells accumulating in hosts bearing immunogenic tumors to cause rejection of the growing tumor, although they may eradicate a small tumor. The suppressor cells may appear after the point of no return of tumor progression, and therefore, the fate of the tumor is not affected by the immunodepression. If, however, the immune cells are still able to slow the tumor progression and the spread of metastases, the appearance of suppressor cells may accelerate these malignant processes.

6. Immunotherapy Based on Suppressor Cells Eradication

On showing that suppressor cells may aid the growth of tumors in the face of potential immunity and characterizing the properties of such suppressor cells, a rational immunotherapy strategy, based on the elimination of the suppressor cells, may be planned. Kurashige and associates (824) found that suppressor cells induced in mice bearing an EL4 tumor are sensitive to the combined treatment of Salmonella typhimurium and MMC, but were not sensitive to each agent alone. After this treatment, the splenocytes of the treated mice were no longer able to enhance tumor growth in the Winn assay or to suppress the mitogen-induced proliferative responses of coculativated normal spleen cells.

The immunosuppressive properties of PGs may cause a state of immunodepression that could be followed by either a carcinogenetic process or acceleration of the growth of an already established tumor. Consequently, inhibitors of PG synthesis such as indomethacin or aspirin may have an antitumor therapeutic effect (reviewed in 1). An impressive effect of indomethacin on a pristane-induced plasmacytoma was reported by Potter and associates (825). Mice treated with indomethacin (given continuously in their drinking water) even 60 d after pristane injection developed a considerable resistance to the tumor growth. Pope (826) presented evidence that activation of suppressor T cells, but not of coexisting suppressor macrophages, is inhibited by indomethacin. Splenic T cells from DBA/2J mice bearing MCA tumor (M-1) and treated with indomethacin (given in the drinking water) lost their ability to suppress the in vitro primary anti-SRBC PFC response of cocultivated normal spleen cells. It was demonstrated in a separate experiment that a factor released from the TBH spleen cells activated appearance of suppressor cells in normal splenocytes when the two populations were separated by a dialysis membrane. The activation of the suppressor cells was inhibited by addition of indomethacin and coaddition of PG reversed the inhibitory effect, suggesting that PG activates directly or indirectly the suppressor cells.

More evidence has been published concerning the role of H_2 antagonists (214,215) in blocking TBH suppressor cells bearing histamine H_2 receptors. Gorczynski and colleagues (827) suggest that activation of H_2-receptor-positive suppressor cells in BALB/c mice can be conditioned by the provision of a novel taste (saccharin) in their drinking water. Immunosuppressed BALB/c mice whose drinking water was supplemented with saccharin exhibited accelerated mortality after challenge with plasmacytoma (TEPC-15) only if their drinking water was resupplemented with saccharin immediately after the challenge and thereafter. Evidence was presented that suppressor cells bearing H_2 receptors were activated in these conditioned and tumor-challenged mice. Furthermore, the mortality of immunosuppressed mice that were conditioned by the saccharin was not accelerated after tumor challenge and reexposure to saccharin if cimetidine (H_2 receptor antagonist) was also given to the mice after the tumor challenge. The clinical application of this observation should be considered.

The effect of cytotoxic drugs, especially those with alkylating properties, on tumor-induced suppressor cells has been extensively investigated (reviewed in 1). Nagarkatti and Kaplan (828) demonstrated that 1,3-bis(2-chloroethyl)-1-nitrosourea (BCNU), an alkylating agent, cured most C57BL/6 mice bearing a spontaneous thymic lymphoma (LSA). A proportion of these cured animals were, however, killed by a new challenge of viable tumor cells if they also received spleen cells from tumor-bearing mice, suggesting that suppressor cells mediated the enhancement of the tumor growth were the target of the drug. This assumption was confirmed in a direct experiment showing that the drug eliminated completely the activity of tumor-specific suppressor T cells (Thy-1$^+$, Lyt-1$^-$,2$^+$) and partially eliminated the tumor nonspecific suppressor T cells (Thy-1$^+$, Lyt-1$^+$,2$^+$) in the TBH spleens.

The effect of Cy, another aklylating agent, on the TBH suppressor cells was discussed in detail previously (1); there are, however, some recent interesting findings in this field. Spleen cells from BALB/c mice bearing a large plasmacytoma inhibited tumor growth in the Winn assay, and this effect was further enhanced if the donor TBH were treated with Cy (829), suggesting that the drug eliminates suppressor cells that interfere with the killing function of the immune cells.

Cyclophosphamide-sensitive suppressor cells have also been shown to prevent the induction of TNP-specific helper cell function that can support the immunological rejection of TNP-modified tumor cells. BALB/c mice that were treated with Cy in order to eliminate the suppressor cells, and then sensitized with trinitrochlorobenzene (TNCB) rejected a subsequent challenge of Rous sarcoma virus-induced tumor, if TNCB was injected into the tumor site (830). In the absence of interfering suppressor cells, the TNP recognizing helper cells (induced with TNCB) supported the immunological rejection of TNP-modified tumors and possibly unmodified neighboring tumor cells. The same experimental protocol has been used before by a different group (*831*) in order to obtain a regression of X5563 tumor from C3H/He mice.

North and associates (reviewed in *820*) presented evidence that resident suppressor cells interfered with cell-mediated adoptive immunotherapy in TBH. Elimination of the suppressor cells from the TBH either by Cy treatment or by ionizing radiation enabled the rejection of the tumors from these animals by transplanted immune cells. The therapeutic effect of the immune cells was prevented, however, if the TBH also received splenic T cells from mice bearing homologous large tumors. This finding suggests that suppressor cells (Lyt-2$^-$, L3T4a$^+$, relatively Cy resistant) antagonize the adoptive immunity possibly by blocking the generation of cytotoxic cells (*832*). Interestingly, animals bearing early small tumors (Meth A Fibrosarcoma) contain suppressor cells that are different by character (Lyt-1$^-$2$^+$; Cy sensitive) and function (suppress DTH rather than cell-mediated adoptive immunity) from the suppressor cells of animals bearing late-appearing large tumors (*833*).

Using the same experimental principle, Greenberg and colleagues (*834*) cured adult thymectomized, irradiated, and bone-marrow-reconstituted C57BL/6 mice with disseminated FBL-3 leukemia by treating the mice with Cy and immune T cells. Similarly, Shu and Rosenberg (*835*) cured C57BL/6 mice bearing newly emerged MCA tumors by exposing the mice to 500 rad and injecting them with immune cells. It is not known if the drug treatment of FBL-3 TBH or the irradiation treatment of the MCA TBH affected the tumors, the suppressor cells, or both. In a different study, North (*823*) presented, however, evidence that 500 rad X-irradiation caused rejection of Meth A fibrosarcoma from BALB/c mice because of elimination of the suppressor cells with no effect on the immune cells or the tumor cells.

7. Immunoregulation of Antitumor Autoimmunity by Suppressor T Cells

The antigenic repertoire of tumor cells may include, in addition to the tumor-specific antigens, antigens that appear on normal cells some time during their maturation. Natural spontaneously arising tumors, in contrast to experimentally induced tumors, may exclusively express such normal antigen (e.g., differentiation antigens), and immune responses against them might be considered as autoimmune responses. If so, it is not surprising that the immune responses against such normal tumor antigens are strictly controlled to prevent what looks to the immune system as inappropriate autoimmunity. Suppressor cells may be involved in such downregulation. Examples that support this concept were reviewed previously (1), but recently more information has come to light. Kölsch and associates (791,836) induced suppressor cells in CBA/J mice by injecting them with a plasmacytoma of BALB/c mice. These suppressor cells inhibited the MLC of CBA/J responder cells against BALB/c, BALB.K, or BALB.B stimulator cells, but not the MLC of the same responder cells against B10.D₂ or C57BL/6 stimulator cells. These results suggest that the tumor-induced suppressor cells were activated in the in vitro culture by normal cellular antigens coded by non-H-2 genes of the BALB/c mice. The results further suggest that the suppressor cells were induced by normal antigens of the plasmacytoma, which also appear in cells of mice carrying the BALB/c background. An accidental cross-reaction between tumor-associated antigens and the BALB/c mouse background antigens cannot, however, be excluded. Grooten and colleagues (238) similarly suggest that EL4 cells contain normal antigens that induce upon injection into syngeneic hosts suppressor T cells (Lyt-1⁺). These cells suppress the proliferative immune response of autoreactive clones against syngeneic spleen cells.

We described in our previous review (1) the elegant experiment of Tilkin and colleagues (837) demonstrating the ability of T lymphocytes derived from normal mice to suppress the in vitro secondary cytotoxic responses against tumor cells induced with endogenous viruses (Gross leukemia virus), but not the responses against tumor cells induced with exogenous viruses (M-MuLV). Because the genome of the endogenous virus is integrated into the normal cellular genome, the immune responses against tumor cells induced by such viruses may be considered as immune responses against self, which are strictly controlled by suppressor cells. This assumption is further supported by a recent finding of the same authors (838). Thymocytes of Mov-13 (V⁺) mice, in which the exogenous M-MuLV was artificially introduced into the germ line, and which express the virus during embryonal life, suppressed the secondary cytotoxic response against the tumor induced with this exogenous virus. Thus, once antigens of a tumor (in this case viral antigens) are expressed during embryonal development, they are considered by the immune system as self, and the immune response against them is controlled by suppressor cells.

General Conclusions

The purpose of this book is to examine whether the immuno-depression mediated by suppressor cells has any influence on the carcinogenetic process or on the promotion of tumor progression and metastatic spread. The experimental approaches used to resolve this question must cope, however, with limitations imposed by deriving data from humans rather than from experimental animals. First, unlike using experimental animals, it is not always possible to reduce the "noise" of irrelevant factors such as the activity of drug-induced suppressor cells (*see* chapter on Induction of Suppressor Cells by Immunostimulants, p. 5) or immunosuppression related to aging (449). Secondly, again unlike in experimental animals, the suppressor-cell function of the cancer patients is always measured by tests in vitro while it is clear that such tests do not always reflect the immunological status in vivo (4). Furthermore, the use of an in vitro test permits the introduction of artifacts, such as induction of suppressor cells by the serum supplementing the culture medium (195). Such tests, if not appropriately controlled, can easily lead to wrong conclusions attributing the suppressor-cell activity to the malignant state rather than to environmental factors.

Conscious of these limitations, informative data should be obtained from untreated patients, if possible at the time of their disease diagnosis. In addition, measuring suppressor-cell activity in aged-matched healthy subjects must always be determined simultaneously with similar assessment in cancer patients to avoid being misled by age-associated immunodepression. The suppressor-cell activity of cancer patients is often measured by mixing the patients' MNC with cells derived from normal allogeneic individuals, and stimulating the cellular mixture with antigen or mitogen. In order to avoid misinterpretation of the suppressor-cell activity actually induced by the allogeneic stimuli (839), the suppressor-cell activity of the healthy subjects' MNC must also be tested on allogeneic cells. Another source of misinterpretation is cells inhibiting MLC by cytolyzing either the stimulator cells or the responder cells. Such cells, if not directly tested for cytolytic activity, may be mistakenly described as suppressor cells. Possibly the most reliable indicator of suppressor function associated with malignant development would be the observation of suppressor-cell activity concomitant with the disease activity, being reduced during remission and reappearing during relapse.

The information described in this book and summarized in Tables 1, 2, 4, and 5 clearly indicates that many investigators carefully considered the above-mentioned factors, validating the inclusion of their data in an analysis of the relationship between suppressor-cell function and malignancy. Further information may be found in a recent review article by Von Roenn et al. (*840*), who emphasized some aspects of suppressor-cell function in solid tumor cancer patients that were not emphasized herein. In order to evaluate these aspects from a slightly different point of view, the reader is advised to read this paper carefully.

The heterogeneity of the immunological capabilities of cancer patients, exhibiting the same type of disease, is the dominant feature of the reports reviewed in this book. In some patients, an immunodepression is observed that may or may not be associated with excessive suppressor-cell activity, whereas other patients display a lack of suppressor-cell activity or a normal immunological capacity either in all or part of the compartments of their immune system. This inconsistency was found in both solid and circulating malignancies, such as HD (*344,348*), B-CLL (Table 3), head and neck cancer (*552*), lung cancer (*344,575,582,583*), gastric cancer (*609,611*), colorectal cancer (*610*), and ovarian cancer (*657*). In fact, the inability to find an immunodepression or an increased suppressor-cell activity may provide more information than the positive findings, since it would indicate that immunosuppression is not an obligatory factor in the carcinogenetic process or the promotion of tumor growth. Furthermore, some investigators have clearly found a lack of correlation between the disease activity and the intensity of the immune suppression mediated by suppressor cells (e.g., in HD, ref. *348*; CML, ref. *506*; head and neck cancer, ref. *551*). Taking such negative correlation to an extreme, one report claims that patients with advanced gastric cancer who presented increased suppressor-cell activity survived longer than similar patients with less suppressive activity (*611*). Although other investigators have found a correlation between the disease activity and the intensity of suppressor-cell function (e.g., refs. *593* and *598*), the lack of correlation in this instance is again more informative, since it shows that the disease activity can be completely independent of the suppressor-cell function.

It should also be pointed out that, in those cases where the activity of suppressor cells has been demonstrated, the suppressor cells may appear after the tumor has reached a stage of irreversible progression; thus, the fate of the tumor is not affected by the immunodepression. The excessive activity of the suppressor cells in such patients is possibly secondary to the tumor, the accumulation of factors associated with the malignant state deciding whether suppressor cells will be induced. Thus, the observation of suppression may occur in some patients but not in others.

The conclusion claiming that, in many cases, the suppressor-cell activity does not significantly influence the carcinogenetic process or the tumor progression is based mostly on assays measuring nonspecific immunological responses (exceptions are refs. 582,594,599,619,695 and 696). Whereas such assays detect the activity of nonspecific suppressor cells, the activity of tumor-specific suppressor cells is not determined. It is possible that the effect of tumor-specific suppressor cells on the immunological rejection of the neoplasm is more significant than that of nonspecific suppressor cells, but the data is not yet available to support such a proposal.

While in most cases no firm evidence supports the concept that the carcinogenetic process or tumor progression are dependent upon an immunosuppression, some immunomodulators (e.g., BCG, C. parvum, or INF) employed in therapy of cancer induce, under certain conditions, excessive suppressor-cell activity that may cause complications (e.g., opportunistic infections) associated with the immunodeficiency (see chapter on Induction of Suppressor Cells by Immunostimulants, p. 5, refs. 383 and 653). Thus, not only is the benefit of such agents still uncertain, but they may also cause undesirable consequences.

The activity of NK cells is efficiently controlled by positive and negative signals; among the latter, suppressor cells are significant factors (see chapter on Control of Natural Killer Cells by Suppressor Cells, p. 15). Such suppressor cells have been shown to develop excessive activity in the pleural effusions of patients with lung cancer, and this may be associated with the inability to detect appreciable NK-cell activity at this site (587,588,595). Intrapleural administration of streptococcal preparation OK432 caused a regression and disappearance of the tumor that was accompanied by an increase in NK-cell activity of the pleural effusion and a simultaneous decrease in its suppressor-cell function (589,590). These interesting findings are, however, balanced by the observation that the proportions of suppressor cells with anti-NK-cell activity among patients with epidermoid carcinomas of the upper respiratory tract, adenocarcinomas of the kidney, and ovarian carcinomas were somewhat lower than among healthy subjects (188). One might expect just the reverse if anti-NK suppressor cells were associated with the promotion of malignancy. Nevertheless, discussing the function of anti-NK suppressor cells, we should remember that the significance of NK cells in the control of malignancy has not yet been established.

Although a firm association cannot be demonstrated between immunosuppression and human malignancy, there are still some findings that do not concur with this conclusion, and some of them may even offer practical implications. Prostaglandins produced by cancer patients' suppressor monocytes are clearly associated with the defective immunological functions of MNC derived from the same patients (see Tables 1 and 5). Prostaglandins produced by the tumors themselves (161,162) may also be involved in the immunodeficient state observed in some malignant diseases. Although immunodepression mediated by PGs is not a general phenomenon (e.g., ref. 587), this defect is widely distributed among patients with HD (Table 1), head and neck cancer, lung cancer, colon cancer, renal cell cancer, breast cancer, and CNS malignancies (Table 5). In many cases, the weak immunological responses of the patients' MNC were augmented or even restored to normal levels after addition of indomethacin or other PG synthetase inhibitors. Furthermore, it has been claimed that indomethacin administration caused regression of head and neck cancer (756), skin cancer in xeroderma pigmentosum (757), and metastases in breast cancer (758). These findings suggest that administration of indomethacin alone or in combination with other drugs may be beneficial to patients expressing a PG mediated immunosuppression.

Another point of interest is demonstrated in multiple myeloma. The suppressor cells found in the active stages of the disease do not influence the Ig synthesis by the B cells, since these cells contain an intrinsic defect that is independent of the T cell function (517). In contrast, in the early stages of the disease (526) or when the disease is stable and well controlled (522,542,543), the absolute or relative representation of the suppressor-cell phenotype is increased, suggesting an attempt of suppressor cells to control the malignant cells at the onset of the disease, as well as an involvement of such cells in controlling the malignant cells when the disease is stable (a similar control mechanism may successfully operate in infectious mononucleosis, 390). If this assumption is correct, chemotherapy should be carefully used when the malignant cells are sensitive to regulatory signals (i.e., during the early stages of the disease or when the disease is under control), in order to avoid damage to the suppressor cells. Furthermore, it may be possible to increase the effectiveness of this resident suppressor-cell function, using techniques that have been successfully employed in animal models of myeloma (see our discussion about experimental myeloma in our previous review paper; 1). If malignant B cells present in B cell lymphomas and leukemias are sensitive to regulatory signals, then the considerations suggested in multiple myeloma may be extended to other such malignancies of B-cell phenotype.

Melanoma is another exceptional malignancy where the immune system may successfully control the disease, demonstrated in some instances by spontaneous regression of the tumor and late recurrence of the disease, sometimes 25 y after the removal of the initial primary tumor (674). An efficient activity of suppressor cells is a consistent finding in melanoma patients (Table 5), and their elimination may aid the immune cells to optimally control the disease.

In line with this concept, melanoma tumor regression was found in six out of 20 patients injected with INF who were subsequently orally administered with cimetidine (712). Antitumor responses were not recorded when INF was administered alone. It is possible that suppressor cells bearing H_2-receptors interfere with the activity of immune cells or NK cells induced with INF, and their removal may allow maximal activity of the immune system. If correct, the immune system of melanoma patients, both active and disease free, should be carefully monitored in order to detect increased suppressor-cell function. By observing such a change, elimination of the suppressor cells by cimetidine or other drugs (see our previous review; 1) may be beneficial for the patients.

A further aspect of practical implication is the expression of helper and suppressor T cell phenotypes by lymphoid malignancies. The leukemic cells of most Sézary syndrome and ATL patients display the phenotype $T4^+, T8^-$ (Table 4). In addition, most of the $T4^+, T8^-$ leukemic cells of ATL patients express suppressor-cell function (Table 4), indicating that they belong to the T4$^+$ suppressor-cell subtype (*266,405,406*). In contrast, the leukemic cells of most patients with T-cell lymphocytosis with neutropenia (TγLPD) display the phenotype Tγ$^+$,T4$^-$,T8$^+$, but they usually do not express suppressor-cell function (Table 4). The distinct cell phenotypes and functions of these patients may support the diagnosis of their diseases. Such an approach, however, should be used with caution, since T-CLL or T-PLL patients may express a helper-cell phenotype (T4$^+$,T8$^-$), suppressor-cell phenotype (T4$^-$,T8$^+$), or both phenotypes (T4$^+$,T8$^+$), and in most cases, they display either suppressor-cell function (Table 4) or both helper- and suppressor-cell functions (*468,841,842*).

In answering the question of whether regulatory cells of the immune system directly or indirectly contribute towards the growth of tumors in humans, it is clear from this review that there is a real scarcity of evidence, despite positive evidence for such a phenomenon in animal models (*1*). However, it is worth remembering that many of the laboratory-induced tumors display distinct tumor-associated antigens, of which some express appreciable immunogenic features (*1*). The spontaneous tumors of animals (*219*) and probably humans do not appear to exhibit such characteristics, at least not during the early critical stages of the disease. Thus, at that time they do not induce immune cells.

Although the spontaneous tumors of humans may not display distinct tumor-associated antigens, they may present normal differentiation antigens that are not expressed in the same amount, at the same time or in the same location as they are on normal cells. Any immune response against the "normal" antigens of the tumor ought to be strictly controlled, perhaps by suppressor cells, in order to avoid autoimmunity. This postulate gains support from some animal experimental models described in the previous chapter of this book (*836–838*). Thus, the same type of suppressor cells that may prevent an autoimmune response may also prevent a response against the tumor. Clearly, in this instance, an assay of nonspecific suppressor-cell activity would not detect such a self-protective suppressor cell. In any event, since this type of cell would be part of the normal immunoregulatory system, one might not even expect an increase in suppressor-cell activity, yet tumor growth would still proceed.

In addition, the immunogenic potential of "normal" antigens of the spontaneous tumors may never be detected because of the dominant activity of specific suppressor cells induced by the same tumor. If, however, the immune cells and the suppressor cells are induced by distinct antigens of the same tumor (immunogens and suppressogens, respectively), it may be possible to isolate the immunogen by conventional biochemical methods, or its gene by more recent molecular biological techniques and test the ability of the isolated immunogen or the gene product to induce specific immune responses in the absence of interfering suppressor cells. This approach has been successfully tested in experimental tumors, and the findings are described in a separate chapter of this book. (Antigenic Entities of the Tumor That Induce Suppressor Cells May Prevent the Functional Expression of Coexpressed Immunogenic Entities, p. 41).

Recently, our understanding of the T cell receptor (TCR) of both helper and cytotoxic cells has increased considerably (843). The TCR of helper T cells (mostly CD4) recognizes and binds the antigen in conjunction with HLA class II (DR, DP, and DQ) molecules of the antigen presenting cells, whereas the TCR of cytotoxic T cells (mostly CD8) recognizes and binds the antigen in conjunction with HLA class I molecules (A, B, and C) on the target cells (844). The TCR of both helper and cytotoxic cells consists of a disulphic-linked α and β chain. The tremendous diversity of the TCR expressed on helper and cytotoxic cells (more than 10^7 different sequences) is generated by a rearrangement mechanism similar to that used by B cells, although they employ different genes for this purpose (843). Accordingly, at least 50 different v (variable) region gene segments of α chain can randomly associate with at least 50 different J (Joining) region gene segments, and when combined with c (constant) region genes, they produce a mature α chain gene. Therefore, at least 2500 different sequences of α-chain are possible. Similarly, 50 different V region gene segments of β chain can randomly associate with two D (diversity) region gene segments and 13 J region gene segments, and when combined with C region genes, they produce a full-length active β chain gene (843,844). Using additional mechanism of diversity (for example, the two D-region gene segments can be read in any frame), the β chain can be represented by at least 4000 different sequences. Thus, the combination between the α and β chains may produce at least 10^7 different receptors.

Recently, a phenotypically different TCR has been detected on a small fraction of peripheral T cells and thymocytes (845–848). This TCR consists of a dimer of γ and δ chains, rather than α and β chains (843,849). The function of the γδ TCR, which may have fewer potential sequences than the αβ TCR (850), has not yet been elucidated. Both the αβ and γδ TCR are associated on plasma membrane with a set of three polypeptides represented by the T3 complex on human T cells (845,851–853). It has been suggested that occupation of the TCR by antigen delivers a signal to the T3 complex, which can then initiate a series of intracellular events. Initially, it seems that Ca^{2+} is mobilized from a nonmitochondrial pool, and the cytoplasmic concentration of Ca^{2+} increases. The interaction of TCR and T3 complex additionally activates protein kinase C, which together with the elevated concentration of Ca^{2+} induces the appearance of IL-2 and γ-INF transcripts. The translation products of these mRNAs then permit the activation and the proliferation of the T cells (851).

Whereas much information has accumulated concerning the structure and function of the TCR of helper and cytotoxic T cells, our knowledge of the suppressor T cell TCR is limited and contradictory. It is still unknown whether the suppressor T cells recognize free antigen or antigen associated with MHC products, particularly as both alternatives have been documented in the literature (e.g., 854,855). Moreover, we know almost nothing of the type of receptors used by suppressor T cells. Some workers have claimed that suppressor T cell receptors use α and β chains similar to those expressed on helper and cytotoxic T cells (856,857), whereas others found that suppressor T cells have deleted the β chain genes (858,859) or do not rearrange the β chain germ line genes and therefore do not present an active β chain gene (855). A further report describes a suppressor T cell line that transcribes the β chain gene, but not the α or the γ chain genes, while a different line transcribes the β and γ chain genes (860). Our ignorance is compounded further by our lack of understanding the mechanism of action of suppressor cells, as the vast literature reported in this book clearly demonstrates.

These conflicting findings and the fact that it is much more difficult to clone suppressor T cells than their helper and cytotoxic counterparts has led several immunologists to question the entire existence of these cells. Although the literature reported in this book documents evidence that suppression mediated by macrophages and T cells does exist in malignant diseases and tumors bearing experimental animals, it has not yet provided answers to the questions raised above. In fact, research at the level of molecular biology and genetics on suppressor cells obtained from cancer patients or animals bearing tumors is surprisingly sparse. The fact that several investigators have succeeded in cloning suppressor cells from TBH (*see* chapter on experimental animal models, p. 165) may provide the basis for such research, because cloned cells only can be used for molecular studies. Thus, suppressor T cells derived from TBH may provide an important contribution to the understanding of the structure and the function of the suppressor cell TCR. Furthermore, detailed analysis of suppressor cell TCR may reveal a distinct structure, which may be used as a target for a specific antibody, in an attempt to eliminate the cells or block their activity.

The many inconclusive findings described in this review may simply reflect the fact that we are still missing the relevant questions because of our lack of understanding of the interrelationships between the immune system and the malignant process. We must also substantially change our manner of thinking and create new ideas (*see* aphorism of this book). Doing so, we must remember that the immune system does not necessarily operate according to the logic of human beings, and efforts to impose on the immune system rules that are easily accepted by the human brain may cause selection of experimental artifacts. It is hoped that the recent technical and conceptual advances in the fields of basic immunology and molecular biology will help to overcome the obstacles, and consequently, new avenues of investigation in cancer research will be opened.

References

1. Naor D. and Duke-Cohan J. S. (1986) Suppressor cells and malignancy. I suppressor macrophages and suppressor T cells in experimental animals, in: *Advances in Immunity and Cancer Therapy* (Vol 2) (Ray P. K., ed.), Springer-Verlag, New York, pp. 1–129.
2. Naor D. (1979) Suppressor cells permitters and promoters of malignancy? (1979) *Adv. Cancer Res.* **29,** 45–125.
3. Gillette R. W. and Boone C. W. (1975) Changes in the mitogen response of lymphoid cells with progressive tumor growth. *Cancer Res.* **35,** 3774–3779.
4. Hanna N. and Kripke M. L. (1979) Immunologic significance of nonspecific suppressor cells in spleens of tumor-bearing mice. *Cell Immunol.* **43,** 293–303.
5. Parthenais E. and Haskill S. (1979) Specific T-cell reactivity in mice bearing autochthonous tumors or early-generation trans-

planted spontaneous mammary tumors. *J. Natl. Cancer Inst.* **62,** 1569–1574.

6. Herberman R. B. and Holden H. T. (1978) Natural cell-mediated immunity. *Adv. Cancer Res.* **27,** 305–377.

7. Naor D. (1983) Coexistence of immunogenic and suppressogenic epitopes in tumor cells and various types of macromolecules. *Cancer Immunol. Immunother.* **16,** 1–10.

8. Asherson G. L. and Zembala M. (1976) Suppressor T-cells in cell mediated immunity. *Br. Med. Bull.* **32,** 158–164.

9. Mathé G. (1976) Cancer active immunotherapy. *Recent Results Cancer Res.* **55,** 54–55, 91–95.

10. Sinkovics J. G. (1976) Suppressor cells and human malignant disease. *Br. Med. J.* **2,** 1072–1073.

11. Waldmann T. A. and Broder S. (1977) Suppressor cells in the regulation of the immune response. *Prog. Clin. Immunol.* **3,** 155–199.

12. Broder S., Muul L., and Waldmann T. A. (1978) Suppressor cells in neoplastic disease. *J. Natl. Cancer Inst.* **61,** 5–11.

13. Waldmann T. A., Broder S., Blaese R. M., Durm M., Goldman C., and Muul L. (1980) Disorders of suppressor T cells in immunodeficiency and malignancy. in: *Regulatory T lymphocytes* (Pernis B. and Vogel H. J., eds.), Academic Press, New York, pp. 381–402.

14. Bukowski R. M. (1981) Suppressor cells in oncology, in *Suppressor Cells and Their Factors* (Krakauer R. S. and Clough J. D., eds.): CRC Press, Boca Raton, Florida, pp. 103–122.

15. Stutman O. (1982) Suppressor cells in tumor-host interactions, in *Biological Responses in Cancer* (Mihich E., ed.), Plenum, New York, pp. 23–87.

16. Wheelock E. F., and Robinson M. K. (1983) Biology of disease. Endogenous control of the neoplastic process. *Lab. Invest.* **48,** 120–139.

17. Siegel B. V. (1985) Immunology and oncology. *Int. Rev. Cytol.* **96,** 89–120.

18. Baldwin R. W. and Pimm M. V. (1978) BCG in tumor immunotherapy. *Adv. Cancer Res.* **28,** 91–147.

19. Mitchell M. S. and Murahata R. I. (1979) Modulation of immunity by Bacillus Calmette-Guérin (BCG). *Pharmacol. Ther.* **4,** 329–353.

20. Milas L. and Scott M. T. (1978) Antitumor activity of Corynebacterium parvum. *Adv. Cancer Res.* **26,** 257–306.

21. Mitchell M. S., Kirkpatrick D., Mokyr M. B., and Gery I. (1973) On the mode of action of BCG. *Nature [New Biol.]* **243,** 216–218, 1973.

22. Chapes S. K. and Haskill S. (1983) Role of Corynebacterium

parvum in the activation of peritoneal macrophages. II. Identification of distinguishable anti-tumor activities by macrophage subpopulations. *Cell Immunol.* **76**, 49–57.

23. Herberman R. B. and Santoni A. (1984) Regulation of natural killer cell activity, in *Biological Responses in Cancer* (Vol. 2) (Mihich E., ed.) Plenum, New York, pp. 121–144.

24. Yashphe D. J. (1971) Immunological factors in nonspecific stimulation of host resistance to syngeneic tumors. *Isr. J. Med. Sci.* **7**, 90–107.

25. Smith S. E. and Scott M. T. (1972) Biological effects of Corynebacterium parvum: III Amplification of resistance and impairment of active immunity to murine tumors. *Br. J. Cancer* **26**, 361–367.

26. Terry W. D. (1978) Concluding remarks, in *Immunotherapy of Cancer: Present Status of Trials in Man* (Vol. 6) (Terry W. D. and Windhorst D. eds.), Raven Press, New York, pp. 669–671.

27. Scott M. T. (1974) Corynecbacterium parvum as a therapeutic antitumor agent in mice. II. Local injection. *J. Natl. Cancer Inst.* **53**, 861–865.

28. Chee D. O. and Bodurtha A. J. (1974) Facilitation and inhibition of B16 melanoma by BCG in vivo and by lymphoid cells from BCG-treated mice in vitro. *Int. J. Cancer* **14**, 137–143.

29. Piessens W. F., Campbell M., and Churchill W. H. (1977) Inhibition or enhancement of rat mammary tumor dependent on dose of BCG. *J. Natl. Cancer Inst.* **59**, 207–211.

30. Jacobs D. M. and Kripke M. L. (1974) Accelerated development of transplanted mammary tumors in mice pretreated with the methanol extraction residue of BCG and prevention of acceleration by concomitant specific immunization. *J. Natl. Cancer Inst.* **52**, 219–224.

31. Geffard M. and Orbach-Arbouys S. (1976) Enhancement of T suppressor activity in mice by high doses of BCG. *Cancer Immunol. Immunother.* **1**, 41–43.

32. Orbach-Arbouys S. and Poupon M-F. (1978) Active suppression of in vitro reactivity of spleen cells after BCG treatment. *Immunology* **34**, 431–437.

33. Castés M. and Orbach-Arbouys S. (1980) A role for BCG-induced suppressor cells in the antitumor activity of this agent, in *Abstracts of the Fourth International Congress of Immunology*, Theme 10, Workshop 5, Paper 10 (Preud'homme J. L. and Hawken V. A., eds.), Paris.

34. Orbach-Arbouys S. and Castés M. (1980) Suppression of T-cell responses to histocompatibility antigens by BCG pretreatment. *Immunology* **39**, 263–268.

35. Castés M., Lynch N. R., Lespinats G., and Orbach-Arbouys S. (1981) Possible role of macrophage-like suppressor cells in the anti-tumor activity of BCG. *Br. J. Cancer* **44**, 828–837.

36. Collins F. M. and Watson S. R. (1979) Suppressor T cells in BCG-infected mice. *Infect. Immun.* **25**, 491–496.

37. Payelle B., Bruley-Rosset M., Poupon M. F., and Lespinats G. (1984) Suppressor T cells in BCG-treated mice interfere with an in vivo specific antitumoral immune response. *Br. J. Cancer* **49**, 759–768.

38. Florentin I., Huchet R., Bruley-Rosset M., Halle-Pannenko O., and Mathé G. (1976) Studies on the mechanisms of action of BCG. *Cancer Immunol. Immunother.* **1**, 31–39.

39. Bennett J. A. and Mitchell M. S. (1978) Intravenous Bacillus Calmette-Guérin (BCG) induces splenic suppressor cells that inhibit in vitro immunization. *Proc. Am. Assoc. Cancer Res.* **19**, 22.

40. Bennett J. A., Rao V. S., and Mitchell M. S. (1978) Systemic Bacillus Calmette-Guérin (BCG) activates natural suppressor cells. *Proc. Natl. Acad. Sci. (USA)* **75**, 5142–5144.

41. Bennett J. A. and Mitchell M. S. (1979) Induction of suppressor cells by intravenous administration of Bacillus Calmette-Guérin and its modulation by cyclophosphamide. *Biochem. Pharmacol.* **28**, 1947–1952.

42. Bennett J. A. and Marsh J. C. (1980) Relationship of Bacillus Calmette-Guérin-induced suppressor cells to hematopoietic precursor cells. *Cancer Res.* **40**, 80–85.

43. Wepsic H. T., Harris S., Sander J., Alaimo J., and Morris H. (1976) Enhancement of tumor growth following immunization with Bacillus Calmette-Guérin cell walls. *Cancer Res.* **36**, 1950–1953.

44. Druker B. J., Wepsic H. T., Alaimo J., and Murray W. (1981) The negative systemic effect of BCGcw inoculated intraperitoneally. II. In vitro demonstration of the presence of suppressor cells in BCGcw-immunized rats. *Cancer Immunol. Immunother.* **10**, 227–237.

45. Wepsic H. T., Alaimo J., Druker B. J., Murray W., and Morris H. P. (1981) The negative systemic effect of BCGcw inoculated intraperitoneally. I. In vivo demonstration of intramuscular tumor growth enhancement with Morris hepatomas. *Cancer Immunol. Immunother.* **10**, 217–225.

46. Druker B.-J. and Wepsic H. T. (1983) BCG induced macrophages as suppressor cells. *Cancer Invest.* **1**, 151–161.

47. Wren S. M., Wepsic H. T., Larson C. H., De Silva M. A., and Mizushima Y. (1983) Inhibition of the graft-versus-host response

by BCGcw-induced suppressor cells or prostaglandin E_1. *Cell Immunol.* **76**, 361–371.

48. Mizushima Y., Wepsic T., De Silva M. A., Janns G., and Larson C. H. (1984) Comparative studies on tumor and adjuvant BCG cell wall induced nonspecific suppressor cells in rats. *Tohoku J. Exp. Med.* **143**, 295–304.

49. Mizushima Y., Wepsic H. T., Yamamura Y., DeSilva M. A., Janns G., and Larson C. H. (1984) Negative and positive immunobiological responses in mice pretreated with Bacillus Calmette-Guérin cell wall. *Cancer Res.* **44**, 20–24.

50. DeSilva M. A., Wepsic H. T., Mizushima Y., Nikcevich D. A., and Larson C. H. (1985) Modification of in vitro and in vivo BCG cell wall-induced immunosuppression by treatment with chemotherapeutic agents or indomethacin. *J. Natl. Cancer Inst.* **74**, 917–921.

51. Klimpel G. R. and Henney C. S. (1978) BCG-induced suppressor cells. I. Demonstration of macrophage-like suppressor cell that inhibits cytotoxic T cell generation in vitro. *J. Immunol.* **120**, 563–569.

52. Klimpel G. R. and Henney C. S. (1978) A comparison of the effect of T and macrophage-like suppressor cells on memory cell differentiation in vivo. *J. Immunol.* **121**, 749–754.

53. Klimpel G. R., Okada M., and Henney C. S. (1979) Inhibition of in vitro cytotoxic responses by BCG-induced macrophage-like suppressor cells. II. Suppression occurs at the level of a "helper" T cell. *J. Immunol.* **123**, 350–357.

54. Allen E. M. and Moore V. L. (1979) Suppression of phytohemagglutinin and lipopolysaccharide responses in mouse spleen cells by Bacillus Calmette-Guérin. *J. Reticuloendothel. Soc.* **26**, 349–356.

55. Schrier D. J., Allen E. M., and Moore V. L. (1980) BCG-induced macrophage suppression in mice: Suppression of specific and nonspecific antibody-medicated and cellular immunologic responses. *Cell Immunol.* **56**, 347–356.

56. Allen E. M., Sternick J. L., Schrier D. J., and Moore V. L. (1981) BCG-induced chronic pulmonary inflammation and splenomegaly in mice: Suppression of PHA-induced proliferation, delayed hypersensitivity to sheep erythrocytes, and chronic pulmonary inflammation by soluble factors from adherent spleen cells. *Cell Immunol.* **58**, 61–71.

57. Colizzi V., Ferluga J., Garreau F., Malkovsky M., and Asherson G. L. (1984) Suppressor cells induced by BCG release non-specific factors in vitro which inhibit DNA synthesis and interleukin-2 production. *Immunology* **51**, 65–71.

58. Bomford R. (1977) An analysis of the factors allowing promotion (rather than inhibition) of tumor growth by Corynebacterium parvum. *Int. J. Cancer* **19**, 673–679.

59. Berd D. and Mitchell M. S. (1976) Immunological enhancement of leukemia L1210 by Corynebacterium parvum in allogeneic mice. *Cancer Res.* **36**, 4119–4124.

60. Scott M. T. (1972) Biological effects of the adjuvant Corynebacterium parvum. I. Inhibition of PHA, mixed lymphocyte and GVH reactivity. *Cell Immunol.* **5**, 459–468.

61. Scott M. T. (1972) Biological effects of the adjuvant Corynebacterium parvum. II. Evidence for macrophage-T-cell interaction. *Cell Immunol.* **5**, 469–479.

62. Scott M. T. (1974) Depression of delayed-type hypersensitivity by Corynebacterium parvum: Mandatory role of the spleen. *Cell Immunol.* **13**, 251–263.

63. Kirchner H., Holden H. T., and Herberman R. B. (1975) Splenic suppressor macrophages induced in mice by injection of Corynebacterium parvum. *J. Immunol.* **115**, 1212–1216.

64. Varesio L. and Holden H. T. (1980) Suppression of lymphokine production. I. Macrophage-mediated inhibition of MIF production. *Cell Immunol.* **56**, 16–28.

65. Varesio L., Holden H. T., and Taramelli D. (1981) Suppression of lymphokine production. II. Macrophage-dependent inhibition of production of macrophage activating factor. *Cell Immunol.* **63**, 279–292.

66. Varesio L. and Holden H. T. (1980) Regulation of lymphocyte activation: macrophage-dependent suppression of T lymphocyte protein synthesis. *J. Immunol.* **125**, 1694–1701.

67. Lotzová E. C. (1980) Parvum-mediated suppression of the phenomenon of natural killing and its analysis, in *Natural Cell-Mediated Immunity Against Tumors* (Herberman R. B., ed.) Academic Press, New York, pp. 735–752.

68. Milisauskas V. K., Cudkowicz G., and Nakamura I. (1983) Cellular suppression of murine ADCC and NK activities induced by Corynebacterium parvum. *Cancer Immunol. Immunother.* **15**, 149–154.

69. Ojo E., Haller O., Kimura A., and Wigzell H. (1978) An analysis of conditions allowing Corynebacterium parvum to cause either augmentation or inhibition of natural killer cell activity against tumor cells in mice. *Int. J. Cancer* **21**, 444–452.

70. Farzad A., Penneys N. S., Ghaffar A., Ziboh V. A., and Schlossberg J. (1977) PGE_2 and $PGF_{2\alpha}$ biosynthesis in stimulated and nonstimulated peritoneal preparations containing macrophages. *Prostaglandins* **14**, 829–837.

71. Grimm W., Seitz M., Kirchner H. and Gemsa D. (1978) Prostaglandin synthesis in spleen cell cultures of mice injected with Corynebacterium parvum. *Cell Immunol.* **40,** 419–426.

72. Baird L. G., and Kaplan A. M. (1977) Macrophage regulation of mitogen-induced blastogenesis. I. Demonstration of inhibitory cells in the spleens and peritoneal exudates of mice. *Cell Immunol.* **28,** 22–35.

73. Hanna N., Blanc S., and Nelken D. (1980) Adjuvant-induced nonspecific suppressor cells: in vitro and in vivo studies. *Cell Immunol.* **53,** 225–235.

74. Glaser M. (1978) Adjuvant-induced thymus-derived suppressor cells of cell-mediated tumor immunity. *Nature* **275,** 654–656.

75. Koyama S., Yoshioka T., and Sakita T. (1982) Suppression of cell-mediated antitumor immunity by complete Freund's adjuvant. *Cancer Res.* **42,** 3215–3219.

76. Koyama S., Fujimoto S., Tada T., and Sakita T. (1981) Effect of Bacillus Calmette-Guérin cell wall skeleton on the induction of the cytotoxic and suppressor T cells against syngeneic tumor in the mouse. *Int. J. Cancer* **27,** 829–835.

77. Bennett J. A. Kemp J. D. Rao V. S., and Mitchell M. S. (1981) Selectivity in the effects of indomethacin on BCG-activated suppressor cell populations. *J. Immunopharmacol.* **3,** 221–239.

78. Lynch N. R. and Salomon J. C. (1979) Tumor growth inhibition and potentiation of immunotherapy by indomethacin in mice. *J. Natl. Cancer Inst.* **62,** 117–121.

79. Herberman R. B. (ed.) (1980) *Natural Cell Mediated Immunity Against Tumors.* Academic Press, New York.

80. Herberman R. B. (ed.) (1982) *NK Cells and Other Natural Effector Cells.* Academic Press, New York.

81. Cudkowicz G. and Hochman P. S. (1979) Regulation of natural killer activity by macrophage-like and other types of suppressor cells, in Developmental Immunobiology (Siskind G. W., Litwin, S. D., and Weksler M. E., eds.) Grune and Stratton, New York, pp. 1–21.

82. Riccardi C., Barlozzari T., Santoni A., Herberman R. B., and Cesarini C. (1981) Transfer to cyclophosphamide-treated mice of natural killer (NK) cells and in vivo natural reactivity against tumors. *J. Immunol.* **126** 1284–1289.

83. Bolhuis R. (1980) Characteristics of NK and related cells, in *Natural Cell Mediated Immunity Against Tumors* (Herberman R. B., ed.) Academic Press, New York, pp. 7–18.

84. Abo T., Cooper M. D., and Balch C. M. (1982) Characterization of HNK-1$^+$ (Leu-7) human lymphocytes. I. Two distinct phenotypic

of human NK cells with different cytotoxic capability. *J. Immunol.* **129**, 1752–1757.

85. Abo T. and Balch C. M. (1982) Characterization of HNK-1⁺ (Leu-7) human lymphocytes. III. Interferon effects on spontaneous cytotoxicity and phenotypic expression of lymphocyte subpopulations delineated by the monoclonal HNK-1 antibody. *Cell Immunol.* **73**, 376–384.

86. Lanier L. L., Le A. M., Phillips J. H., Warner N. L., and Babcock G. F. (1983) Subpopulations of human natural killer cells defined by expression of the Leu-7 (HNK-1) and Leu-11 (NK-15) antigens. *J. Immunol.* **131**, 1789–1796.

87. Nunn M. E., Herberman R. B., and Holden H. T. (1977) Natural cell-mediated cytotoxicity in mice against non-lymphoid tumor cells and some normal cells. *Int. J. Cancer* **20**, 381–387.

88. Hansson M., Kiessling R., Anderson B., Kärre K., and Roder J. (1979) NK cell-sensitive T-cell subpopulation in thymus: Inverse correlation to host NK activity. *Nature* **278**, 174–176.

89. Riccardi C., Santoni A., Barlozzari T., and Herberman R. B. (1981) In vivo reactivity of mouse natural killer (NK) cells against normal bone marrow cells. *Cell Immunol.* **60**, 136–143.

90. Santoni A., Riccardi C., Barlozzari T., Herberman R. B. (1982) Natural suppressor cells for murine NK activity, in *NK Cells and Other Natural Effector Cells* (Herberman R. B., ed.), Academic Press, New York, pp. 527–533.

91. Nasrallah A. G., Gallagher M. T., Datta S. K., Priest E. L., and Trentin J. J. (1982) Lack of suppressor cell activity for natural killer cells in infant, aged and low responder strain of mice, in *NK Cells and Other Natural Effector Cells* (Herberman R. B., ed.), Academic Press, New York, pp. 557–561.

92. Riccardi C., Santoni A., Barlozzari T., Cesarini C., and Herberman R. B. (1981) Suppression of natural killer (NK) activity by splenic adherent cells of low NK-reactive mice. *Int. J. Cancer* **28**, 811–818.

93. Migliorati G., Herberman R. B., and Riccardi C. (1986) Low frequency of NK-cell progenitors and development of suppressor cells in IL-2-dependent cultures of spleen cells from low NK-reactive SJL/J mice. *Int. J. Cancer* **38**, 117–125.

94. Riccardi C., Barlozzari T., Santoni A., Cesarini C., and Herberman R. B. (1982) Regulation of in vivo reactivity of natural killer (NK) cells, in *NK Cells and Other Natural Effector Cells* (Herberman R. B., ed.) Academic Press, New York, pp. 549–556.

95. Nair M. P. N., Schwartz S. A., Fernandes G., Pahwa R., Ikehara S., and Good R. A. (1981) Suppression of natural killer (NK) cell activity of spleen cells by thymocytes. *Cell Immunol.* **58**, 9–18.

96. Zöller M., Matzku S., Andrighetto G., and Wigzell H. (1982) Regulation of NK reactivity by suppressor cells, in *NK Cells and Other Natural Effector Cells* (Herberman R. B., ed.), Academic Press, New York, pp. 541–548.

97. Zöller M. and Wigzell H. (1982) Normally occurring inhibitory cells for natural killer cell activity. I. Organ distribution. *Cell Immunol.* **74**, 14–26.

98. Zöller M. and Wigzell H. (1982) Normally occurring inhibitory cells for natural killer cell activity. II. Characterization of the inhibitory cell. *Cell Immunol.* **74**, 27–39.

99. Brooks C. G. and Flannery G. R. (1980) Quantitative studies of natural immunity to solid tumors in rats. Persistence of natural immunity throughout reproductive life, and absence of suppressor cells in infant rats. *Immunology* **39**, 187–194.

100. Brunda M. J., Taramelli D., Holden H. T., and Varesio L. (1981) Peritoneal macrophages from normal mice suppress natural killer cell activity. *Fed. Proc.* **40**, 1094.

101. Brunda M. J., Taramelli D., Holden H. T., and Varesio L. (1981) Effects of resting and activated macrophages on natural killer cell activity and lymphoproliferation. *Proc. Am. Assoc. Cancer Res.* **22**, 310.

102. Brunda M. J., Taramelli D., Holden H. T., and Varesio L. (1982) Suppression of murine natural killer cell activity by normal peritoneal macrophages. in *NK cells and Other Natural Effector Cells* (Herberman R. B., ed.), Academic Press, New York, pp. 535–540.

103. Brunda M. J., Taramelli D., Holden H. T., and Varesio L. (1983) Suppression of in vitro maintenance and interferon-mediated augmentation of natural killer cell activity by adherent peritoneal cells from normal mice. *J. Immunol.* **130**, 1974–1979.

104. Welsh R. M., Jr., Zinkernagel R. M., and Hallenbeck L. A. (1979) Cytotoxic cells induced during lymphocytic choriomeningitis virus infection of mice. *J. Immunol.* **122**, 475–481.

105. Anderson R. E. and Warner N. L. (1976) Ionizing radiation and the immune response. *Adv. Immunol.* **24**, 215–335.

106. Bennett M., Baker E. E., Eastcott J. W., Kumar V., and Yonkosky D. (1976) Selective elimination of marrow precursors with the bone-seeking isotope [89]Sr: Implications for hemopoiesis, lymphopoiesis, viral leukemogenesis and infection. *J. Reticuloendothel. Soc.* **20**, 71–87.

107. Cudkowicz G. and Hochman P. S. (1979) Do natural killer cells engage in regulated reactions against self to ensure homeostasis? *Immunol. Rev.* **44**, 13–41.

108. Merluzzi V. J., Levy E. M., Kumar V., Bennett M., and Cooperband S. R. (1978) In vitro activation of suppressor cells from

spleens of mice treated with radioactive strontium. *J. Immunol.*
121, 505–512.

109. Morecki S., Weigensberg M., and Slavin S. (1985) Lectin separation of nonlymphoid suppressor cells induced by total lymphoid
irradiation. *Eur. J. Immunol.* **15**, 138–148.

110. Kumar V., Caruso T., and Bennett M. (1976) Mechanisms of genetic resistance to Friend virus leukemia. III. Susceptibility of
mitogen-responsive lymphocytes mediated by T cells. *J. Exp.
Med.* **143**, 728–740.

111. Hochman P. S., Cudkowicz G., and Dausset J. (1978) Decline of
natural killer cell activity in sublethally irradiated mice. *J. Natl.
Cancer Inst.* **61**, 265–268.

112. Kumar V., Ben-Ezra J., Bennett M., and Sonnenfeld G. (1979)
Natural killer cells in mice treated with [89]strontium: Normal
target-binding cell numbers but inability to kill even after interferon administration. *J. Immunol.* **123**, 1832–1838.

113. Levy E. M., Bennett M., Kumar V., Fitzgerald P., and Cooperband S. R. (1980) Adoptive transfer of spleen cells from mice
treated with radioactive strontium: Suppressor cells, natural
killer cells, and "hybrid resistance" in recipient mice. *J. Immunol.*
124, 611–618.

114. Kumar V., Mellen P. F., Lust J. A., and Bennett M. (1982) Suppressor cells active against NK-B but not NK-A cells in mice
treated with radioactive strontium, in *NK Cells and Other Natural
Effector Cells* (Herberman R. B., ed.), Academic Press, New York,
pp. 563–568.

115. Levy E. M., Kumar V., and Bennett M. (1981) Natural killer activity and suppressor cells in irradiated mice repopulated with a
mixture of cells from normal and ^{89}Sr-treated donors. *J. Immunol.*
127, 1428–1432.

116. Levy E. M., Kumar V., and Bennett M. (1982) Does a marrow de-
pendent cell regulate suppressor cell activity, in *NK Cells and
Other Natural Effector Cells* (Herberman R. B., ed.), Academic
Press, New York, pp. 569–573.

117. Mellen P. F., Lust J. A., Bennett M., and Kumar V. (1982) Analysis of low natural killer cell activity in ^{89}Sr-treated mice. *Eur. J.
Immunol.* **12**, 442–445.

118. Kumar V., Luevano E., and Bennett M. (1979) Hybrid resistance
to EL-4 lymphoma cells. I. Characterization of natural killer cells
that lyse EL-4 cells and their distinction from marrow-dependent
natural killer cells. *J. Exp. Med.* **150**, 531–547.

119. Luevano E., Kumar V., and Bennett M. (1981) Hybrid resistance
to EL-4 lymphoma cells. II. Association between loss of hybrid

resistance and detection of suppressor cells after treatment of mice with ^{89}Sr. *Scand. J. Immunol.* **13**, 563–571.

120. Lust J. A., Bennett M., and Kumar V. (1984) Lysis of FLD-3 Friend erythroleukemia cells in vitro and in vivo effect of ^{89}Sr treatment and Friend virus. *Int. J. Cancer* **33**, 107–113.

121. Seaman W. E., Gindhart T. D., Greenspan J. S., Blackman M. A., and Talal N. (1979) Natural killer cells, bone, and the bone marrow: Studies in estrogen-treated mice and in congenitally osteopetrotic (mi/mi) mice. *J. Immunol.* **122**, 2541–2547.

122. Seaman W. E. and Talal N. (1980) The effect of 17 β-estradiol on natural killing in the mouse, in *Natural Cell-Mediated Immunity Against Tumors* (Herberman R. B., ed.), Academic Press, New York, pp. 765–777.

123. Milisauskas V. K., Cuckowicz G., and Nakamura I (1983) Role of suppressor cells in the decline of natural killer cell activity in estrogen-treated mice. *Cancer Res.* **43**, 5240–5243.

124. Seaman W. E., Blackman M. A., Gindhart T. D., Roubinian J. R., Loeb J. M., and Talal N. (1978) β-Estradiol reduces natural killer cells in mice. *J. Immunol.* **121**, 2193–2198.

125. Santoni A., Riccardi C., Barlozzari T., and Herberman R. B. (1982) C. parvum-induced suppressor cells for mouse NK activity, *NK Cells and Other Natural Effector Cells* (Herberman R. B., ed.), Academic Press, New York, pp. 519–526.

126. Pollack S. B. and Herrick M. V. (1977) Inhibition of antibody-dependent cellular cytotoxicity by autologous lymph node cells. *J. Immunol.* **119**, 2172–2178.

127. Landazuri M. O., Silva A., Alvarez J., and Herberman R. B. (1979) Evidence that natural cytotoxicity and antibody-dependent cellular cytotoxicity are mediated in humans by the same effector cell populations. *J. Immunol.* **123**, 252–258.

128. Ito M., Ralph P., and Moore M. A. S. (1980) Suppression of spleen natural killing activity induced by BCG. *Clin. Immunol. Immunopathol.* **16**, 30–38.

129. Kasai M., Iwamori M., Nagai Y., Okumura K., and Tada T. (1980) A glycolipid on the surface of natural killer cells. *Eur. J. Immunol.* **10**, 175–180.

130. Kasai M., Yoneda T., Habu S., Maruyama Y., Okumura K., and Tokunaga T. (1981) In vivo effect of anti-asialo GM1 antibody on natural killer activity. *Nature* **291**, 334–335.

131. Wolfe S. A., Tracey D. E., and Henney C. S. (1976) Induction of "natural killer" cells by BCG. *Nature* **262**, 584–586.

132. Santoni D., Trinchieri G., and Koprowski H. (1978) Cell-mediated cytotoxicity against virus-infected target cells in hu-

mans. II. Interferon induction and activation of natural killer cells. *J. Immunol.* **121** 532–538.

133. Djeu J. Y., Heinbaugh J. A., Holden H. T., and Herberman R. B. (1979) Augmentation of mouse natural killer cell activity by interferon and interferon inducers. *J. Immunol.* **122,** 175–181.

134. Puccetti P. and Giampietri A. (1978) Immunopharmacology of pyran copolymer. *Pharmacol. Res. Commun.* **10,** 489–501.

135. Merigan T. C. (1967) Induction of circulating interferon by synthetic anionic polymers of known composition. *Nature* **214,** 416–417.

136. Santoni A., Riccardi C., Barlozzari T., and Herberman R. B. (1980) Inhibition as well as augmentation of mouse NK activity by pyran copolymer and adriamycin, in *Natural Cell-Mediated Immunity Against Tumors* (Herberman R. B., ed.), Academic Press, New York, pp. 753–763.

137. Riccardi C., Santoni A., Barlozzari T., Puccetti P., Sorci V., and Herberman R. B. (1979) Stimulatory and inhibitory effects on mouse natural killer (NK) activity by in vivo treatment with pyran copolymer. *Proc. Am. Assoc. Cancer Res.* **20,** 251.

138. Santoni A., Puccetti P., Riccardi C., Herberman R. B., and Bonmassar E. (1979) Augmentation of natural killer activity by pyran copolymer in mice. *Int. J. Cancer* **24,** 656–661.

139. Puccetti P., Santoni A., Riccardi C., Holden H. T., and Herberman R. B. (1979) Activation of mouse macrophages by pyran copolymer and role in augmentation of natural killer activity. *Int. J. Cancer* **24,** 819–825.

140. Santoni A., Riccardi C., Barlozzari T., and Herberman R. B. (1980) Suppression of activity of mouse natural killer (NK) cells by activated macrophages from mice treated with pyran copolymer. *Int. J. Cancer* **26,** 837–843.

141. Migliorati G., Frati L., Pastore S., Bonmassar E., and Riccardi C. (1984) Increase of natural killer activity of mouse lymphocytes following in vitro treatment with cytosine arabinoside. *Int. J. Immunopharmacol.* **6,** 433–444.

142. Santoni A., Riccardi C., Sorci V., and Herberman R. B. (1980) Effects of adriamycin on the activity of mouse natural killer cells. *J. Immunol.* **124,** 2329–2335.

143. Hochman P. S., Cudkowicz G., and Evans P. D. (1981) Carrageenan-induced decline of natural killer activity. II. Inhibition of cytolysis by adherent non-T Ia-negative suppressor cells activated in vivo. *Cell Immunol.* **61,** 200–212.

144. Hochman P. S. and Cudkowicz G. (1979) Suppression of natural cytotoxicity by spleen cells of hydrocortisone-treated mice. *J. Immunol.* **123,** 968–976.

145. Cudkowicz G. and Hochman P. S. (1980) Carrageenan-induced decline of natural killer activity. I. In vitro activation of adherent non-T-suppressor cells. *Cell Immunol.* **53**, 395–404.

146. Yung Y. P. and Cudkowicz G. (1978) Suppression of cytotoxic T lymphocytes by carrageenan-activated macrophage-like cells. *J. Immunol.* **121**, 1990–1997.

147. Herberman R. B., Ortaldo J. R., Djeu J. Y., Holden H. T., Jett J., Lang N. P., Rubinstein M., and Pestka S. (1980) Role of interferon in regulation of cytotoxicity by natural killer cells and macrophages. *Ann. NY Acad. Sci.* **350**, 63–71.

148. Riccardi C., Vose B. M., and Herberman R. B. (1983) Modulation of IL 2-dependent growth of mouse NK cells by interferon and T lymphocytes. *J. Immunol.* **130**, 228–232.

149. Riccardi C., Vose B. M., and Herberman R. B. (1982) Regulation by interferon and T cells of IL-2 dependent growth of NK progenitor cells. A limiting dilution analysis, in *NK Cells and Other Natural Effector Cells* (Herberman R. B., ed.), Academic Press, New York, pp. 909–915.

150. Toy S. T. and Wheelock E. F. (1975) In vitro depression of cellular immunity by friend virus leukemic spleen cells. *Cell Immunol.* **17**, 57–73.

151. Garaci E., Migliorati G., Jezzi T., Bartocci A., Gioia L., Rinaldi C., and Bonmassar E. (1981) Impairment of in vitro generation of cytotoxic or T suppressor lymphocytes by Friend leukemia virus infection in mice. *Int. J. Cancer* **28**, 367–373.

152. Migliorati G., Jezzi T., Favalli C., Garaci E., Rossi G. B., and Bonmassar E. (1982) Impairment of splenic natural killer cell activity of mice infected with polycythemic strain of Friend leukemia virus. *Cancer Immunol. Immunother.* **12**, 177–179.

153. Migliorati G., Jezzi T., Frati L., Bonmassar E., Rossi G. B., Garaci E., and Riccardi C. (1983) Modulation of natural killer (NK) cell activity during FLV-P virus infection of mice. *Int. J. Cancer* **31**, 81–90.

154. Pettey C. L. and Collins J. J. (1984) Immunotherapy of murine leukemia. XI. Differential susceptibility of spleen cells from serum-protected mice to the in vitro immunosuppressive effects on Friend leukemia virus-infected splenocytes. *Int. J. Cancer* **34**, 269–276.

155. Moody D. J. Specter S., Bendinelli M., and Friedman H. (1984) Suppression of natural killer cell activity by Friend murine leukemia virus. *J. Natl. Cancer Inst.* **72**, 1349–1356.

156. Moody D. J., Specter S., and Friedman H. (1986) Suppression of natural killer cell activity by splenic macrophages from Friend leukemia virus infected mice, unpublished manuscript.

157.   Young M. R., Wheeler E., and Newby M. (1986) Macrophage-mediated suppression of natural killer cell activity in mice bearing Lewis lung carcinoma. *J. Natl. Cancer. Inst.* **76,** 745–750.

158.   Leung K. H., Fischer D. G., and Koren H. S. (1983) Erythromyeloid tumor cells (K562) induce PGE synthesis in human peripheral blood monocytes. *J. Immunol.* **131,** 445–449.

159.   Young M. R., and Knies S. (1984) Prostaglandin E production by Lewis lung carcinoma: Mechanism for tumor establishment in vivo. *J. Natl. Cancer Inst.* **72,** 919–922.

160.   Plescia O. J. Smith A. H., and Grinwich K. (1975) Subversion of immune system by tumor cells and role of prostaglandins. *Proc. Natl. Acad. Sci. USA* **72,** 1848–1851.

161.   Goodwin J. S. and Webb D. R. (1980) Review: Regulation of the immune response by prostaglandins. *Clin. Immunol. Immunopathol.* **15,** 106–122.

162.   Goodwin J. S., Husby G., and Williams R. C. (1980) Prostaglandin E and cancer growth. *Cancer Immunol. Immunother.* **8,** 3–7.

163.   Gerson J. M., Holden H. T., Bonnard G. D., and Herberman R. B. (1979) Natural killer cell (NK) activity in murine and human tumors. *Proc. Am. Assoc. Cancer Res.* **20,** 238.

164.   Gerson J. M. (1980) Systemic and in situ natural killer activity in tumor-bearing mice and patients with cancer, in *Natural Cell-Mediated Immunity Against Tumors* (Herberman R. B., ed.), Academic Press, New York, pp. 1047–1062.

165.   Gerson J. M. Varesio L., and Herberman R. B. (1981) Systemic and in situ natural killer and suppressor cell activities in mice bearing progressively growing murine sarcoma-virus-induced tumors. *Int. J. Cancer* **27,** 243–248.

166.   Tanino T. and Egawa K. (1985) Suppression of natural cytotoxicity in tumor-bearing mice and inhibition of the suppression by D-mannose. *Jpn. J. Exp. Med.* **55,** 155–160.

167.   Herberman R. B. (1980) Summary: Suppression or inhibition of NK activity, in *Natural Cell-Mediated Immunity Against Tumors* (Herberman R. B. (ed.), Academic Press, New York, pp. 779–784.

168.   Djeu J. Y., Heinbaugh J. A., Vieira W. D., Holden H. T., and Herberman R. B. (1979) The effect of immunopharmacological agents on mouse natural cell-mediated cytotoxicity and on its augmentation by poly I:C. *Immunopharmacology* **1,** 231–244.

169.   Kendall R. A. and Targan S. (1980) The dual effect of prostaglandin (PGE$_2$) and ethanol in the natural killer cytolytic process: Effector activation and NK-cell-target cell conjugate lytic inhibition. *J. Immunol.* **125,** 2770–2777.

170.   Allison A. C. (1978) Mechanisms by which activated macrophages inhibit lymphocyte responses. *Immunol. Rev.* **40,** 3–27.

171. Stenson W. F. and Parker C. W. (1980) Opinion: prostaglandins, macrophages, and immunity. *J. Immunol.* **125,** 1–5.

172. Droller M. J., Perlmann P., and Schneider M. U. (1978) Enhancement of natural and antibody-dependent lymphocytes cytotoxicity by drugs which inhibit prostaglandin production by tumor target cells. *Cell Immunol.* **39,** 154–164.

173. Droller M. J., Schneider M. U., and Perlmann P. (1978) A possible role of prostaglandins in the inhibition of natural and antibody-dependent cell mediated cytotoxicity against tumor cells. *Cell Immunol.* **39,** 165–177.

174. Roder J. C. and Klein M. (1979) Target-effector interaction in the natural killer cell system. IV. Modulation by cyclic nucleotides. *J. Immunol.* **123,** 2785–2790.

175. Brunda M. J., Herberman R. B., and Holden H. T. (1980) Inhibition of murine natural killer cell activity by prostaglandins. *J. Immunol.* **124,** 2682–2687.

176. Brunda M. J. and Holden H. T. (1980) Prostaglandin-mediated inhibition of murine natural killer cell activity, in *Natural Cell-Mediated Immunity Against Tumors* (Herberman R. B., ed.), Academic Press, New York, pp. 721–734.

177. Humes J. L., Bonney R. J., Pelus L., Dahlgren M. E., Sadowski S. J., Kuehl F. A., Jr., and Davies P. (1977) Macrophages synthesis and release prostaglandins in response to inflammatory stimuli. *Nature* **269,** 149–151.

178. Brune K., Glatt M., Kälin H., and Peskar B. A. (1978) Pharmacological control of prostaglandin and thromboxane release from macrophages. *Nature* **274,** 261–263.

179. Kurland J. I., and Bockman R. (1978) Prostaglandin E production by human blood monocytes and mouse peritoneal macrophages. *J. Exp. Med.* **147,** 952–957.

180. Pelus L. M. and Bockman R. S. (1979) Increased prostaglandin synthesis by macrophages from tumor-bearing mice. *J. Immunol.* **123,** 2118–2125.

181. Tracey D. E. and Adkinson N. F. (1980) Prostaglandin synthesis inhibitors potentiate the BCG induced augmentation of natural killer cell activity. *J. Immunol.* **125,** 136–141.

182. Humes J. L., Cupo J. J., Jr., and Strausser H. R. (1974) Effects of indomethacin on Moloney sarcoma virus induced tumors. *Prostaglandins* **6,** 463–473.

183. Strausser H. R. and Humes J. L. (1975) Prostaglandin synthesis inhibition: Effect on bone changes and sarcoma tumor induction in BALB/c mice. *Int. J. Cancer* **15,** 724–730.

184. Herberman R. B., Nunn M. E., and Lavrin D. H. (1975) Natural cytotoxic reactivity of mouse lymphoid cells against syngeneic

and allogeneic tumors. I. Distribution of reactivity and specificity. *Int. J. Cancer* **16**, 216–229.

185. Becker S. and Klein E. (1976) Decreased "natural killer" effect in tumor-bearing mice and its relation to the immunity against oncorna virus determined cell surface antigens. *Eur. J. Immunol.* **6**, 892–898.

186. Parhar R. S., and Lala P. K. (1985) Changes in host natural killer cell population in mice during tumor development. 2. The mechanism of suppression of NK activity. *Cell Immunol.* **93**, 265–279.

187. Egawa K. and Tanino T. (1985) Suppression and abrogation of suppression of induced nonspecific cytotoxicity against tumor cells. *Jpn. J. Exp. Med.* **55**, 143–153.

188. Tarkkanen J. and Saksela E. (1982) Suppressor lymphocytes of human NK activity, in *NK Cells and Other Natural Effector Cells*, (Herberman R. B., ed.), Academic Press, New York, 575–580.

189. Tarkkanen J. and Saksela E. (1982) Umbilical-cord-blood-derived suppressor cells of the human natural killer cell activity are inhibited by interferon. *Scand. J. Immunol.* **15**, 149–157.

190. DeBoer K. P., Kleinman R., and Teodorescu M. (1981) Identification and separation by bacterial adherence of human lymphocytes that suppress natural cytotoxicity. *J. Immunol.* **126**, 276–281.

191. Kay H. D. and Smith D. (1981) Natural killer (NK) cell activity against K-562 cells: Regulation in vitro by blood granulocytes. *Fed. Proc.* **40**, 987.

192. Kay H. D. and Smith D. (1981) Regulation in vitro of human natural killer (NK) cells by peripheral blood granulocytes: suppressive and enhancing effects. *Immunobiology* **159**, 136–137.

193. Kay H. D. and Smith D. L. (1983) Regulation of human lymphocyte-mediated natural killer (NK) cell activity. I. Inhibition in vitro by peripheral blood granulocytes. *J. Immunol.* **130**, 475–483.

194. Nair M. P. N. and Schwartz S. A. (1981) Suppression of natural killer activity and antibody-dependent cellular cytotoxicity by cultured human lymphocytes. *J. Immunol.* **126**, 2221–2229.

195. Kedar E., Schwartzbach M., Unger E., and Lupu T. (1978) Characteristics of suppressor cells induced by fetal bovine serum in murine lymphoid cell cultures. *Transplantation* **26**, 63–65.

196. Uchida A. (1984) Lack of spontaneous and inducible natural killer cell activity in human bone marrow: Presence of adherent suppressor cells. *Nat. Immun. Cell Growth Regul.* **3**, 181–192.

197. Uchida A., Yagita M., Sugiyama H., Hoshino T., and Moore M. (1984) Strong natural killer (NK) cell activity in bone marrow of myeloma patients: Accelerated maturation of bone marrow NK cells and their interaction with other bone marrow cells. *Int. J. Cancer* **34**, 375–381.

198. Hoshino T., Uchida A., and Yagita M. (1984) Human bone marrow natural killer cell activity: Lack of reactivity in normal subjects and high activity in patients with myeloma, in *Natural Killer Activity and Its Regulation*, (Hoshino T., Koren H. S., and Uchida A., eds.), Excerpta Medica, Amsterdam, pp. 432–439.

199. Bordignon C., Villa F., Vecchi A., Giavazzi M., Introna M., Avallone R., and Mantovani A. (1982) Natural cytotoxic activity in human lungs. *Clin. Exp. Immunol.* **47**, 437–444.

200. Bordignon C., Allavena P., Introna M., Biondi A., Bottuzzi B., and Mantovani A. (1982) Modulation of NK activity by human mononuclear phagocytes: Suppressive activity of broncho-alveolar macrophages, in *NK Cells and Other Effector Cells*, (Herberman R. B., ed.), Academic Press, New York, pp. 581–588.

201. Bordignon C., Villa F., Allavena P., Introna M., Biondi A., Avallone R., and Mantovani A. (1982) Inhibition of natural killer activity by human broncho-alveolar macrophages. *J. Immunol.* **129**, 587–591.

202. De Boer K. P., Braun D. P., and Harris J. E. (1982) Natural cytotoxicity and antibody-dependent cytotoxicity in solid tumor cancer patients: Regulation by adherent cells. *Clin. Immunol. Immunopathol.* **23**, 133–144.

203. Uchida A., and Micksche M. (1982) Suppression of natural killer cell activity by adherent cells in cancer patients after surgery, in *Current Concepts in Human Immunology and Cancer Immunomodulation* (Serrou B., Rosenfeld C., Daniels J. C., and Saunders J. P., eds.), Elsevier Biomedical Press B.V., Amsterdam, pp. 365–370.

204. Bankhurst A. D. (1982) The modulation of human natural killer cell activity by prostaglandins. *J. Clin. Lab. Immunol.* **7**, 85–91.

205. Nair M. P. N. and Schwartz S. A. (1982) Suppression of human natural and antibody-dependent cytotoxicity by soluble factors from unstimulated normal lymphocytes. *J. Immunol.* **129**, 2511–2518.

206. Koren H. S., Anderson S. J., Fischer D. G., Constance S., Copeland C. S., and Jensen P. J. (1981) Regulation of human natural killing. 1. The role of monocytes, interferon and prostaglandins. *J. Immunol.* **127**, 2007–2013.

207. Leung K. H. and Koren H. S. (1982) Regulation of cytotoxic reactivity of NK cells by interferon and PGE_2, in *NK Cells and Other Natural Effector Cells*, (Herberman R. B., ed.), Academic Press, New York, pp. 615–620.

208. Leung K. H. and Koren H. S. (1982) Regulation of human natural killing. II. Protective effect of interferon on NK cells from suppression by PGE_2. *J. Immunol.* **129**, 1742–1747.

209. Targan S. R. (1981) The dual interaction of prostaglandin E_2

(PGE$_2$) and interferon (IFN) on NK lytic activation: Enhanced capacity of effector-target lytic interactions (recycling) and blockage of pre-NK cell recruitment. *J. Immunol.* **127,** 1424–1428.

210. Hiserodt J. C., Britvan L. J., and Targan S. R. (1982) Differential effects of various pharmacologic agents on the cytolytic reaction mechanism of the human natural killer lymphocyte: Further resolution of programming for lysis and KCIL into discrete stages. *J. Immunol.* **129,** 2266–2270.

211. Zielinski C. C., Gisinger C., Binder C., Mannhalter J. W., Eibl M. M. (1984) Regulation of NK cell activity by prostaglandin E$_2$: The role of T cells. *Cell Immunol.* **87,** 65–72.

212. Seaman W. E., Gindhart T. D., Blackman M. A., Dalal B., Talal N., and Werb Z. (1981) Natural killing of tumor cells by human peripheral blood cells. Suppression of killing in vitro by tumor-promoting phorbol diesters. *J. Clin. Invest.* **67,** 1324–1333.

213. Seaman W. E., Gindhart T. D., Blackman M. A., Dalal B., Talal N., and Werb Z. (1982) Suppression of natural killing in vitro by monocytes and polymorphonuclear leukocytes. *J. Clin. Invest.* **69,** 876–888.

214. Ogden B. E. and Hill H. R. (1980) Histamine regulates lymphocyte mitogenic responses through activation of specific H$_1$ and H$_2$ histamine receptors. *Immunology* **41,** 107–114.

215. Rocklin R. E., Breard J., Gupta S., Good R. A., and Melmon K. L. (1980) Characterization of the human blood lymphocytes that produce a histamine-induced suppressor factor (HSF). *Cell Immunol.* **51,** 226–237.

216. Nair M. P. N. and Schwartz S. A. (1983) Effect of histamine and histamine antagonists on natural and antibody-dependent cellular cytotoxicity of human lymphocytes in vitro. *Cell Immunol.* **81,** 45–60.

217. Flodgren P., and Sjögren O. (1985) Influence in vitro on NK and K cell activities by cimetidine and indomethacin with and without simultaneous exposure to interferon. *Cancer Immunol. Immunother.* **19,** 28–34.

218. Ruiz-Argüelles A., Seroogy K. B., and Ritts R. E. (1982) In vitro effect of cimetidine on human cell mediated cytotoxicity. 1. Inhibition of natural killer cell activity. *Cell Immunol.* **69,** 1–12.

219. Hewitt H. B., Blake E. R., and Walder A. S. (1976) A critique of the evidence for active host defence against cancer, based on personal studies of 27 murine tumours of spontaneous origin. *Br. J. Cancer* **33,** 241–250.

220. Burnet F. M. (1970) The concept of immunological surveillance. *Prog. Exp. Tumor Res.* **13,** 1–27.

221. Wicker L. S., Katz M., Sercarz E. E., and Miller A. (1984) Immunodominant protein epitopes. I. Induction of suppression to hen egg white lysozyme is obliterated by removal of the first three N-terminal amino acids. *Eur. J. Immunol.* **14**, 442–447.

222. Oki A., and Sercarz E. (1985) T cell tolerance studied at the level of antigenic determinants. I. Latent reactivity to lysozyme peptides that lack suppressogenic epitopes can be revealed in lysozyme-tolerant mice. *J. Exp. Med.* **161**, 897–911.

223. Krzych U., Fowler A. V., and Sercarz E. E. (1985) Repertoires of T cells directed against a large protein antigen, β-galactosidase. II. Only certain T helper or T suppressor cells are relevant in particular regulatory interactions. *J. Exp. Med.* **162**, 311–323.

224. Corradin G. and Chiller J. M. (1981) Lymphocyte specificity to protein antigens. III. Capacity of low responder mice to beef cytochrome c to respond to a peptide fragment of the molecule. *Eur. J. Immunol.* **11**, 115–119.

225. Fresno M., Nabel G., McVay-Boudreau L., Furthmayer H., and Cantor H. (1981) Antigen-specific T lymphocyte clones. I. Characterization of a T lymphocyte clone expressing antigen-specific suppressive activity. *J. Exp. Med.* **153**, 1246–1259.

226. Muckerheide A., Pesce A. J., and Michael J. G. (1977) Immunosuppressive properties of a peptic fragment of BSA. *J. Immunol.* **119**, 1340–1345.

227. Fainboim L., Jaraquemada D., Festenstein H., and Sachs J. A. (1981) MHC-specified lymphocyte activating and suppressor activating determinants in human mixed lymphocyte reactions. *Scand. J. Immunol.* **14**, 655–667.

228. Swanborg R. H. (1975) Antigen-induced inhibition of experimental allergic encephalomyelitis. III. Localization of an inhibitory site distinct from the major encephalitogenic determinant of myelin basic protein. *J. Immunol.* **114**, 191–194.

229. Sette A., Collizzi V., Appella E., Doria G., and Adorini L. (1986) Analysis of lysozyme-specific immune responses by synthetic peptides. 1. Characterization of antibody and T cell mediated responses to the N-terminal peptide of hen egg-white lysozyme. *Eur. J. Immunol.* **16**, 1–6.

230. Goodman J. W., and Sercarz E. E. (1983) The complexity of structures involved in T-cell activation. *Annu. Rev. Immunol.* **1**, 465–498.

231. Asano Y. and Hodes R. J. (1984) T cell regulation of B cell activation. An antigen-mediated tripartite interaction of Ts cells, Th cells, and B cells is required for suppression. *J. Immunol.* **133**, 2864–2867.

232. Greene M. I., and Perry L. L. (1978) Regulation of the immune response to tumor antigen. VI. Differential specificities of suppressor T cells or their products and effector T cells. *J. Immunol.* **121,** 2363–2366.

233. Fujimoto S. and Tada T. (1978) I region expression on cytotoxic and suppressor T cells against syngeneic tumors in the mouse. *Gann Monograph on Cancer Research* **21,** 11–20.

234. Yamauchi K., Fujimoto S., and Tada T. (1979) Differential activation of cytotoxic and suppressor T cells against syngeneic tumors in the mouse. *J. Immunol.* **123,** 1653–1658.

235. Romerdahl C. A. and Kripke M. L. (1986) Regulation of the immune response against UV-induced skin cancers: specificity of helper cells and their susceptibility to UV-induced suppressor cells. *J. Immunol.* **137,** 3031–3035.

236. Kripke M. L. (1981) Immunologic mechanisms in UV radiation carcinogenesis. *Adv. Cancer Res.* **34,** 69–106.

237. Caignard A., Martin M. S., Michel M. F., and Martin F. (1985) Interaction between two cellular subpopulations of a rat colonic carcinoma when inoculated to the syngeneic host. *Int. J. Cancer* **36,** 273–279.

238. Grooten J., Leroux-Roels G., and Fiers W. (1987) Specific suppression elicited by EL4 lymphoma cells in syngeneic mice. Specificity includes self-antigens on EL4. *Eur. J. Immunol.* **17,** 605–611.

239. Pellis N. R., Yamagishi H., Macek C. M., and Kahan B. D. (1980) Specificity and biological activity of extracted murine tumor-specific transplantation antigens. *Int. J. Cancer* **26,** 443–449.

240. Pellis N. R., Yamagishi H., Shulan D. J., and Kahan B. D. (1981) Use of preparative isoelectric focusing in a Sephadex gel slab to separate immunizing and growth facilitating moieties in crude 3 M KCl extracts of a murine fibrosarcoma. *Cancer Immunol. Immunother.* **11,** 53–58.

241. Yamamoto H. (1984) Isolation of immunogenic and suppressogenic glycoproteins from adenovirus type 12 hamster tumor cells. *Microbiol. Immunol.* **28,** 339–348.

242. Kahan B. D., Tanaka T., and Pellis N. R. (1980) Immunotherapy of a carcinogen-induced murine sarcoma with soluble tumor-specific transplantation antigens. *J. Natl. Cancer Inst.* **65,** 1001–1004.

243. Saunders T. L., Kahan B. D., and Pellis N. R. (1985) The effect of purification on the immunogenicity of tumor-specific transplantation antigens. *Cancer Immunol. Immunother.* **19,** 22–27.

244. Saunders T. L. Kahan B. D., and Pellis N. R. (1983) Purification of

immunoprotective tumor antigens by preparative isotachophoresis. *Cancer Immunol. Immunother.* **16**, 101–108.

245. Jessup J. M., Kahan B. D., LeGrue S. J., Rutzky L., and Pellis N. R. (1984) Soluble factors from murine and human tumors induce suppressor cells. *J. Surg. Res.* **36**, 631–638.

246. Jessup J. M., LeGrue S. J., Kahan B. D., and Pellis N. R. (1985) Induction of suppressor cells by a tumor-derived suppressor factor. *Cell Immunol.* **93**, 9–25.

247. Jessup J. M., Kahan B. D., LeGrue S. J., Rutzky L. R., and Pellis N. R. (1984). Soluble factors from murine and human tumor induced suppressor cells. *J. Surg. Res.* **36**, 631–638.

248. Klein G., Klein E., and Haughton G. (1966) Variation of antigenic characteristics between different mouse lymphomas indued by the Moloney virus. *J. Natl. Caner Inst.* **36**, 607–621.

249. Galili N., Naor D., Åsjö B., and Klein G. (1976) Induction of immune responsiveness in a genetically low-responsive tumor-host combination by chemical modification of the immunogen. *Eur. J. Immunol.* **6**, 473–476.

250. Galili N., Devens B., Naor D., Becker S., and Klein E. (1978) Immune responses to weakly immunogenic virally induced tumors. I. Overcoming low responsiveness by priming mice with a syngeneic in vitro tumor line or allogeneic cross-reactive tumor. *Eur. J. Immunol.* **8**, 17–22.

251. Devens B., Deutsch O., Avraham Y., and Naor D. (1981) Immune response to weakly immunogenic virally induced tumors. IX. Mice injected with the in vitro variant of YAC tumor (YAC-1) resist lethal doses of the tumorgenic YAC cells. *Immunobiology* **159**, 432–443.

252. Devens B., Galili N., Deutsch O., Naor D., and Klein E. (1978) Immune responses to weakly immunogenic virally induced tumors. II. Suppressive effects of the in vivo carried tumor YAC. *Eur. J. Immunol.* **8**, 573–578.

253. Kobrin B. J., Naor D., and Klein B. Y. (1981) Immunogenicity of subcellular fractions and molecular species of MuLV-induced tumors. II. Stimulation of syngeneic anti-tumor cell-mediated immune responses by subcellular fractions and molecular species of the Rauscher-virus-induced RBL5 tumor. *J. Immunol.* **126**, 1874–1882.

254. Ahituv A., Naor D., Sharon R., Tarcic N., and Klein B. Y. (1982) Immunogenicity of subcellular fractions and molecular species of MuLV-induced tumors. III. Stimulation of syngeneic antitumor responses by subcellular fractions and molecular species of Moloney virus-induced tumors in CBA and A mice. *Cancer Immunol. Immunother.* **14**, 16–26.

255. Klein B. Y., Frenkel S., Ahituv A., and Naor D. (1980) Immuno-genicity of subcellular fractions and molecular species of MuLV-induced tumors. I. Screening of immunogenic components by isopycnic ultracentrifugation and polyacrylamide electrophoresis of a tumor homogenate. *J. Immunol. Methods* **38**, 325–341.

256. Klein B. Y., Devens B., Deutsch O., Ahituv A., Frenkel S., Kobrin B. J., and Naor D. (1981) Isolation of immunogenic and suppressogenic determinants of the nonimmunogenic YAC tumor and the change in its immunogenic repertoire after in vitro cultivation. *Transplant Proc.* **13**, 790–797.

257. Klein B. Y., Sharon R., Tarcic N., and Naor D. (1982) Induction of antitumor reactive cells or suppressor cells by different molecular species isolated from the same nonimmunogenic tumor. *Immuno-biology* **163**, 7–21.

258. Sharon R., and Naor D. (1984) The isolation of immunogenic molecular entities from immunogenic and nonimmunogenic tumor homogenates by sodium dodecyl sulfate polyacrylamide gel electrophoresis (SDS-PAGE). *Cancer Immunol. Immunother.* **18**, 203–208.

259. Klein B. Y., Sharon R., Avraham Y., Ahituv A., and Naor D. (1983) Isolation of immunogenic entitles from nonimmunogenic transplantable tumors and their normal cell counterparts. *Transplant Proc.* **15**, 225–231.

260. Yefenof E., Goldapfel M., and Ber R. (1982) Nonimmunogenic radiation-induced lymphoma: Immunity induction by a somatic cell hybrid. *J. Natl. Cancer Inst.* **68**, 841–849.

261. Klein B. Y., Frenkel S., and Naor D. (1984) Isolated soluble fractions from the murine B16 melanoma induce primary in vitro syngeneic antitumor responses. *Cancer Immunol. Immunother.* **18**, 195–202.

262. Srivastava P. K., DeLeo A. B., and Old L. J. (1986) Tumor rejection antigens of chemically induced sarcomas of inbred mice. *Proc. Natl. Acad. Sci. USA* **83**, 3407–3411.

263. Harvey M. A., Adorini L., Miller A., and Sercarz E. E. (1979) Lysozyme-induced T-suppressor cells and antibodies have a predominant idiotype. *Nature* **281**, 594–596.

264. Maier T., Kilburn D. G., and Levy J. G. (1981) Properties of syngeneic and allogeneic antisera raised to tumor specific suppressor factor from DBA/2J mice. *Cancer Immunol. Immunother.* **12**, 49–56.

265. Ballieux R. E. and Heijnen C. J. (1983) Immunoregulatory T cell subpopulations in man: Dessection by monoclonal antibodies and Fc-receptors. *Immunol. Rev.* **74**, 5–28.

266. Thomas Y., Rogozinski L., and Chess L. (1983) Relationship between human T cell functional heterogeneity and human T cell surface molecules. *Immunol. Rev.* **74**, 113–128.

267. Lanier L. L., Engleman E. G., Gatenby P., Babcock G. F., Warner N. L., and Herzenberg L. A. (1983) Correlation of functional properties of human lymphoid cell subsets and surface marker phenotypes using multiparameter analysis and flow cytometry. *Immunol. Rev.* **74**, 143–160.

268. Farrar J. J., Benjamin W. R., Hilfiker M. L., Howard M., Farrar W. L., and Fuller-Farrar J. (1982). The biochemistry, biology, and role of interleukin 2 in the induction of cytotoxic T cell and antibody-forming B cell responses. *Immunol. Rev.* **63**, 129–166.

269. Durum S. K., Schmidt J. A., and Oppenheim J. J. (1985) Interleukin 1: An immunological perspective. *Annu. Rev. Immunol.* **3**, 263–287.

270. Heijnen C. J., Uytdehaag F., Pot K. H., and Ballieux R. E. (1981) Antigen-specific human T cell factors. I. T cell helper factor: Biologic properties. *J. Immunol.* **126**, 497–502.

271. Reinherz E. L., Meuer S. C., and Schlossman S. F. (1983) The human T cell receptor: Analysis with cytotoxic T cell clones. *Immunol. Rev.* **74**, 83–112.

272. Lipton J. M., Reinherz E. L., Kudisch M., Jackson P. L., Schlossman S. F., and Nathan D. G. (1980) Mature bone marrow erythroid burst-forming units do not require T cells for induction of erythropoietin-dependent differentiation. *J. Exp. Med.* **152**, 350–360.

273. Pick E., Cohen S., and Oppenheim J. J. (1979) The lymphokine concept, in *Biology of the Lymphokines* (Cohen S., Pick E., and Oppenheim J. J., eds.), Academic Press, New York, pp. 1–12.

274. Thomas Y., Rogozinski L., Rothman P., Rabbani L. E., Andrews S., Irigoyen O. H., and Chess L. (1982) Further dissection of the functional heterogeneity within the OKT4⁺ and OKT8⁺ human T cell subsets. *J. Clin. Immunol.* **2**, 85–145.

275. Reinherz E. L., Moretta L., Roper M., Breard J. M., Mingari M. C., Cooper M. D., and Schlossman S. F. (1980) Human T lymphocyte subpopulations defined by Fc receptors and monoclonal antibodies. A comparison. *J. Exp. Med.* **151**, 969–974.

276. Lehner T. (1986) Antigen presenting, contrasuppressor human T cells. *Immunol. Today* **7**, 87–92.

277. Kaplan H. S. (1980) Hodgkin's disease: Unfolding concepts concerning its nature, management and prognosis. *Cancer* **45**, 2439–2474.

278. Rosenberg S. A. (1982) Hodgkin's disease, in *Cancer Medicine* (Holland J. F., and Frei E. III, eds.), Lea and Febiger, Philadelphia, pp. 1478–1502.

279. Poppema S., Bhan A. K., Reinherz E. L., Posner M. R., and Schlossman S. F. (1982) In situ immunologic characterization of cellular constituents in lymph nodes and spleens involved by Hodgkin's disease. *Blood* **59,** 226–232.

280. Fisher R. I., Cossman J., Diehl V., and Volkman D. J. (1985) Antigen presentation by Hodgkin's disease cells. *J. Immunol.* **135,** 3568–3571.

281. Steiner P. E. (1934) Etiology of Hodgkin's disease. II. Skin reactions to avian and human tuberculin proteins in Hodgkin's disease. *Arch. Intern. Med.* **54,** 11–17.

282. Schier W. W., Roth A., Ostroff G., and Schrift M. H. (1956) Hodgkin's disease and immunity. *Am. J. Med.* **20,** 94–99.

283. Sokal J. E. and Primikirios N. (1961) The delayed skin test response in Hodgkin's disease and lymphosarcoma. Effect of disease activity. *Cancer* **14,** 597–607.

284. De Gast G. C., Halie M. R., and Nieweg H. O. (1975) Immunological responsiveness against two primary antigens in untreated patients with Hodgkin's disease. *Eur. J. Cancer* **11,** 217–224.

285. Miller D. G., Lizardo J. G., and Snyderman R. K. (1961) Homologous and heterologous skin transplantation in patients with lymphomatous disease. *J. Natl. Cancer Inst.* **26,** 569–583.

286. Brown R. S., Haynes H. A., Foley H. T., Godwin H. A., Berard C. W., and Carbone P. P. (1967) Hodgkin's disease. Immunologic, clinical, and histologic features of 50 untreated patients. *Ann. Intern. Med.* **67,** 291–302.

287. Fuks Z., Strober S., Bobrove A. M., Sasazuki T., McMichael A., and Kaplan H. S. (1976) Long term effects of radiation on T and B lymphocytes in peripheral blood of patients with Hodgkin's disease. *J. Clin. Invest.* **58,** 803–814.

288. Holm G., Mellstedt H., Björkholm M., Johansson B., Killander D., Sundblad R., and Söderberg G. (1976) Lymphocyte abnormalities in untreated patients with Hodgkin's disease. *Cancer* **37,** 751–762.

289. Minassian A. A. (1986) Suppressor cells in the peripheral blood and spleen of patients with Hodgkin's disease. *Cancer* **57,** 1756–1761.

290. Rühl H., Vogt W., Bochert G., Schmidt S., Moelle R., and Schaoua H. (1975) Mixed lymphocyte culture stimulatory and responding capacity of lymphocytes from patients with lymphoproliferative diseases. *Clin. Exp. Immunol.* **19,** 55–65.

291. Churchill W. H., Rocklin R. R., Moloney W. C., and David J. R. (1973) In vitro evidence of normal lymphocyte function in some patients with Hodgkin's disease and negative delayed cutaneous hypersensitivity. *Natl. Cancer Inst. Monogr.* **36**, 99–106.

292. Golding B., Golding H., Lomnitzer R., Jacobson R., Koornhof H. J., and Rabson A. R. (1977) Production of leukocyte inhibitory factor (LIF) in Hodgkin's disease. Spontaneous production of an inhibitor of normal lymphocyte transformation. *Clin. Immunol. Immunopathol.* **7**, 114–122.

293. Holm G., Perlmann P., and Johansson B. (1967) Impaired phyto-haemagglutinin-induced cytotoxicity in vitro of lymphocytes from patients with Hodgkin disease or chronic lymphatic leukaemia. *Clin. Exp. Immunol.* **2**, 351–360.

294. Bobrove A. M., Fuks Z., Strober S., and Kaplan H. S. (1975) Quantitation of T and B lymphocytes and cellular immune function in Hodgkin's disease. *Cancer* **36**, 169–179.

295. Levy R. and Kaplan H. S. (1974) Impaired lymphocyte function in untreated Hodgkin's disease. *N. Engl. J. Med.* **290**, 181–186.

296. Twomey J. J., Good R. A., and Chase D. C. (1978) Immunologic changes with Hodgkin's disease, in *The Immunopathology of Lymphoreticular Neoplasms* (Twomey J. J. and Good R. A., eds.), Plenum, New York, pp. 585–608.

297. Björkholm M., Holm G., and Mellstedt H. (1977) Immunologic profile of patients with cured Hodgkin's disease. *Scand. J. Haematol.* **18**, 361–368.

298. Case D. C., Hansen J. A., Corrales E., Young C. W., Dupont B., Pinsky C. M., and Good R. A. (1977) Depressed in vitro lymphocyte responses to PHA in patients with Hodgkin's disease in continuous long remission. *Blood* **49**, 771–778.

299. Gobbi M., Fiacchini M., Tomasini I., Ruggero D., Lauria F., and Tura S. (1977) Immunological study of patients with Hodgkin's disease in long lasting, not maintained, complete remission. *Boll Ist Sieroter Milan* **56**, 144–150.

300. Desser R. K. and Ultmann J. E. (1972) Risk of severe infection in patients with Hodgkin's disease or lymphoma after diagnostic laparotomy and splenectomy. *Ann. Intern. Med.* **77**, 143–146.

301. Lauria F., Fiacchini M., Gobbi M., and Tura S. (1974) Herpes zoster and total therapy in Hodgkin's disease. *Haematologica* **59**, 375–376.

302. Hall T. C. (1978) Leukemia in patients treated for Hodgkin's disease. *N. Engl. J. Med.* **298**, 853–854.

303. Moretta L., Mingari M. C., and Moretta A. (1979) Human T cell subpopulations in normal and pathologic conditions. *Immunol. Rev.* **45**, 163–193.

304. Romagnani S., Maggi E., Biagiotti R., Giudizi M. G., Amadori A., and Ricci M. (1978) Altered proportion of Tμ - and Tγ-cell subpopulations in patients with Hodgkin's disease. *Scand. J. Immunol.* **7**, 511–514.

305. Sibbitt W. L., Jr., Bankhurst A. D., Williams R. C., Jr. (1978) Studies of cell subpopulations mediating mitogen hyporesponsiveness in patients with Hodgkin's disease. *J. Clin. Invest.* **61**, 55–63.

306. Gupta S. (1980) Subpopulations of human T lymphocytes. XVI. Maldistribution of T cell subsets associated with abnormal locomotion of T cells in untreated adult patients with Hodgkin's disease. *Clin. Exp. Immunol.* **42**, 186–195.

307. Gupta S. and Tan C. (1980) Subpopulations of human T lymphocytes. XIV. Abnormality of T-cell locomotion and of distribution of subpopulations of T and B lymphocytes in peripheral blood and spleen from children with untreated Hodgkin's disease. *Clin. Immunol. Immunopathol.* **15**, 133–143.

308. Kaszubowski P. A., Husby G., Tung K. S. K. and Williams R. C. (1980) T lymphocyte subpopulations in peripheral blood and tissues of cancer patients. *Cancer Res.* **40**, 4648–4657.

309. Schulof R. S., Bockman R. S., Garofalo J. A., Cirrincione C., Cunningham-Rundles S., Fernandes G., Day N. K., Pinsky C. M., Incefy G. S., Thaler H. T., Good R. A., and Gupta S. (1981) Multivariate analysis of T-cell functional defects and circulating serum factors in Hodgkin's disease. *Cancer* **48**, 964–973.

310. Reinherz E. L. and Schlossman S. F. (1980) The differentiation and function of human T lymphocytes. *Cell* **19**, 821–827.

311. Acuto O. and Reinherz E. L. (1985) The human T cell receptor. *J. N. Engl. Med.* **312**, 1100–1111.

312. Posner M. R., Reinherz E. L., Breard J., Nadler L. M., Rosenthal D. S. and Schlossman S. F. (1981) Lymphoid subpopulations of peripheral blood and spleen in untreated Hodgkin's disease. *Cancer* **48**, 1170–1176.

313. Dorreen M. S., Habeshaw J. A., Wrigley P. F. M., and Lister T. A. (1982) Distribution of T-lymphocyte subsets in Hodgkin's disease characterized by monoclonal antibodies. *Br. J. Cancer* **45**, 491–499.

314. Lauria F., Foa R., Gobbi M., Camaschella C., Lusso P., Raspadori D., and Tura S. (1983) Increased proportion of suppressor/cytotoxic (OKT8+) cells in patients with Hodgkin's disease in long-lasting remission. *Cancer* **52**, 1385–1388.

315. Lauria F., Raspadori D., Foa R., Tazzari P. L., Lusso P., Fierro M. T., Matera L., Baccarani M., and Tura S. (1986) Normal T-lymphocyte function in patients with Hodgkin's disease in long-lasting remission. *Tumori* **72**, 75–80.

316. Romagnani S., Del Prete G. F., Maggi E., Bosi A., Bernardi F., Ponticelli P., Di Lollo S., and Ricci M. (1983) Displacement of T lymphocytes with the "helper/inducer" phenotype from peripheral blood to lymphoid organs in untreated patients with Hodgkin's disease. *Scand. J. Haematol.* **31**, 305–314.

317. Maggi E., Parronchi P., Del Prete G., Ricci M., Bosi A., Moretta L., and Romagnani S. (1986) Frequent T4-positive cells with cytolytic activity in spleens of patients with Hodgkin's disease (a clonal analysis). *J. Immunol.* **136**, 1516–1520.

318. Aisenberg A. C., and Wilkes B. M. (1982) Lymph node T cells in Hodgkin's disease: Analysis of suspensions with monoclonal antibody and rosetting techniques. *Blood* **59**, 522–527.

319. Knowles II D. M., Halper J. P., and Jakobiec F. A. (1984) T-lymphocyte subpopulations in B-cell-derived non-Hodgkin's lymphomas and Hodgkin's disease. *Cancer* **54**, 644–651.

320. Martin J. M. E. and Warnke R. A. (1984) A quantitative comparison of T-cell subsets in Hodgkin's disease and reactive hyperplasia. Frozen section immuno histochemistry. *Cancer* **53**, 2450–2455.

321. Abdulaziz Z., Mason D. Y., Stein H., Gatter K. C., and Nash J. R. (1984) An immuno histological study of the cellular constituents of Hodgkin's disease using a monoclonal antibody panel. *Histopathology* **8**, 1–25.

322. Thomas Y., Sosman J., Irigoyen O. H., Rogozinski L., Friedman S. M., and Chess L. (1981) Interactions among human T cell subsets. *Int. J. Immunopharmacol.* **3**, 193–201.

323. Schechter G. P. and Soehnlen F. (1978) Monocyte-mediated inhibition of lymphocyte blastogenesis in Hodgkin's disease. *Blood* **52**, 261–271.

324. Twomey J. J., Laughter A. H., Rice L., and Ford R. (1980) Spectrum of immunodeficiencies with Hodgkin's disease. *J. Clin. Invest.* **66**, 629–637.

325. Passwell J., Levanon M., Davidsohn J., and Ramot B. (1983) Monocyte PGE_2 secretion in Hodgkin's disease and its relation to decreased cellular immunity. *Clin. Exp. Immunol.* **51**, 61–68.

326. Hillinger S. M. and Herzig G. P. (1978) Impaired cell-mediated immunity in Hodgkin's disease mediated by suppressor lymphocytes and monocytes. *J. Clin. Invest.* **61**, 1620–1627.

327. Schechter G. P., Wahl L. M., and Oppenheim J. J. (1980) Suppressor monocytes in human disease: A review, in *Macrophages and Lymphocytes. Nature, Functions, and Interaction. Part B.* (Escobar M. R. and Friedman H., eds.), Plenum, New York, pp. 283–298.

328. Twomey J. T., Laughter A. H., Farrow S., and Douglass C. C.

(1975) Hodgkin's disease. An immunodepleting and immuno-suppressive disorder. *J. Clin. Invest.* **56**, 467–475.

329. Schechter G. P. and Soehnlen F. (1976) Monocyte-mediated inhibition of lymphocyte blastogenesis associated with peripheral blood monocytosis in Hodgkin's disease and tuberculosis. *Blood* **48**, 988.

330. Sheagren J. N., Block J. B., and Wolff S. M. (1967) Reticuloendothelial system phagocytic function in patients with Hodgkin's disease. *J. Clin. Invest.* **46**, 855–862.

331. Han T. (1980) Role of suppressor cells in depression of T lymphocyte proliferative response in untreated and treated Hodgkin's disease. *Cancer* **45**, 2102–2108.

332. Sieber G., Herrmann F., and Rüehl H. (1984) Suppression of B-lymphocyte differentiation in vitro by mononuclear peripheral blood and spleen cells from a patient with active Hodgkin's disease. *Immunol. Clin. Sper.* **3**, 131–137.

333. Goodwin J. S., Messner R. P., Bankhurst A. D., Peake G. T., Saiki J. H., and Williams R. C., Jr. (1977) Prostaglandin-producing suppressor cells in Hodgkin's disease. *N. Engl. J. Med.* **297**, 963–968.

334. Goodwin J. S., Bankhurst A. D., and Messner R. P. (1977) Suppression of human T-cell mitogenesis by prostaglandin. Existence of a prostaglandin-producing suppressor cell. *J. Exp. Med.* **146**, 1719–1734.

335. Han T. (1980) Indomethacin-mediated enhancement of lymphocyte response to mitogens in treated and untreated Hodgkin's disease (HD) and non-Hodgkin's lymphoma (NHL). *Proc. Am. Assoc. Cancer Res.* **21**, 374.

336. Fisher R. I. and Bostick-Bruton F. (1982) Depressed T cell proliferative responses in Hodgkin's disease: Role of monocyte-mediated suppression via prostaglandins and hydrogen peroxide. *J. Immunol.* **129**, 1770–1774.

337. DeShazo R. D. (1980) Indomethacin-responsive mononuclear cell dysfunction in Hodgkin's disease. *Clin. Immunol. Immunopathol.* **17**, 66–75.

338. Han T. and Winnicki M. S. (1980) Indomethacin-mediated enhancement of lymphocyte response to mitogens in treated and untreated Hodgkin's disease and non-Hodgkin's lymphoma. *NY State J. Med.* **80**, 1070–1075.

339. DeShazo R. D., Ewel C., Londono S., Metzger Z., Hoffeld J. T., and Oppenheim J. J. (1981) Evidence for the involvement of monocyte-derived toxic oxygen metabolites in the lymphocyte dysfunction of Hodgkin's disease. *Clin. Exp. Immunol.* **46**, 313–320.

340. Haim N., Meidav A., Samuelly B., Segal R., Mekori T., and Robinson E. (1984) Prostaglandin related and adherent cell suppressor system in apparently cured Hodgkin's disease patients. *J. Biol. Resp. Modif.* **3,** 219–225.

341. Bockman R. S. (1979) Prostaglandins and T-lymphocyte colonies in Hodgkin's disease. *Clin. Res.* **27,** 381A.

342. Bochman R. S. (1980) Stage-dependent reduction in T colony formation in Hodgkin's disease. Coincidence with monocyte synthesis of prostaglandins. *J. Clin. Invest.* **66,** 523–531.

343. Bochman R. S., and Rothschild M. (1979) Prostaglandin E inhibition of T-lymphocyte colony formation. A possible mechanism of monocyte modulation of clonal expansion. *J. Clin. Invest.* **64,** 812–819.

344. Thomas Y., Huchet R., and Grandjon D. (1981) Role of adherent suppressor cells in the depression of cell-mediated immunity in Hodgkin's disease and lung carcinoma. *Ann. Immunol. (Paris)* **132C,** 167–180.

345. Metzger Z., Hoffeld J. T., and Oppenheim J. J. (1980) Macrophage-mediated suppression. I. Evidence for participation of both hydrogen peroxide and prostaglandins in suppression of murine lymphocyte proliferation. *J. Immunol.* **124,** 983–988.

346. Weidemann M. J., Peskar B. A., Wrogemann K., Rietschel E. T., Staudinger H., and Fischer H. (1978) Prostaglandin and thromboxane synthesis in a pure macrophage population and the inhibition, by E-type prostaglandins, of chemiluminescence. *FEBS Lett.* **89,** 136–140.

347. Engleman E. G., Hoppe R., Kaplan H., Comminskey J., and McDevitt H. O. (1978) Suppressor cells of the mixed lymphocyte reaction in healthy subjects and patients with Hodgkin's disease and sarcoidosis. *Clin. Res.* **26,** 513A.

348. Engleman E. G., Benike C., Hoppe R. T., and Kaplan H. S. (1979) Suppressor cells of the mixed lymphocyte reaction in patients with Hodgkin's disease. *Transplant Proc.* **11,** 1827–1829.

349. Strober S., Slavin., Gottleib M., Zan-Bar I., King D. P., Hoppe R. T., Fuks Z., Grumet F. C., and Kaplan H. S. (1979) Allograft tolerance after total lymphoid irradiation (TLI). *Immunol. Rev.* **46,** 87–112.

350. Zarling J. M., Berman C., and Raich P. C. (1980) Depressed cytotoxic T-cell responses in previously treated Hodgkin's and non-Hodgkin's lymphoma patients. Evidence for histamine receptor-bearing suppressor cells. *Cancer Immunol. Immunother.* **7,** 243–249.

351. Schulof R. S., Lee B. J., Lacher M. J., Straus D. J., Clarkson B. D., Good R. A., and Gupta S. (1980) Concanavalin A-induced sup-

pressor cell activity in Hodgkin's disease. *Clin. Immunol. Immunopathol.* **16,** 454–462.

352. Akbar A. N., Jones D. B., and Wright D. H. (1984) Spontaneous and Concanavalin A-induced suppressor activity in control and Hodgkin's disease patients. *Br. J. Cancer* **49,** 349–356.

353. Vanhaelen C. P. J., and Fischer R. I. (1981) Increased sensitivity of lymphocytes from patients with Hodgkin's disease to Concanavalin A-induced suppressor cells. *J. Immunol.* **127,** 1216–1220.

354. Fisher R. I., Vanhaelen C., and Bostick F. (1981) Increased sensitivity to normal adherent suppressor cells in untreated advanced Hodgkin's disease. *Blood* **57,** 830–835.

355. Vanhaelen C. P. J., and Fisher R. I. (1982) Increased sensitivity of T cells to regulation by normal suppressor cells persists in long-term survivors with Hodgkin's disease. *Am. J. Med.* **72,** 385–390.

356. Kabakow B., Mines M. F., and King F. H. (1957) Hypercalcaemia in Hodgkin's disease. *N. Engl. J. Med.* **256,** 59–62.

357. Davies M., Mawer E. B., Hayes M. E., and Lumb G. A. (1985) Abnormal vitamin D metabolism in Hodgkin's lymphoma. *Lancet* **1,** 1186–1188.

358. Bar-Shavit Z., Teitelbaum S. L., Reitsma P., Hall A., Pegg L. E., Trial J., and Kahn A. J. (1983) Induction of monocytic differentiation and bone resorption by 1, 25 dihydroxyvitamin D_3. *Proc. Natl. Acad. Sci. USA* **80,** 5907–5911.

359. Bar-Shavit Z., Noff D., Edelstein S., Meyer M., Shibolet S., and Goldman R. (1981) 1, 25- dihydroxyvitamin D_3 and the regulation of macrophage function. *Calcif. Tissue Int.* **33,** 673–676.

360. Lemire J. M., Adams J. S., Kermani-Arab V., Bakke A. C., Sakai R., and Jordan S. C. (1985) 1, 25- dihydroxyvitamin D_3 suppresses human T helper/inducer lymphocyte activity in vitro. *J. Immunol.* **134,** 3032–3035.

361. Tsoukas C. D., Provvedini D. M., and Manolagas S. C. (1984) 1, 25-dihydroxyvitamin D_3: A novel immunoregulatory hormone. *Science* **224,** 1438–1440.

362. Fisher R. I., Bostick-Bruton F., Sauder D. N., Scala G., and Diehl V. (1983) Neoplastic cells obtained from Hodgkin's disease are potent stimulators of human primary mixed lymphocyte cultures. *J. Immunol.* **130,** 2666–2670.

363. Fisher R. I., Bates S. E., Bostick-Bruton F., Tuteja N., and Diehl V. (1984) Neoplastic cells obtained from Hodgkin's disease function as accessory cells for mitogen-induced human T cell proliferative responses. *J. Immunol.* **132,** 2672–2677.

364. Lukes R. J., Butler J. J., and Hicks E. B. (1966) Natural history of Hodgkin's disease as related to its pathologic picture. *Cancer* **19,** 317–344.

365. Burchenal J. H. (1982) Hematologic neoplasms. Introduction, in *Cancer Medicine* (Holland J. F. and Frei E. III, eds.), Lea and Febiger, Philadelphia pp. 1373–1378.

366. Foon K. A., Schroff R. W., and Gale R. P. (1982) Surface markers on leukemia and lymphoma cells: Recent advances. *Blood* **60**, 1–19.

367. Stein H., Lennert K., Feller A. C., Mason D. Y. (1984) Immunohistological analysis of human lymphoma: Correlation of histological and immunological categories. *Adv. Cancer Res.* **42**, 67–147.

368. Koeffler H. P., and Golde D. W. (1981) Chronic myelogenous leukemia—new concepts. *N. Engl. J. Med.* **304**, 1201–1209.

369. DeVita V. T., Jr., Fisher R. I., Johnson R. E., and Berard C. W. (1982) Non-Hodgkin's lymphomas, *Cancer Medicine*, (Holland J. F. and Frei E. III, eds.), Lea & Febiger, Philadelphia, pp, 1502–1537.

370. Devita V. T., Jr., Jaffe E. S., and Hellman S. (1985) Hodgkin's disease and the non-Hodgkin's lymphomas, in *Cancer Principles and Practice of Oncology* (DeVita V. T., Jr., Hellman S., and Rosenberg and S. A., eds.) J.B. Lippincott, Philadelphia, pp. 1623–1709.

371. Cossman J., Jaffe E. S., and Fisher R. I. (1984) Immunologic phenotypes of diffuse, aggressive, non-Hodgkin's lymphomas. Correlation with clinical features. *Cancer* **54**, 1310–1317.

372. Rubinstein A. and Dauber L. G. (1983) Lymphoma of cytotoxic suppressor T cell phenotype T-8 following angio immuno blastic lymph adenopathy. *Oncology* **40**, 195–199.

373. Durham J. C., Stephens D. S., Rimland D., Nassar V. H., and Spira T. J. (1987) Common variable hypogammaglobulinemia complicated by an unusual T-suppressor/cytotoxic cell lymphoma. *Cancer* **59**, 271–276.

374. Jones S. E., Griffith K., Dombrowski P., and Gaines J. A. (1977) Immunodeficiency in patients with non-Hodgkin's lymphomas. *Blood* **49**, 335–344.

375. Advani S. H., Dinshaw K. A., Nair C. N., Gopal R., Talwalker G. V., Iyyer Y. S., Bhatia H. M., and Desai P. B. (1980) Immune dysfunction in non-Hodgkin's lymphoma. *Cancer* **45**, 2843–2848.

376. Miller D. G. (1962) Patterns of immunological deficiency in lymphomas and leukemias. *Ann. Intern. Med.* **57**, 703–716.

377. Gattringer C., Huber H., Radaszkiewicz T., Pfaller W., and Braunsteiner H. (1984) Imbalance of helper and suppressor T lymphocytes in malignant non-Hodgkin's lymphomas: An in situ morphometric analysis. *Int. J. Cancer* **33**, 751–757.

378. Raziuddin S., Hussain N. K., and Latif A. B. A. (1987) A monoclonal antibody and functional study of malignant T cells of a pa-

tient with suppressor-T-cell lymphoma. *Clin. Immunol. Immunopathol.* **45**, 230–234.

379. Whisler R. L., Balcerzak S. P., and Murray J. L. (1981) Heteroge-
      neous mechanisms of impaired lymphocyte responses in non-
      Hodgkin's lymphoma. *Blood* **57**, 1081–1087.

380. Whisler R. L., Murray J. L., Roach R. W., and Balcerzak S. P.
      (1984) Characterization of multiple immune defects in human
      malignant lymphoma. *Cancer* **53**, 2628–2634.

381. Shohat B., Shaklai M., Nemes L., and Trainin N. (1984) Immune
      modulation of a T-suppressor cell lymphoma by thymic humoral
      factor, a thymic hormone. *Cancer* **54**, 2122–2126.

382. Rümke H. C., Miedema F., ten Berge I. J. M., Terpstra F., van der
      Reijden H. J., van de Griend R. J., de Bruin H. G., Von dem
      Borne A. E. Gk., Smit J. W., Zeijlemaker W. P., and Melief C. J.
      M. (1982) Functional properties of T cells in patients with chronic
      T γ lymphocytosis and chronic T cell neoplasia. *J. Immunol.* **129**,
      419–426.

383. Mangan K. F., Zidar B., Shadduck R.K., Zeigler Z., and
      Winkelstein A. (1985) Interferon-induced aplasia: Evidence for
      T-cell-mediated suppression of hematopoiesis and recovery after
      treatment with horse antihuman thymocyte globulin. *Am. J.
      Hematol.* **19**, 401–413.

384. Borden E. C. and Ball L. A. (1981) Interferons: Biochemical cell
      growth inhibitory and immunological effects. *Prog. Hematol.* **12**,
      299–339.

385. Stiehm E. R., Kronenberg L. H., Rosenblatt H. M., Bryson Y.,
      and Merigan T. C. (1982) Interferon: Immunobiology and clinical
      significance. *Ann. Intern. Med.* **96**, 80–93.

386. Mangan K. F., Hartnett M. E., Matis S. A., Winkelstien A., and
      Abo T. (1984) Natural killer cells suppress human erythroid stem
      cell proliferation in vitro. *Blood* **63**, 260–269.

387. Hooks J. J., Haynes B. F., Detrick-Hooks B., Diehl L. F., Gerrard
      T. L., and Fauci A. S. (1982) Gamma (immune) interferon produc-
      tion by leukocytes from a patient with a Tγ cell proliferative dis-
      ease. *Blood* **59**, 198–201.

388. Zoumbos N., Gascon P., Djeu J., and Young N. (1983) Interferon
      is the mediator of hematopoeitic suppression in aplastic anemia
      in vitro and possibly in vivo. *Blood (Suppl)* **62**, 52.

389. Whittle H. C., Brown J., Marsh K., Greenwood B. M., Seidelin
      P., Tighe H., and Wedderbrun L. (1984) T cell control of Epstein-
      Barr virus-infected B cells is lost during P. falciparum malaria.
      Nature **312**, 449–450.

390. Tosato G., Magrath I., Koski I., Dooley N., and Blaese M. (1979)
      Activation of suppressor T cells during Epstein-Barr-virus-

induced infectious mononucleosis. *N. Engl. J. Med.* **301,** 1133–1137.

391. Wang F., Blaese R. M., Zoon K. C., and Tosato G. (1987) Suppressor T cell clones from patients with acute Epstein-Barr virus-induced infectious mononucleosis. *J. Clin. Invest.* **79,** 7–14.

392. Sundar S. K. and Menezes J. (1985) Generation of Epstein-Barr virus antigen-specific suppressor T cells in vitro. *Int. J. Cancer.* **35,** 351–357.

393. Henderson E. S. and Jones B. (1982) Acute lymphoblastic leukemia, in *Cancer Medicine* (Holland J. F. and Frei E. III, eds.) Lea and Febiger, (1986) Philadelphia, pp. 1379–1406.

394. Knowles D. M. II (1986) The human T-cell leukemias: Clinical, cytomorphologic, immunophenotypic, and genotypic characteristics. *Hum. Pathol.* **17,** 14–33.

395. Cossman J., Neckers L. M., Arnold A., and Korsmeyer S. J. (1982) Induction of differentiation in a case of common, acute lymphoblastic leukemia. *N. Engl. J. Med.* **307,** 1251–1254.

396. Poplack D. G., Cassady J. R., and Pizzo P. A. (1985) Leukemias and lymphomas of childhood, in *Cancer Principles and Practice of Oncology* (DeVita V. T., Jr., Hellman S., Rosenberg S. A., eds.), J.B. Lippincott, Philadelphia, pp. 1591–1622.

397. Reinherz E. L., Nadler L. M., Sallan S. E., and Schlossman S. F. (1979) Subset derivation of T-cell acute lymphoblastic leukemia in man. *J. Clin. Invest.* **64,** 392–397.

398. Evans R. L., Lazarus H., Penta A. C. and Schlossman S. F. (1978) Two functionally distinct subpopulations of human T cells that collaborate in the generation of cytotoxic cells responsible for cell-mediated lympholysis. *J. Immunol.* **120,** 1423–1428.

399. Reinherz E. L. and Scholossman S. F. (1979) Con A-inducible suppression of MLC: Evidence for mediation by the H_2^+ cell subset in man. *J. Immunol.* **122,** 1335–1341.

400. Reinherz E. L., Kung P. C., Goldstein G., Levey R. H., and Schlossman S. F. (1980) Discrete stages of human intrathymic differentiation: Analysis of normal thymocytes and leukemic lymphoblasts of T-cell lineage. *Proc. Natl. Acad. Sci. USA* **77,** 1588–1592.

401. Roper M., Crist W. M., Metzgar R., Ragab A. H., Smith S., Starling K., Pullen J., Leventhal B., Bartolucci A. A., and Cooper M. D. (1983) Monoclonal antibody characterization of surface antigens in childhood T-cell lymphoid malignancies. *Blood* **61,** 830–837.

402. Nasrallah A. G. and Miale T.D. (1983) Decreased natural killer cell activity in children with untreated acute leukemia. *Cancer Res.* **43,** 5580–5585.

403. Gorski A., Rokicka-Milewska R., Madalinski K., Jagielski P., Derulska D., Litwin J., Gaciong Z., and Korczak-Kowalska G. (1983) Deficiency of short-lived suppressor cells controlling T lymphocyte colony formation in acute lymphoblastic leukemia. *Arch. Immunol. Ther. Exp.* **31**, 93–98.

404. Ballieux R. E., Heijnen C. J., Uytdehaag F., and Zegers B. J. M. (1979) Regulation of B cell activity in man: Role of T cells. *Immunol. Rev.* **45**, 3–39.

405. Thomas Y., Rogozinski L., Irigoyen O. H., Friedman S. M., Kung P. C., Goldstein G., and Chess L. (1981) Functional analysis of human T cell subsets defined by monoclonal antibodies. IV. Induction of suppressor cells within the OKT4$^+$ population. *J. Exp. Med.* **154**, 459–467.

406. Thomas Y., Rogozinski L., Irigoyen O. H., Shen H. H., Talle M. A., Goldstein G., and Chess L. (1982) Functional analysis of human T cell subsets defined by monoclonal antibodies. V. Suppressor cells within the activated OKT4$^+$ population belong to a distinct subset. *J. Immunol.* **128**, 1386–1390.

407. Broder S., Uchiyama T., Muul L. M., Goldman C., Sharrow S., Poplack D. G., and Waldmann T. A. (1981) Activation of leukemic pro-suppressor cells to become suppressor-effector cells. Influence of cooperating normal T cells. *N. Engl. J. Med.* **304**, 1382–1387.

408. Canellos G. P. (1985) Chronic leukemias, in *Cancer Principles and Practice of Oncology* (DeVita V. T., Jr., Hellman S., and Rosenberg S. A., eds.) J.B. Lippincott, Philadelphia, pp. 1739–1752.

409. Dameshek W. (1967) Chronic lymphocytic leukemia—an accumulative disease of immunologically incompetent lymphocytes. *Blood* **29**, 566–584.

410. Aisenberg A. C. (1981) Cell-surface markers in lymphoproliferative disease. *N. Engl. J. Med.* **304**, 331–336.

411. Catovsky D., Pittman S., O'Brien M., Cherchi M., Costello C., Foa R., Pearce E., Hoffbrand A. V., Janossy G., Ganeshaguru K., and Greaves M. F. (1979) Multiparameter studies in lymphoid leukemias. *Am. J. Clin. Pathol.* **72**, 736–745.

412. Klein E. and Schwartz R. A. (1982) Cancer and the skin, in *Cancer Medicine* (Holland J. F. and Frei E. III, eds.), Lea and Febiger, Philadelphia, pp. 2057–2108.

413. Bakri K., Ezdinli E. Z., Wasser L. P., Han T., Sinclair T., Singh S., Ozer H., and Minowada J. (1984) T-suppressor cell chronic lymphocytic leukemia. Phenotypic characterization by monoclonal antibodies. *Cancer* **54**, 284–292.

414. Reynolds C. W. and Foon K. A. (1984) Tγ -lymphoproliferative disease and related disorders in humans and experimental ani-

mals: A review of the clinical, cellular, and functional characteristics. *Blood* **64**, 1146–1158.

415. Uchiyama T., Yodoi J., Sagawa K., Takatsuki K., and Uchino H. (1977) Adult T-cell leukemia: Clinical and hematologic features of 16 cases. *Blood* **50**, 481–492.

416. Gunz F. W. (1982) Chronic lymphocytic leukemia, in *Cancer Medicine* (Holland J. F. and Frei E. III, eds.), Lea and Febiger, Philadelphia, pp. 1460–1477.

417. Platsoucas C. D., Kempin S., Karanas A., Clarkson B., and Good R. A. (1980) Receptors for immunoglobulin isotype of T and B lymphocytes from untreated patients with chronic lymphocytic leukaemia. *Clin. Exp. Immunol.* **40**, 256–263.

418. Lauria F., Foa R., and Catovsky D. (1980) Increase in Tγ lymphocytes in B-cell chronic lymphocytic leukaemia. *Scand. J. Haematol.* **24**, 187–190.

419. Catovsky D., Lauria F., Matutes E., Foa R., Mantovani V., Tura S., and Galton D. A. G. (1981) Increase in Tγ lymphocytes in B-cell chronic lymphocytic leukaemia. II. Correlation with clinical stage and findings in B-prolymphocytic leukaemia. *Br. J. Haematol.* **47**, 539–544.

420. Inoshita T. and Whiteside T. L. (1981) Imbalance of T-cell subpopulations does not result in defective helper function in chronic lymphocytic leukemia. *Cancer* **48**, 1754–1760.

421. Dainer P. M. and Spiegelberg H. L. (1978) Fc receptors for IgG, IgM and IgE on human leukemic lymphocytes. *Clin. Res.* **26**, 513A.

422. Kay N. E., Johnson J. D., Stanek R., and Douglas S. D. (1979) T-cell subpopulations in chronic lymphocytic leukemia: Abnormalities in distribution and in in vitro receptor maturation. *Blood* **54**, 540–544.

423. McCann S. R., Whelan C. A., Willoughby R., Lawlor E., Greally J., and Temperley I. J. (1980) T-lymphocyte function in B-chronic lymphatic leukemia (CLL). *Br. J. Haematol.* **46**, 331–332.

424. Kay N. E. (1981) Abnormal T-cell subpopulation function in CLL: Excessive suppressor (Tγ) and deficient helper (Tμ) activity with respect to B-cell proliferation. *Blood* **57**, 418–420.

425. Semenzato G., Pezzutto A., Agostini C., Albertin M., and Gasparotto G. (1981) T-lymphocyte subpopulations in chronic lymphocytic leukemia: A quantitative and functional study. *Cancer* **48**, 2191–2197.

426. Semenzato G., Pezzutto A., Foa R., Lauria F., and Raimondi R. (1983) T lymphocytes in B-cell chronic lymphocytic leukemia: characterization by monoclonal antibodies and correlation with Fc receptors. *Clin. Immunol. Immunopathol.* **26**, 155–161.

427. Samarut C. and Revillard J.-P. (1980) Active passive re-expression of Fcγ receptors on human lymphocytes. *Eur. J. Immunol.* **10,** 352–358.

428. Davis S. (1981) Characterization of the phytohemagglutinin-induced proliferating lymphocyte subpopulations in chronic lymphocytic leukemia patients using a clonogenic agar technique and monoclonal antibodies. *Blood* **58,** 1053–1055.

429. Matutes E., Wechsler A., Gomez R., Cherchi M., and Catovsky D. (1981) Unusual T-cell phenotype in advanced B-chronic lymphocytic leukaemia. *Br. J. Haematol.* **49,** 635–642.

430. Herrmann F., Lochner A., Philippen H., Jauer B., and Rühl H. (1982) Imbalance of T cell subpopulations in patients with chronic lymphocytic leukaemia of the B cell type. *Clin. Exp. Immunol.* **49,** 157–162.

431. Mangan K. F., Chikkappa G., and Farley P. C. (1982) T gamma (Tγ) cells suppress growth of erythroid colony-forming units in vitro in the pure red cell aplasia of B-cell chronic lymphocytic leukemia. *J. Clin. Invest.* **70,** 1148–1156.

432. Mills K. H. G., Worman C. P., and Cawley J. C. (1982) T-cell subsets in B-chronic lymphocytic leukaemia (CLL). *Br. J. Haematol.* **50,** 710–712.

433. Platsoucas C. D., Galinski M., Kempin S., Reich L., Clarkson B., and Good R. A. (1982) Abnormal T lymphocyte subpopulations in patients with B cell chronic lymphocytic leukemia: An analysis by monoclonal antibodies. *J. Immunol.* **129,** 2305–2312.

434. Lahat N., Aghai E., Quitt M., Nir E., and Froom P. (1985) A subpopulation of suppressor cells in Richter's syndrome with both monocytic and T-lymphocytic characteristics. *Am. J. Haematol.* **20,** 293–296.

435. Mangan K. F. and D'Allessandro L. (1985) Hypoplastic anemia in B cell chronic lymphocytic leukemia: Evolution of T cell-mediated suppression of erythropoiesis in early-stage and late-stage disease. *Blood* **66,** 533–541.

436. Rai K. R., Cronkite E. P., Sawitsky A., Chandra P., and Steinberg J. (1985) Studies in chronic lymphocytic leukemia: blood lymphocyte surface characteristics and immunologic functional status of patients and correlation with clinical stage. *Ann. NY Acad. Sci.* **459,** 336–343.

437. Silber R. and Conklyn M. (1984) Decreased 5'-nucleotidase activity in a T lymphocyte subpopulation from patients with B cell chronic lymphocytic leukemia. *Blood* **64,** 479–481.

438. Hersey P., Wotherspoon J., Reid G., and Gunz F. W. (1980) Hypogammaglobulinaemia associated with abnormalities of both

B and T lymphocytes in patients with chronic lymphocytic leukaemia. *Clin. Exp. Immunol.* **39**, 698–707.

439. Faguet G. B. (1979) Mechanisms of lymphocyte activation. The role of suppressor cells in the proliferative responses of chronic lymphatic leukemia lymphocytes. *J. Clin. Invest.* **63**, 67–74.

440. Bloem A. C., Heijnen C. J., Bast B. J. E. G., and Ballieux R. E. (1985) T cells in B cell chronic lymphocytic leukemia. II. Lack of antigen-specific T suppressor cells and their progenitors. *J. Immunol.* **135**, 4261–4265.

441. Ayanlar-Batuman O., Ebert E., and Hauptman S. P. (1986) Defective Interleukin-2 production and responsiveness by T cells in patients with chronic lymphocytic leukemia of B cell variety. *Blood* **67**, 279–284.

442. Fu S. M., Chiorazzi N., Kunkel H. G., Halper J. P., and Harris S. R. (1978) Induction of in vitro differentiation and immunoglobulin synthesis of human leukemic B lymphocytes. *J. Exp. Med.* **148**, 1570–1578.

443. Chiorazzi N., Fu S. M., Montazeri G., Kunkel H. G., Rai K., and Gee T. (1979) T cell helper defect in patients with chronic lymphocytic leukemia. *J. Immunol.* **122**, 1087–1090.

444. Wolos J. A. and Davey F. R. (1979) Depressed stimulation in the MLR by B lymphocytes in chronic lymphocytic leukemia: Failure to demonstrate suppressor cell. *Clin. Immunol. Immunopathol.* **14**, 77–85.

445. Fernandez L. A., MacSween J. M., and Langley G. R. (1981) Impaired T-cell responses in chronic lymphocytic leukemia: Lack of suppressor cell effect. *Clin. Immunol. Immunopathol.* **18**, 168–175.

446. Fauci A. S., Pratt K. R., and Whalen G. (1977) Intrinsic B cell defect in the immunoglobulin deficiency of chronic lymphocytic leukemia. *Clin Res.* **25**, 482A.

447. Fernandez L. A., MacSween J. M., and Langley G. R. (1983) Immunoglobulin secretory function of B cells from untreated patients with chronic lymphocytic leukemia and hypogammaglobulinemia: Role of T cells. *Blood* **62**, 767–774.

448. Andersson J. and Melchers F. (1974) Maturation of mitogen-activated bone marrow-derived lymphocytes in the absence of proliferation. *Eur. J. Immunol.* **4**, 533–539.

449. Makinodan T. and Kay M. M. B. (1980) Age influence on the immune system. *Adv. Immunol.* **29**, 287–330.

450. Mangan K. F., Chikkappa G., Bieler L. Z., and Scharfman W. B. (1981) The role of T lymphocytes bearing Fc receptors for IgM or IgG in the pathogenesis of pure red cell aplasia in a patient with chronic lymphocytic leukemia, in *Experimental Hematology Today*

(Baum S. J., Ledney G. D., and Khan A. eds.), S. Karger, Basel pp. 161–168.

451. Mangan K. F. (1983) Hypoplastic anemia in B cell chronic lymphocytic leukemia (CLL): Correlation of erythroid progenitor cell (CFU-E) growth with RAI stage and marrow T gamma (Tγ) cell frequency. *Exp. Hematol.* **11,** 83.

452. Hoffman R., Kopel S., Hsu S. D., Dainiak N., and Zanjani E. D. (1978) T cell chronic lymphocytic leukemia: Presence in bone marrow and peripheral blood of cells that suppress erythropoiesis in vitro. *Blood* **52,** 255–260.

453. Nagasawa T., Abe T., and Nakagawa T. (1981) Pure red cell aplasia and hypogammaglobulinemia associated with Tr-cell chronic lymphocytic leukemia. *Blood* **57,** 1025–1031.

454. Jansen J., Schuit H. R. E., Meijer C. J. L. M., Le Bein T. W., Hijmans W., and Kersey J. H. (1981) Cell markers in hairy-cell leukemia, in *Leukemia Markers* (Knapp W., ed.), Academic Press, London, p. 179).

455. Cawley J. C., Burns G. F., Worman C. P., Roberts B. E., and Hayhoe F. G. J. (1980) Clinical and hematologic fluctuations in hairy-cell leukemia: A sequential surface-marker analysis. *Blood* **55,** 784–791.

456. Worman C. P. and Cawley J. C. (1982) Monoclonal antibody-defined T-cell subsets in hairy-cell leukemia. *Scand. J. Haematol.* **29,** 338–344.

457. Planas A. T., Zamkoff K. W., Poiesz B. J., Kurec A. S., and Davey F. R. (1983) T-cell prolymphocytic leukemia with a suppressor phenotype. *Ann. Clin. Lab. Sci.* **13,** 193–200.

458. Pandolfi F., De Rossi G., Semenzato G., Quinti I., Ranucci A., De Sanctis G., Lopez M., Gasparotto G., and Aiuti F. (1982) Immunologic evaluation of T chronic lymphocyte leukemia cells: correlations among phenotype, functional activities, and morphology. *Blood* **59,** 688–695.

459. Catovsky D., Wechsler A., Matutes E., Gomez R., Bourikas G., Cherchi M., Pepys E. O., Pepys M. B., Kitani T., Hoffbrand A. V., and Greaves M. F. (1982) The membrane phenotype of T-prolymphocytic leukaemia. *Scand. J. Haematol.* **29,** 398–404.

460. Shimoyama M., Tobinai K., Hirose M., and Minato K. (1982) Cellular origin of T cell malignancies. *Gann Monograph on Cancer Research* **28,** 23–35.

461. Krajewski A. S., Dewar A. E., Seidelin P. H., and Murray R. (1983) Colony formation and interleukin 2 production by leukaemic human T cells. *Clin. Exp. Immunol.* **54,** 103–109.

462. Koubek K., Hrodek O., Stary J., Chudomel V., and Malasková V.

(1985) Immunologic characterization of T-lymphoproliferative disorders by monoclonal antibodies. *Folia Haematol.* **112**, 649–657.

463. Thien S. L., Catovsky D., Oscier D., Goldman J. M., van der Reijden H. J., Melief C. J. M., Rümke H. C., ten Berge R. J. M., and von dem Borne A. E. G. K. R. (1982) T-chronic lymphocytic leukaemia presenting as primary hypogammaglobulinaemia— evidence of a proliferation of T-suppressor cells. *Clin. Exp. Immunol.* **47**, 670–676.

464. Geisler C., Ralfkiaer E., Astrup L., Christensen I., Dickmeiss E., Hansen M. M., Larsen J. K., Petersen J., and Plesner T. (1983) Chronic lymphocytic leukaemia of T cell origin. Clinical variation possibly due to involvement of different T lymphocyte subpopulations. *Scand. J. Haematol.* **31**, 109–121.

465. Volk J. R., Kjeldsberg C. R., Eyre H. J., and Marty J. (1983) T-cell prolymphocytic leukemia. Clinical and immunologic characterization. *Cancer* **52**, 2049–2054.

466. Crosier P. S. (1986) In vitro function of a T-cell chronic lymphocytic leukemia with suppressor cell phenotype. *Aust. NZ J. Med.* **16**, 389–392.

467. Hui P. K., Feller A. C., Pileri S., Gobbi M., and Lennert K. (1987) New aggresive variant of suppressor/cytotoxic T-CLL. *Am. J. Clin. Pathol.* **87**, 55–59.

468. Hofman F. M., Smith D., and Hocking W. (1982) T cell chronic lymphocytic leukaemia with suppressor phenotype. *Clin Exp. Immunol.* **49**, 401–409.

469. Stavem P., Førre O., Brandtzaeg P., and Nyberg H. (1983) T-lymphocytes with both helper- and suppressor markers on the same cell in chronic lymphocytic leukaemia. *Scand. J. Haematol.* **30**, 177–182.

470. Simpkins H., Kiprov D. D., Davis J. L., Morand P., Puri S., and Grahn E. P. (1985) T cell chronic lymphocytic leukemia with lymphocytes of unusual immunologic phenotype and function. *Blood* **65**, 127–133.

471. Pandolfi F., Strong D. M., Slease R. B., Smith M. L., Ortaldo J. R., and Herberman R. B. (1980) Characterization of a suppressor T-cell chronic lymphocytic leukemia with ADCC but not NK activity. *Blood* **56**, 653–660.

472. Kai S., Hamano T., Fujita S., Nakamuta K., Hara H., and Nagai K. (1980) Suppression of mitogen- and alloantigen-induced proliferation by chronic lymphocytic leukemia. Cells of T-cell origin. *Clin. Immunol. Immunopathol.* **17**, 427–438.

473. Zamkoff K. W., Poiesz B. J., Ruscetti F. W., Moore J. L., Davey F. R., Planas A. T., and Lamberson H. (1984) Functional diversity

within the suppressor phenotype as defined by monoclonal anti-body in T-cell prolymphocytic leukemia. *Am. J. Hematol.* **16,** 409–417.

474. Mangan K. F., Volkin R., and Winkelstein A. (1986) Autoreactive erythroid progenitor-T suppressor cells in the pure red cell apla-sia associated with thymoma and panhypogammaglobulinemia. *Am. J. Hematol.* **23,** 167–173.

475. Lutzner M. R., Edelson R., Schein P., Green I., Kirkpatrick C., and Ahmed A. (1975) Cutaneous T-cell lymphomas: The Sézary syndrome, mycosis fungoides, and related disorders. *Ann. Intern. Med.* **83,** 534–552.

476. Gupta S., Safai B., and Good R. A. (1978) Subpopulations of hu-man T lymphocytes. IV. Quantitation and distribution in patients with mycosis fungoides and Sézary syndrome. *Cell Immunol.* **39,** 18–26.

477. Greaves M., Delia D., Sutherland R., Rao J., Verbi W., Kemshead J., Hariri G., Goldstein G., and Kung P. (1981) Expression of the OKT monoclonal antibody defined antigenic determinants in ma-lignancy. *Int. J. Immunopharmacology* **3,** 283–300.

478. Farnarier-Seidel C., Kaplanski S., Golstein M.-M., Jancovici E., Sayag J., and Depieds R. (1983) An OKT4+ T-cell population with suppressor activity in Sézary syndrome. *Scand. J. Immunol.* **18,** 389–398.

479. Broder S., Edelson R. L., Lutzner M. A., Nelson D. L., MacDermott R. P., Durm M. E., Goldman C. K., Meade B. D., and Waldmann T. A. (1976) The Sézary syndrome. A malignant proliferation of helper T cells. *J. Clin. Invest.* **58,** 1297–1306.

480. Lawrence E. C., Broder S., Jaffe E. S., Braylan R. C., Dobbins W. O., Young R. C., and Waldmann T. A. (1978) Evolution of a lym-phoma with helper T cell characteristics in Sézary syndrome. *Blood* **52,** 481–492.

481. Kansu E. and Hauptman S. P. (1979) Suppressor cell population in Sézary syndrome. *Clin. Immunol. Immunopathol.* **12,** 341–350.

482. Hopper J. E. and Haren J. M. (1980) Studies on a Sézary lympho-cyte population with T-suppressor activity. Suppression of Ig synthesis of normal peripheral blood lymphocytes. *Clin. Immunol. Immunopathol.* **17,** 43–54.

483. Goldstein M. M., Farnarier-Seidel C., Daubney P., and Kaplanski S. (1986) An OKT4+ T-cell population in Sézary syndrome: At-tempts to elucidate its lack of proliferative capacity and its sup-pressive effect. *Scand. J. Immunol.* **23,** 53–64.

484. Catovsky D., Greaves M. F., Rose M., Galton D. A. G., Goolden A. W. G., McCluskey D. R., White J. M., Lampert I., Bourikas G., Ireland R., Brownell A. I., Bridges J. M., Blattner W. A., and

Gallo R. C. (1982) Adult T-cell lymphoma-leukaemia in blacks from the West Indies. *Lancet* **1**, 639–643.

485. Blayney D. W., Blattner W. A., Robert-Guroff M., Jaffe E. S., Fisher R. I., Bunn P. A., Jr., Patton M. G., Rarick H. R., and Gallo R. C. (1983) The human T-cell leukemia-lymphoma virus (HTLV) in the southeastern United States. *J. Am. Med. Assoc.* **250**, 1048–1052.

486. Gallo R. C. and Wong-Staal F. (1982) Retroviruses as etiologic agents of some animal and human leukemias and lymphomas and as tools for elucidating the molecular mechanism of leukemogenesis. *J. Am. Soc. Hematol.* **60**, 545–557.

487. Hattori T., Uchiyama T., Toibana T., Takatsuki K., and Uchino H. (1981) Surface phenotype of Japanese adult T-cell leukemia cells characterized by monoclonal antibodies. *Blood* **58**, 645–647.

488. Nakahara K, Òhashi T., Ichimaru M., Amagasaki T., Shimoyama M., Nakauchi H., and Okumura K. (1982) Analyses of adult T-cell leukemia using the monoclonal (anti-Leu-1, anti-Leu-2a, and anti-Leu-3a) and heterologous anti-glycolipid (anti-asialo GM_1) antibodies. *Clin. Immunol. Immunopathol.* **25**, 43–52.

489. Blayney D. W., Jaffe E. S., Blattner W. A., Cossman J., Robert-Guroff M., Longo D. L., Bunn P. A., Jr., and Gallo R. C. (1983) The human T-cell leukemia/lymphoma virus associated with American adult T-cell leukemia/lymphoma. *Blood* **62**, 401–405.

490. Yamada Y. (1983) Phenotypic and functional analysis of leukemic cells from 16 patients with adult T-cell leukemia/lymphoma. *Blood* **61**, 192–199.

491. Miedema F., Terpstra F. G., Smit J. W., Daenen S., Gerrits W., Hegde U., Matutes E., Catovsky D., Greaves M. F., and Melief C. J. M. (1984) Functional properties of neoplastic T cells in adult T cell lymphoma/leukemia patients from the Caribbean. *Blood* **63**, 477–481.

492. Waldmann T. A., Greene W. C., Sarin P. S., Saxinger C., Blayney D. W., Blattner W. A., Goldman C. K., Bongiovanni K., Sharrow S., Depper J. M., Leonard W., Uchiyama T., and Gallo R. C. (1984) Functional and phenotypic comparison of human T cell leukemia/lymphoma virus positive adult T cell leukemia with human T cell leukemia/lymphoma virus negative Sézary leukemia, and their distinction using anti-Tac. Monoclonal antibody identifying the human receptor for T cell growth factor. *J. Clin. Invest.* **73**, 1711–1718.

493. Morimoto C., Matsuyama T., Oshige C., Tanaka H., Hercend T., Reinherz E. L., and Schlossman S. F. (1985) Functional and phenotypic studies of Japanese adult T cell leukemia cells. *J. Clin. Invest.* **75**, 836–843.

494. Yamada Y., Amagasaki T., Kamihira S., Kinoshita K., Ikeda S., Kusano M., Suzuyama J., Toriya K., Tomonaga Y., and Ichimaru M. (1985) T lymphomas associated with human T-cell leukemia-lymphoma virus may show phenotypic and functional differences from adult T-cell leukemias. *Clin. Immunol. Immunopathol.* **36**, 306–319.

495. Okawa H., Takase K., Takagi S., Yata J., Matsumoto M., and Matsumoto T. (1986) Immunoregulatory function and expression of OKT17 antigen of adult T-cell leukemia cells. *Cancer* **57**, 732–736.

496. Tatsumi E., Takiuchi Y., Domae N., Shirakawa S., Uchino H., Baba M., Yasuhira K., and Morikawa S. (1980) Suppressive activity of some leukemic T cells from adult patients in Japan. *Clin. Immunol. Immunopathol.* **15**, 190–199.

497. Uchiyama T., Sagawa K., Takatsuki K., and Uchino H. (1978) Effect of adult T-cell leukemia cells on pokeweed mitogen-induced normal B-cell differentiation. *Clin. Immunol. Immunopathol.* **10**, 24–34.

498. Hattori T., Uchiyama T., Takatsuki K., and Uchino H. (1980) Presence of human B-lymphocyte antigens on adult T-cell leukemia cells. *Clin. Immunol. Immunopathol.* **17**, 287–295.

499. Brouet J.-C. (1980) Proliferation of Tγ cells with killer-cell activity in patients with neutropenia. *N. Engl. J. Med.* **303**, 882.

500. Melief C., van de Griend R., Rümke H., de Bruin H., Astaldi A., Bom-van Noorloos A., Pegels H., van Oers R., Goudsmit R., Zeijlemaker W., von dem Borne A. Kr., Silberbusch J., and Feltkamp-Vroom T. (1980) Proliferation of Tγ cells with killer-cell activity in patients with neutropenia. *N. Engl. J. Med.* **303**, 882–883.

501. Semenzato G., Pizzolo G., Ranucci A., Agostini C., Chilosi M., Quinti I., De Sanctis G., Vercelli B., and Pandolfi F. (1984) Abnormal expansions of polyclonal large to small size granular lymphocytes: Reactive or neoplastic process? *Blood* **63**, 1271–1277.

502. Aisenberg A. C., Wilkes B. M., Harris N. L., Ault K. A., and Carey R. W. (1981) Chronic T-cell lymphocytosis with neutropenia: Report of a case sutdy with monoclonal antibody. *Blood* **58**, 818–822.

503. Callard R. E., Smith C. M., Worman C., Linch D., Cawley J. C., and Beverley P. C. L. (1981) Unusual phenotype and function of an expanded subpopulation of T cells in patients with haemopoietic disorders. *Clin. Exp. Immunol.* **43**, 497–505.

504. Bom-van Noorloos A. A., Pegels H. G., van Oers R. H. J., Silberbusch J., Feltkamp-Vroom T. M., Goudsmit R., Zeijlemaker W. P., von dem Borne A. E. G. K.R., and Melief C. J. M. (1980)

Proliferation of Tγ cells with killer-cell activity in two patients with neutropenia and recurrent infections. *N. Engl. J. Med.* **302**, 933–937.

505. Tanzer J. and Frei E. III (1982) Chronic myelocytic leukemia, in *Cancer Medicine* (Holland J. F. and Frei E. III, eds.) Lea and Febiger, Philadelphia, pp. 1446–1460.

506. Somasundaram R., Advani S. H., and Gangal S. G. (1983) Concanavalin A induced suppressor cell activity and autorosette forming cells in chronic myeloid leukemia patients. *Br. J. Cancer* **48**, 783–790.

507. Shubinskii G. Z. and Lozovoi V. P. (1983) T lymphocytes functional properties of patients with chronic lymphocytic leukemia. *Immunologiya* **4**, 62–65.

508. Hamaoka T., Matsuzaki N., Itoh K., Tsuji Y., Izumi Y., Fujiwara H., and Ono S. (1983) Human trophoblast- and tumor cell-derived immunoregulatory factor, in *Reproductive Immunology, 1983. Preceedings of the 2nd International Congress of Reproductive Immunology, Kyoto, 1983* (Isojima S. and Billington W. D. eds.), Elsevier, Amsterdam, pp. 133–146.

509. Fleisher T. A., Greene W. C., Uchiyama T., Goldman C. K., Nelson D. L., Blaese R. M., and Waldmann T. A. (1981) Characterization of a soluble suppressor of human B cell immunoglobin biosynthesis produced by a continuous human suppressor T cell line. *J. Exp. Med* **154**, 156–167.

510. Sacchi N., Fiorini G., Plevani P., Badaracco G., Breviario D., and Ginelli E. (1983) Acquisition of deoxyguanosine resistance by TPA-induced T lymphoid lines. *J. Immunol.* **130**, 1622–1626.

511. Pegoraro L., Flerro M. T., Lusso P., Glovinazzo B., Lanino E., Glovarelli M., Matera L., and Foa R. (1985) A novel leukemia T-cell line (PF-382) with phenotypic and functional features of suppressor lymphocytes. *J. Natl. Cancer Inst.* **75**, 285–289.

512. Bergsagel D. E. (1982) Plasma cell neoplasms, in *Cancer Medicine* (Holland J. F. and Frei E. III, eds.), Lea and Febiger, Philadelphia, pp. 1546–1576.

513. Fahey J. L., Scoggins R., Utz J. P., and Szwed C. F. (1963) Infection, antibody response and gamma globulin components in multiple myeloma and macroglobulinemia. *Am. J. Med.* **35**, 698–707.

514. Cone L. and Uhr J. W. (1964) Immunological deficiency disorders associated with chronic lymphocytic leukemia and multiple myeloma. *J. Clin. Invest.* **43**, 2241–2248.

515. Salmon S. E. (1974) "Paraneoplastic" syndromes associated with monoclonal lymphocyte and plasma cell proliferation. *Ann. NY Acad. Sci.* **230**, 228–239.

516. Han T. and Dadey B. (1979) In vitro functional studies of

mononuclear cells in patients with CLL. Evidence for functionally normal T lymphocytes and monocytes and abnormal B lymphocytes. *Cancer* **43**, 109–117.

517.   Ozer H., Han T., Henderson E. S., Nussbaum A., and Sheedy D. (1981) Immunoregulatory T cell function in multiple myeloma. *J. Clin. Invest.* **67**, 779–789.

518.   Salmon S. E. (1973) Immunoglobulin synthesis and tumor kinetics of multiple myeloma. *Semin. Hematol.* **10**, 135–147.

519.   Bhoopalam N., Yakulis V., Costea N., and Heller P. (1972) Surface immunoglobulins of circulating lymphocytes in mouse plasmacytoma. II. The influence of plasmacytoma RNA on surface immunoglobulins of lymphocytes. *Blood* **39**, 465–471.

520.   Tanapatchaiyapong P. and Zolla S. (1974) Humoral immunosuppressive substance in mice bearing plasmacytomas. *Science* **186**, 748–750.

521.   Hoover R. G., Hickman S., Gebel H. M., Rebbe N., and Lynch R. G. (1981) Expansion of Fc receptor-bearing T lymphocytes in patients with immunoglobulin G and immunoglobulin A myeloma. *J. Clin. Invest.* **67**, 308–311.

522.   Oken M. M. and Kay N. E. (1981) T-cell subpopulations in multiple myeloma: Correlation with clinical disease status. *Br. J. Haematol.* **49**, 629–634.

523.   Pezzutto A., Semenzato G., Agostini C., Raimondi R., and Gasparotto G. (1981) Subpopulations of T-lymphocytes in multiple myeloma. *Scand. J. Haematol.* **26**, 333–338.

524.   Mellstedt H., Holm G., Pettersson D., Björkholm M., Johansson B., Lindemalm C., Peest D., and Åhre A. (1982) T cells in monoclonal gammopathies. *Scand. J. Haematol.* **29**, 57–64.

525.   Mills K. H. G. and Cawley J. C. (1983) Abnormal monoclonal antibody-defined helper/suppressor T-cell subpopulations in multiple myeloma: Relationship to treatment and clinical stage. *Br. J. Haematol.* **53**, 271–275.

526.   Lauria F., Foa R., Cavo M., Gobbi M., Raspadori D., Giubellino M. C., Tazzari P. L., and Tura S. (1984) Membrane phenotype and functional behaviour of T lymphocytes in multiple myeloma: Correlation with clinical stages of the disease. *Clin. Exp. Immunol.* **56**, 653–658.

527.   Massaia M., Dianzani U., Pioppo P., Sibilla E., Boccadoro M., and Pileri A. (1987) Multiple myeloma: Ecto-5' nucleotidase deficiency of suppressor/cytotoxic (CD8) lymphocytes in a marker for the expansion of suppressor T cells. *Clin. Exp. Immunol.* **69**, 426–432.

528.   Massaia M., Ma D. D. F., Boccadoro M., Golzio F., Gavarotti P., Dianzani U., and Pileri A. (1985) Decreased ecto-5' nucleotidase

activity of peripheral blood lymphocytes in human monoclonal gammopathies: Correlation with tumor cell kinetics. *Blood* **65**, 530–534.

529. Pilarski L. M., Mant M. J., Ruether B. A., Carayanniotis G., Otto D., and Krowka J. F. (1985) Abnormal clonogenic potential of T cells from multiple myeloma patients. *Blood* **66**, 1266–1271.

530. Landay A., Gartland G. L., and Clement L. T. (1983) Characterization of a phenotypically distinct sub-populaton of Leu2$^+$ cells that suppresses T cell proliferative responses. *J. Immunol.* **131**, 2757–2761.

531. Barnaba V., Ruberti G., Levrero M., and Balsano F. (1987) *In vitro* induction of HBsAg-specific CD8 CD11 human suppressor T cells. *Immunology* **62**, 431–438.

532. Broder S., Humphrey R., Durm M., Blackman M., Meade B., Goldman C., Strober W., and Waldmann T. (1975). Impaired synthesis of polyclonal (non-paraprotein) immunoglobulins by circulating lymphocytes from patients with multiple myeloma. Role of suppressor cells. *N. Engl. J. Med.* **293**, 887–892.

533. Waldmann T. A., Broder S., Krakauer R., MacDermott R. P., Durm M., Goldman C., and Meade B. (1976) The role of suppressor cells in the pathogenesis of common variable hypogammaglobulinemia and the immunodeficiency associated with myeloma. *Fed Proc.* **35**, 2067–2072.

534. Waldmann T. A., Blaese R. M., Broder S., and Krakauer R. S. (1978) Disorders of suppressor immunoregulatory cells in the pathogenesis of immunodeficiency and autoimmunity. *Ann. Intern. Med.* **88**, 226–238.

535. Knapp W. and Baumgartner G. (1978) Monocyte-mediated suppression of human B lymphocyte differentiation in vitro. *J. Immunol.* **121**, 1177–1183.

536. Paglieroni T. and MacKenzie M. R. (1977) Studies on the pathogenesis of an immune defect in multiple myeloma. *J. Clin Invest.* **59**, 1120–1133.

537. Paglieroni T. and MacKenzie M. R. (1980) Multiple myeloma: An immunologic profile. III. Cytotoxic and suppressive effects of the EA rosette-forming cell. *J. Immunol.* **124**, 2563–2570.

538. MacKenzie M. R., Paglieroni T. G., and Warner N. L. (1987) Multiple myeloma: an immunologic profile. IV. The EA rosette-forming cell is a Leu-1 positive immunoregulatory B cell. *J. Immunol.* **139**, 24–28.

539. Perri R. T., Oken M. M., and Kay N. E. (1982) Enhanced T cell suppression is directed toward sensitive circulating B cells in multiple myeloma. *J. Lab. Clin. Med.* **99**, 512–519.

540. Abbas A. K. (1979) T lymphocyte-mediated suppression of my-

eloma function in vitro. I. Suppression by allogeneically activated T lymphocytes. *J. Immunol.* **123**, 2011–2018.

541.   Lynch R. G., Rohrer J. W., Odermatt B., GeBel H. M., Autry J. R., and Hoover R. G. (1979) Immunoregulation of murine myeloma cell growth and differentiation: A monoclonal model of B cell differentiation. *Immunol. Rev.* **48**, 45–80.

542.   Ludwig C. U., Hicks M. J., Durie B. G. M., and Tabing T. (1982) T lymphocyte subsets in multiple myeloma (MM) patients (PT.S) with active and stable disease. *Proc. Am. Soc. Clin. Oncol.* **1**, 191.

543.   Ludwig C., Hicks M. J., Pena D., and Durie B. G. M. (1983) OKT-8$^+$ suppressor-T-lymphozyten sind bei patienten mit stabilem multiplen myelom vermehrt. *Schweiz. Med. Wochenschr.* **113**, 1451–1454.

544.   Flood P. M., Phillips C., Taupier M. N., and Schreiber H. (1980) Regulation of myeloma growth in vitro by idiotype-specific T lymphocytes. *J. Immunol.* **124**, 424–430.

545.   Million R. R., Cassisi N. J. and Wittes R. E. (1985) Cancer of the head and neck, in *Cancer Principles and Practice of Oncology* (DeVita V. T., Jr., Hellman S., and Rosenberg S. A., eds.), J.B. Lippincott, Philadelphia, pp. 407–506.

546.   Catalona W. J. and Chretien P. B. (1973) Abnormalities of quantitative dinitrochlorobenzene sensitization in cancer patients: Correlation with tumor stage and histology. *Cancer* **31**, 353–356.

547.   Lundy J., Wanebo H., Pinsky C., Strong E., and Oettgen H. (1974) Delayed hypersensitivity reactions in patients with squamous cell cancer of the head and neck. *Am. J. Surg.* **128**, 530–533.

548.   Pinsky C. M., Domeni A. F., and Caron A. S. (1974) Delayed hypersensitivity reactions in patients with cancer: Investigation and stimulation of immunity in cancer patients. *Recent Results Cancer Res.* **47**, 37–41.

549.   Zighelboim J., Dorey F., Parker N. H., Calcaterra T., Ward P., and Fahey J. L. (1979) Immunologic evaluation of patients with advanced head and neck cancer receiving weekly chemoimmunotherapy. *Cancer* **44**, 117–123.

550.   Catalona W. J., Sample W. F., and Chretien P. B. (1973) Lymphocyte reactivity in cancer patients: Correlation with tumor histology and clinical stage. *Cancer* **31**, 65–71.

551.   Balch C. M., Dougherty P. A., and Tilden A. B. (1982) Excessive prostaglandin E$_2$ production by suppressor monocytes in head and neck cancer patients. *Ann. Surg.* **196**, 645–650.

552.   Berlinger N. T., Hilal E. Y., Oettgen H. F., and Good R. A. (1978) Deficient cell-mediated immunity in head and neck cancer patients secondary to autologous suppressive immune cells. *Laryngoscope* **88**, 470–483.

553. Gray W. C., Chretien P. B., Sutter C. M., Revie D. R., Tomazic V. T., Blanchard C. L., Aygun C., Amornmarn R., and Ordonez J. V. (1985) Effects of radiation therapy on T-lymphocyte subpopulations in patients with head and neck cancer. *Otolaryngol. Head Neck Surg* **93**, 650–660.

554. Wolf G. T., Amendola B. E., Diaz R., Lovett E. J. 3d, Hammerschmidt R. M., and Peterson K. A. (1985) Definite vs adjuvant radiotherapy. Comparative effects on lymphocyte subpopulations in patients with head and neck squamous carcinoma. *Arch. Otolaryngol.* **111**, 716–726.

555. Wolf G. T., Lovett E. J., Peterson K. A., Beauchamp M. L., and Baker S. R. (1984) Lymphokine production and lymphocyte subpopulations in patients with head and neck squamous carcinoma. *Arch. Otolaryngol.* **110**, 731–735.

556. Braun D. P., Cobleigh M. A., and Harris J. E. (1980) Multiple concurrent immunoregulatory defects in cancer patients with depressed PHA-induced lymphocyte DNA synthesis. *Clin. Immunol. Immunopathol.* **17**, 89–101.

557. Braun D. P. and Harris J. E. (1981) Relationship of leukocyte numbers, immunoregulatory cell function, and phytohemagglutinin responsiveness in cancer patients. *J. Natl. Cancer Inst.* **67**, 809–814.

558. Berlinger N. T., Lopez C., and Good R. A. (1976) Facilitation or attenuation of mixed leukocyte culture responsiveness by adherent cells. *Nature* **260**, 145–146.

559. Wang B. S., Heacock E. H., Wu A. V. O., and Mannick J. A. (1980) Generation of suppressor cells in mice after surgical trauma. *J. Clin. Invest.* **66**, 200–209.

560. Macca R. and Panje W. (1980) Indomethacin sensitive suppressor cells in patients with head and neck carcinomas. *Proc. Am. Assoc. Cancer Res.* **21**, 211.

561. Vose B. M. and Moore M. (1980) Heterogeneity of suppresors of mitogen responsiveness in human malignancy. *Cancer Immunol. Immunother.* **9**, 163–171.

562. Balch C. M., Dougherty P. A., and Tilden A. B. (1981) Excessive prostaglandin E_2 production by suppressor cells in head and neck cancer patients. *Proc. Am. Assoc. Cancer Res.* **22**, 310.

563. Maca R. D. and Panje W. R. (1982) Indomethacin sensitive suppressor cell activity in head and neck cancer patients pre- and postirradiation therapy. *Cancer* **50**, 483–489.

564. Tarkkanen J., Saksela E., and Paavolainen M. (1983) Suppressor cells of natural killer activity in normal and tumor-bearing individuals. *Clin. Immunol. Immunopathol.* **28**, 29–38.

565. Minna J. D., Higgins G. A., and Glatstein E. J. (1985) Cancer of

the lung, in *Cancer Principles and Practice of Oncology* (DeVita V. T., Jr., Hellman S., Rosenberg S. A., eds.), J.B. Lippincott, Philadelphia, pp. 507–597.

566. Krant M. J., Manskopf G., Brandrup C. S., and Madoff M. A. (1968) Immunologic alterations in bronchogenic cancer. Sequential study. *Cancer* **21**, 623–631.

567. Wagner V., Janků O, Wagnerová M., Mates J., and Koníčková Z. (1972) The production of complete and incomplete antibodies in patients with neoplastic disease. *Neoplasma* **19**, 75–87.

568. Price Evans D. A. (1976) Immunology of bronchial carcinoma. *Thorax* **31**, 493–506.

569. Holmes E. C. (1976, 1977) Immunology of lung cancer. *Ann. Thorac. Surg.* **21**, 250–258, and *Chest* **71**, 643–644.

570. Brugarolas A., Han T., Takita H., and Minowada J. (1973) Immunologic assays in lung cancer: Skin tests, lymphocyte blastogenesis, and rosette-forming cell count. *NY State J. Med.* **73**, 747–750.

571. Uchida A. and Hoshino T. (1980) Clinical studies on cell-mediated immunity in patients with malignant disease. I. Effect of immunotherapy with OK-432 on lymphocyte subpopulation and phytomitogen responsiveness in vitro. *Cancer* **45**, 476–483.

572. Ducos J., Migueres J., Colombies P., Kessous A., and Poujoulet N. (1970) Lymphocyte response to PHA in patients with lung cancer. *Lancet* **1**, 1111–1112.

573. Jerrells T. R., Dean J. H., and Herberman R. B. (1978) Relationship between T lymphocyte levels and lymphoproliferative responses in mitogens and alloantigens in lung and breast cancer patients. *Int. J. Cancer* **21**, 282–290.

574. Han T. and Takita H. (1980) Indomethacin-mediated enhancement of lymphocyte response to mitogens in healthy subjects and lung cancer patients. *Am. Cancer Soc.* **46**, 2416–2420.

575. Venkataraman M., Rao D. S., Levin R. D., and Westerman M. P. (1985) Suppression of B-lymphcyte function by T-lymphocytes in patients with advanced lung cancer. *J. Natl. Cancer Inst.* **74**, 37–41.

576. Straus S. E., Pizzo P. A., and Lutwick L. I. (1983) Infectious complications of lung cancer, in *Lung Cancer Clinical Diagnosis and Treatment* (Strauss M. J., ed.), Grune and Stratton, New York pp. 293–314.

577. Cobleigh M. A., Braun D. P., and Harris J. E. (1980) Quantitation of lymphocytes and T-cell subsets in patients with disseminated cancer. *J. Natl. Cancer Inst.* **64**, 1041–1045.

578. Moretta L., Ferrarini M., and Cooper M. D. (1978) Characteriza-

tion of human T-cell subpopulations as defined by specific receptors for immunoglobulins. *Contemp. Top. Immunobiol.* **8**, 19–53.

579. Ginns, L. C., Goldenheim P. D., Miller L. G., Burton R. C., Gillick L., Colvin R. B., Goldstein G., Kung P. C., Hurwitz C., and Kazemi H. (1982) T-lymphocyte subsets in smoking and lung cancer. Analysis by monoclonal antibodies and flow cytometry. *Am. Rev. Respir. Dis.* **126**, 265–269.

580. Schulof R. S., Chorba T. L., Cleary P. A., Palaszynski S. R., Alabaster O., and Goldstein A. L. (1985) T-cell abnormalities after mediastinal irradiation for lung cancer. The in vitro influence of synthetic thymosin alpha-1. *Cancer* **55**, 974–983.

581. Camacho E. S., Schechter P., and Graham R. (1982) Immune competence evaluation including T-cell subsets in patients with lung or head and neck carcinomas and smokers. *Proc. Am. Soc. Clin. Oncol.* **1**, 40.

582. Akiyama M, Bean M. A., Sadamoto K., Takahashi Y., and Brankovan V. (1983) Suppression of the responsiveness of lymphocytes from cancer patients triggered by coculture with autologous tumor derived cells. *J. Immunol.* **131**, 3085–3090.

583. Hengst J. C. D., Kan-Mitchell J., Kempf R. A., Strumpf I. J., Sharma O. P., Kortes V. L., and Mitchell M. S. (1985) Correlation between cytotoxic and suppressor activities of human pulmonary alveolar macrophages. *Cancer Res.* **45**, 459–463.

584. Uchida A. and Hoshino T. (1980) Clinical studies on cell-mediated immunity in patients with malignant disease. II. Suppressor cells in patients with cancer. *Cancer Immunol. Immunother.* **9**, 153–158.

585. Uchida A. and Hoshino T. (1980) Reduction of suppressor cells in cancer patients treated with OK-432 immunotherapy. *Int. J. Cancer* **26**, 401–404.

586. Uchida A. and Micksche M. (1981) Concanavalin A-inducible suppressor cells in pleural effusions and peripheral blood of cancer patients. *Cancer Immunol. Immunother.* **10**, 203–210.

587. Uchida A. and Micksche M. (1981) Suppressor cells for natural killer activity in carcinomatous pleural effusions of cancer patients. *Cancer Immunol. Immunother.* **11**, 255–263.

588. Uchida A. and Micksche M. (1982) Suppression of NK cell activity by adherent cells from malignant pleural effusions of cancer patients, in *NK Cells and Other Natural Effector Cells* (Herberman, R. B., ed.), Academic Press, New York, pp. 589–594.

589. Uchida A. and Micksche M. (1982) Agumentation of NK cell activity in cancer patients by OK432: Activation of NK cells and reduction of suppressor cells, in *NK Cells and Other Natural Effector*

Cells, (Herberman R. B., ed.), Academic Press, New York. pp. 1303–1308.

590. Uchida A. and Micksche M. (1983) Intrapleural administration of OK432 in cancer patients: Activation of NK cells and reduction of suppressor cells. *Int. J. Cancer* **31**, 1–5.

591. Uchida A., Colot M., and Micksche M. (1984) Suppression of natural killer cell activity by adherent effusion cells of cancer patients. Suppression of motility, binding capacity and lethal hit of NK cells. *Br. J. Cancer* **49**, 17–23.

592. Han T. and Takita H. (1977) Suppressor activity of monocytes on T lymphocyte response to mitogens in lung cancer patients. *IRCS Med. Sci.* **5**, 178.

593. Han T. and Takita H. (1979) Depression of T lymphocyte response by non-T suppressor cells in lung cancer patients. A possible prognostic value of suppressor cell activity. *Cancer* **44**, 2090–2098.

594. Ostenson R. C. and Lum L. G. (1984) In vitro differences in lymphocyte subpopulation reactivity in lung cancer patients: Purified protein derivative-specific suppressor T lymphocytes in patients who have received bacillus Calmette-Guérin. *Clin. Immunol. Immunopathol.* **30**, 233–240.

595. Uchida A. and Micksche M. (1981) Natural killer cells in carcinomatous pleural effusions. *Cancer Immunol. Immunother.* **11**, 131–138.

596. Uchida A. and Micksche M. (1983) Lysis of fresh human tumor cells by autologous large granular lymphocytes from peripheral blood and pleural effusions. *Int. J. Cancer* **32**, 37–44.

597. Sibbitt W. L., Jr., Bankhurst A. D., Jumonville A. J., Saiki J. H., Saiers J. H., and Doberneck R. C. (1984) Defects in natural killer cell activity and interferon response in human lung carcinoma and malignant melanoma. *Cancer Res.* **44**, 852–856.

598. Minassian A. A. and Kadagidze Z. G. (1983) Suppressor cells in melanoma and lung cancer: Correlation with the clinical stage. *Neoplasma* **30**, 153–158.

599. Uchida A. and Klein E. (1986) Suppression of T-cell response in autologous mixed lymphocyte-tumor culture by large granular lymphocytes. *J. Natl. Cancer Inst.* **76**, 389–398.

600. Jerrells T. R., Dean J. H., Richardson G. L., and Herberman R. B. (1979) Influence of BCG immunotherapy on adherent suppressor cell-activity and monocyte-mediated cytostasis in lung cancer patients. *Proc. Amer. Assoc. Cancer Res.* **20**, 231.

601. Jerrells T. R., Dean J. H., Richardson G., Cannon G. B., and Herberman R. B. (1979) Increased monocyte-mediated cytostasis

of lymphoid cell lines in breast and lung cancer patients. *Int. J. Cancer* **23**, 768–776.

602. Vose B. M. and Moore M. (1979) Suppressor cell activity of lymphocytes inflitrating human lung and breast tumours. *Int. J. Cancer* **24**, 579–585.

603. Vose B. M. (1980) Natural killers in human cancer: Activity of tumor-infiltrating and draining node lymphocytes, in *Natural Cell-Mediated Immunity Against Tumors* (Herberman R. B., ed.), Academic Press, New York, pp. 1081–1097.

604. Rosenberg J. C., Roth J. A., Lichter A. S., and Kelsen D. P. (1985) Cancer of the esophagus, in *Cancer Principles and Practice of Oncology* (DeVita V. T., Jr., Hellman S., and Rosenberg S. A., eds.) J.B. Lippincott, Philadelphia, pp. 621–657.

605. Macdonald J. S., Cohen I., Jr., and Gunderson L. L. (1985) Cancer of the stomach, in *Cancer Principles and Practice of Oncology* (DeVita V. T., Jr., Hellman S., and Rosenberg S. A., eds.), J. B. Lippincott, Philadelphia, pp. 659–690.

606. Moertel C. G. and Thynne G. S. (1982) Large bowel, in *Cancer Medicine* (Holland J. F. and Frei E. III, eds.), Lea and Febiger, Philadelphia, pp. 1830–1859.

607. Moertel C. G. (1982) The liver, in *Cancer Medicine* (Holland J. F. and Frei E. III, eds.), Lea and Febiger, Philadelphia, pp. 1774–1781.

608. Sindelar W. F., Kinsella T. J., and Mayer R. J. (1985) Cancer of the pancreas, in *Cancer Principles and Practice of Oncology* (DeVita V. T., Jr., Hellman S., and Rosenberg S. A., eds.), J. B. Lippincott, Philadelphia, pp. 691–739.

609. Koyama S., Fukao K., and Fujimoto S. (1985) The generation of interleukin-2-dependent suppressor T-cells from patients with systemic metastasis of gastric carcinoma and the phenotypic characterization of the cells defined by monoclonal antibodies. *Cancer* **56**, 2437–2445.

610. Balch C. M., Dougherty P. A., Cloud G. A., and Tilden A. B. (1984) Prostaglandin E_2-mediated suppression of cellular immunity in colon cancer patients. *Surgery* **95**, 71–77.

611. Zembala M., Mytar B., Ruggiero I., Uracz W., Popiela T., and Czupryna A. (1983) Suppressor cells and survival of patients with advanced gastric cancer. *J. Natl. Cancer Inst.* **70**, 223–228.

612. Doldi K., Manger B., Koch B., Riemann J., Hermanek P., and Kalden J. R. (1984) Spontaneous suppressor cell activity in the peripheral blood of patients with malignant and chronic inflammatory bowel diseases. *Clin. Exp. Immunol.* **55**, 655–663.

613. Toge T., Yanagawa E., Nakanishi K., Yamada Y., Nimoto M.,

and Hattori T. (1980) Concanavalin A-activated suppressor cell activity in gastric cancer patients. *Gann* **71**, 784–789.

614. Toge T., Hamamoto S., Itagaki E., Yajima K., Tanada M., Nakane H., Kohno H., Nakanishi K., and Hattori T. (1983) Concanavalin A-induced and spontaneous suppressor cell activities in peripheral blood lymphocytes and spleen cells from gastric cancer patients. *Cancer* **52**, 1624–1631.

615. Toge T., Tanada M., Yajima K., Kohno H., Itagaki E., and Hattori T. (1983) Induction of suppressor cell activities in normal lymphocytes by sera from gastric cancer patients. *Clin. Exp. Immunol.* **54**, 80–86.

616. Takiyama W., Toge T., Yanagawa E., Hirai T., Miyoshi Y., and Hattori T. (1982) Clinical studies on cell mediated immunity of patients with thoracic esophageal cancer. *J. Jpn. Assoc. Thorac. Surg.* **30**, 1428–1433.

617. Kurosu Y., Fukamachi S., and Morita K. (1984) The significance of relationship of the presence of nonspecific suppressor cells in spleens with gastric cancer-related pathology. *Jpn. J. Surg.* **14**, 293–298.

618. Kanayama H., Hamazoe R., Osaki Y., Shimizu N., Maeta M., and Koga S. (1985) Immunosuppressive factor from the spleen in gastric cancer patients. *Cancer* **56**, 1963–1966.

619. Koyama S., Yoshioka T., Sakita T., and Fujimoto S. (1982) Tumor antigen-specific suppressor T cells from peripheral blood lymphocytes and spleen cells in gastric cancer patients in *Proc. 13th International Cancer Congress, Seattle WA*, p. 522.

620. Koyama S. and Sakita T. (1983) Clinical significance of immunosuppressor T cells activated in gastric cancer patients. *Jap. J. Med.* **22**, 291.

621. Gibson P. R., Hermanowicz A., and Jewell D. P. (1984) Factors affecting the spontaneous cell-mediated cytotoxicity of intestinal mononuclear cells. *Immunology* **53**, 267–274.

622. Savage D. (1956) A family history of uterine and gastro-intestinal cancer. *Br. Med. J.* **2**, 341–343.

623. Peltokallio P. and Peltokallio V. (1966) Relationship of familial factors to carcinoma of the colon. *Dis. Colon Rectum* **9**, 367–370.

624. Lynch H. T. and Krush A. J. (1967) Heredity and adenocarcinoma of the colon. *Gastroenterology* **53**, 517–527.

625. Lynch H. T. and Krush A. J. (1971) Cancer family "G" revisited: 1895–1970. *Cancer* **27**, 1505–1511.

626. Lynch H. T. (1974) Familial cancer prevalence spanning eight years: Family N. *Arch. Intern. Med.* **134**, 931–938.

627. Berlinger N. T., Lopez C., Lipkin M., Vogel J. E., and Good R. A.

(1977) Defective recognitive immunity in family aggregates of colon carcinoma. *J. Clin. Invest.* **59**, 761–769.

628. Yao E. H., Li D., and Gu H. (1984) T cell subpopulation in hepatoma. *Am. J. Gastroenterol.* **79**, 227–228.

629. Lee C. S. and Lin T. Y. (1984) T lymphocyte subpopulations in peripheral blood of hepato cellular carcinoma patients. *Chin. J. Microbiol. Immunol. (Taipei)* **17**, 92–97.

630. Prout G. R., Jr. and Garnick M. B. (1982) The kidney and ureter, in *Cancer Medicine* (Holland J. F. and Frei E. III, eds.), Lea and Febiger, Philadelphia, pp. 1880–1896.

631. Paulson D. F., Perez C. A., and Anderson T. (1985) Cancer of the kidney and ureter, in *Cancer Principles and Practice of Oncology* (DeVita V. T., Jr., Helman S., and Rosenberg S. A., eds.), J.B. Lippincott, Philadelphia, pp. 895–913.

632. Richie J. P., Shipley W. U., and Yagoda A. (1985) Cancer of the bladder, in *Cancer Principles and Practice of Oncology* (DeVita V. T., Jr., Hellman S., and Rosenberg S. A., eds.), J.B. Lippincott, Philadelphia, pp. 915–928.

633. Perez C. A., Fair W. R., Ihde D. C., and Labrie F. (1985) Cancer of the prostate, in *Cancer Principles and Practice of Oncology* (DeVita V. T., Jr., Hellman S., and Rosenberg S. A., eds.), J.B. Lippincott, Philadelphia, pp. 929–964.

634. Fahey J. L., Brosman S., and Dorey F. (1977) Immunological responsiveness in patients with bladder cancer. *Cancer Res.* **37**, 2875–2878.

635. Brosman S., Elhilali M., Vescera C., and Fahey J. (1979) Immune response in bladder cancer patients. *J. Urol.* **121**, 162–169.

636. Elhilali M. M. Britton S., Brosman S., and Fahey J. L. (1976) Critical evaluation of lymphocyte functions in urological cancer patients. *Cancer Res.* **36**, 132–137.

637. Catalona W. J., Ratliff T. L., and McCool R. E. (1980) Concanavalin A-activated suppressor cell activity in peripheral blood lymphocytes of urologic cancer patients. *J. Natl. Cancer Inst.* **65**, 553–557.

638. Shaw M. W., Rubenstein M., Stuart R., Guinan P. D., and Ablin R. J. (1983) Subpopulation of lymphocytes in the peripheral blood of patients with carcinoma of the prostate. *41st Ann. Meeting of the Amer. Fed. for Clin. Res.* **31**, 742a.

639. Rubenstein M., Shaw M. W., Ablin R. J., Guinan P. D., and McKiel C. F. (1984) Further evaluation and characterization of the mononuclear cell population of patients with prostate cancer. *IRCS Med. Sci.* **12**, 761–762.

640. Shaw M. W., Bhatti R., McKiel C. F., Guinan P. D., and

Rubenstien M. (1986) Leukocytic subset distributions of spleen cells obtained from rats bearing variants of the Dunning prostatic adenocarcinoma. *J. Urol.* **135**, 159–162.

641. Spina C. A., Dorey F., Vescera C., Brosman S., and Fahey J. L. (1981) Depression of the generation of cell-mediated cytotoxicity by macrophage-like suppresor cells in bladder carcinoma patients. *Cancer Res.* **41**, 4324–4330.

642. Spina C. A., Dorey F., Vescera C., Brosman S., and Fahey J.L. (1980) Depressed cell-mediated cytotoxicity in patients with bladder carcinoma: Presence of macrophage-like suppressor cells. *Proc. Am. Assoc. Cancer Res.* **21**, 250.

643. Catalona W. J., Ratliff T. L., and McCool R. S. (1978) Concanavalin A-activated suppressor cells in peripheral blood and lymph nodes of urologic cancer patients. *Surg. Forum* **29**, 621–623.

644. Catalona W. J., Ratliff T. L., and McCool R. E. (1979) Concanavalin A-inducible suppressor cells in regional lymph nodes of cancer patients. *Cancer Res.* **39**, 4372–4377.

645. Bean M. A., Kodera Y., and Cummings K. B. (1978) Genetically restricted thymus-derived (T) suppressor lymphocyte activity in the blood of a bladder cancer (Ca) patient. *Proc. Am. Assoc. Cancer Res.* **19**, 136.

646. Bean M. A., Akiyama M., Kodera Y., Dupont B., and Hansen J. A. (1979) Human blood T lymphocytes that suppress the mixed leukocyte culture reactivity of lymphocytes from HLA-B14 bearing individuals. *J. Immunol* **123**, 1610–1614.

647. Brankovan V., Bean M. A., Martin P. J., Hansen J. A. Sadamoto K., Takahashi Y., and Akiyama M. (1983) The cell surface phenotype of a naturally occurring human suppressor T-cell of restricted specificity: Definition by monoclonal antibodies. *J. Immunol.* **131**, 175–179.

648. McMichael A. J. and Sasazuki T. (1977) A suppressor T-cell in the human mixed lymphocyte reaction. *J. Exp. Med.* **146**, 368–380.

649. Engleman E. G., McMichael A. J., Batey M. E., and McDevitt H. O. (1978) A suppressor T cell of the mixed lymphocyte reaction in man specific for the stimulating alloantigen. Evidence that identity at HLA-D between suppressor and responder is required for suppression. *J. Exp. Med.* **147**, 137–146.

650. Engleman E. G., and McDevitt H. O. (1978) A suppressor T-cell of the mixed lymphocyte reaction specific for the HLA-D region in man. *J. Clin. Invest.* **61**, 828–838.

651. Thomsen M., Dickmeiss E., Jakobsen B. K., Platz P., Ryder L. P. and Svejgaard A. (1978) Low responsiveness in MLC induced by

certain HLA-A antigens on the stimulator cells. *Tissue Antigens* 11, 449–456.

652. Engleman E. G., McMichael A. J., and McDevitt H. O. (1978) Suppresion of the mixed lymphocyte reaction in man by a soluble T-cell factor. Specificity of the factor for both responder and stimulator. *J. Exp. Med.* 147, 1037–1043.

653. Braun D. P., Harris Z. L., Harris J. E., Sandler S., Khandekar J., Locker G., Haid M., Gordon L., Shaw J., Cobleigh M., Gallagher P., Taylor S. G., Showel J., and Bonomi P. D. (1983) Effect of interferon therapy on indomethacin-sensitive immunoregulation in the peripheral blood mononuclear cells of renal cell carcinoma patients. *J. Biol. Res. Modif.* 2, 251–262.

654. Young R. C., Knapp R. C., Fuks Z., and DiSaia P. J. (1985) *Cancer of the Ovary*, in *Cancer Principles and Practice of Oncology* (DeVita V. T., Jr., Hellman S., and Rosenberg S. A., eds.), J.B. Lippincott, Philadelphia pp. 1083–1117.

655. Nelson J. H., Jr. (1982) Uterine cervix, in *Cancer Medicine* (Holland J. F. and Frei E. III eds.), Lea and Febiger, Philadelphia, pp. 1984–1997.

656. Perez C. A., Knapp R. C., Di Saia P. J., and Young R. C. (1985) Gynecologic tumors, in *Cancer Principles and Practice of Oncology* (DeVita V. T., Jr. Hellman S., and Rosenberg S. A., eds.), J.B. Lippincott, Philadelphia, pp. 1013–1081.

657. Haskill S., Koren H., Becker S., Fowler W., and Walton L. (1982) Mononuclear-cell infiltration in ovarian cancer. III. Suppresor-cell and ADCC activity of macrophages from ascitic and solid ovarian tumors. *Br. J. Cancer* 45, 747–753.

658. Mantovani A., Allavena P., Sessa C., Bolis G., and Mangioni C. (1980) Natural killer activity of lymphoid cells isolated from human ascitic ovarian tumors. *Int. J. Cancer* 25, 573–582.

659. Allavena P., Introna M., Mangioni C., and Mantovani A. (1981) Inhibition of natural killer activity by tumor-associated lymphoid cells from ascites ovarian carcinomas. *J. Natl. Cancer Inst.* 67, 319–325.

660. Grzelak I., Olszewski W. L., and Engeset A. (1983) Suppressor cell activity in peripheral blood in cancer patients after surgery. *Clin. Exp. Immunol.* 51, 149–156.

661. Harris, J. R., Hellman S., Canellos G. P., and Fisher B. (1985) Cancer of the breast, in *Cancer Principles and Practice of Oncology* (DeVita, V. T., Jr., Hellman S., and Rosenberg S. A., eds.), J.B. Lippincott, Philadelphia, pp. 1119–1177.

662. Petrini B., Wasserman J., Glas U., and Blomgren H. (1982) T lym-

phocyte subpopulations in blood following radiation therapy for breast cancer. *Eur. J. Cancer Clin. Oncol.* **18**, 921–924.

663. Wasserman J., Petrini B., and Blomgren H. (1982) Radiosensitivity of T-lymphocyte subpopulations. *J. Clin Lab. Immunol.* **7**, 139–140.

664. Petrini B., Wasserman J., Blomgren H., and Glas U. (1983) Changes of blood T cell subsets following radiation therapy for breast cancer. *Cancer Lett.* **19**, 27–31.

665. Petrini B., Wasserman J., Blomgren H., and Rotstein S. (1984) Changes of blood T cell subsets in patients receiving postoperative adjuvant chemotherapy for breast cancer. *Eur. J. Cancer Clin. Oncol.* **20**, 1485–1488.

666. Toivanen A., Granberg I., and Nordman E. (1984) Lymphocyte subpopulations in patients with breast cancer after postoperative radiotherapy. *Cancer* **54**, 2919–2923.

667. Petrini B., Wasserman J., Blomgren H., and Rotstein S. (1983) T helper/suppressor ratios in chemotherapy and radiotherapy. *Clin. Exp. Immunol.* **53**, 255–256.

668. Petrini B., Wasserman J., Rotstein S., and Blomgren H. (1983) Radiotherapy and persistent reduction of peripheral T cells. *J. Clin Lab. Immunol.* **11**, 159–160.

669. Newman G. H., Rees G. J. G., Jones R. S. J., Grove E. A., and Preece A. W. (1987) Changes in helper and suppresor T lymphocytes following radiotherapy for breast cancer. *Clinical Radiology* **38**, 191–193.

670. Wallace J. I., Coral F. S., Rimm I. J., Lane H., Levine H., Reinherz E. L., Schlossman S. F., and Sonnabend J. (1982) T-cell ratios in homosexuals. *Lancet* **1**, 908.

671. Uchida A., Kolb R., and Micksche M. (1982) Generation of suppressor cells for natural killer activity in cancer patients after surgery. *J. Natl. Cancer Inst.* **68**, 735–741.

672. Eremin O., Ashby J., and Stephens J. P. (1978) Human natural cytotoxicity in the blood and lymphoid organs of healthy donors and patients with malignant disease. *Int. J. Cancer* **21**, 35–41.

673. Eremin O. (1980) NK cell activity in the blood, tumour-draining lymph nodes and primary tumours of women with mammary carcinoma, in *Natural Cell-Mediated Immunity Against Tumors* (Herberman R. B., ed.) Academic Press, New York, pp. 1011–1029.

674. Gutterman J. U. and Scher H. I. (1982) Melanoma, in *Cancer Medicine* (Holland J. F. and Frei E. III, eds.), Lea and Febiger, Philadelphia, pp. 2109–2140.

675. Mastrangelo M. J., Baker A. R., and Katz H. R. (1985) Cutaneous melanoma, in *Cancer Principles and Practice of Oncology* (DeVita V.

T., Jr., Hellman S., Rosenberg S. A., eds.), J.B. Lippincott, Philadelphia, pp. 1371–1422.

676. Klein E. and Schwartz R. A. (1982) Cancer of the skin, in *Cancer Medicine* (Holland J. F. and Frei E. III, eds.), Lea and Febiger, Philadelphia, pp. 2057–2108.

677. Haynes H. A., Mead K. W., and Goldwyn R. M. (1985) Cancers of the skin, in *Cancer Principles and Practice of Oncology* (DeVita V. T., Jr., Hellman S., and Rosenberg S. A., eds.), J.B. Lippincott, Philadelphia, pp. 1343–1369.

678. Schwartz R. A. and Klein E. (1982) Ultraviolet light-induced carcinogenesis, in *Cancer Medicine* (Holland J. F. and Frei E. III, eds.), Lea and Febiger, Philadelphia, pp. 109–119.

679. Blattner W. A. and Hoover R. N. (1985) Cancer in the immunodepressed host, in *Cancer Principles and Practice of Oncology* (DeVita V. T., Jr. Hellman S. and Rosenberg S. A., eds.), J.B. Lippincott, Philadelphia, pp. 1999–2006.

680. Rosenberg S. A., Suit H. D., and Baker L. H. (1985) Sarcomas of soft tissues, in *Cancer Princples and Practice of Oncology* (DeVita V. T., Jr., Hellman S., and Rosenberg S. A., eds.), J.B. Lippincott, Philadelphia, pp. 1243–1291.

681. Kripke M. L. (1981) Immunologic mechanisms in UV radiation carcinogenesis. *Adv. Cancer Res.* **34,** 69–106.

682. Kripke M. L. (1986) Photoimmunology: The first decade. *Curr. Probl. Dermatol.* **15,** 164–175.

683. Kripke M. L. (1986) Immunology and photocarcinogenesis. New light on an old problem. *J. Am. Acad. Dermatol.* **14,** 149–155.

684. Daynes R. A., Bernhard E. J., Gurish M. F., and Lynch D. H. (1981) Experimental photoimmunology: Immunologic ramifications of UV-induced carcinogenesis. *J. Invest. Dermatol.* **77,** 77–85.

685. Daynes R. A., Samlowski W. E., Burnham D. K., Gahring L. C., and Roberts L. K. (1986) Immunobiological consequences of acute and chronic UV exposure. *Curr. Probl. Dermatol.* **15,** 176–194.

686. Fisher M. S. and Kripke M. L. (1984) Antigenic similarity between cells transformed by ultraviolet radiation in vitro and in vivo. *Science* **223,** 593–594.

687. Toews G. B., Bergstresser P. R., Streilein J. W., and Sullivan S. (1980) Epidermal Langerhans cell density determines whether contract hypersensitivity or unresponsiveness follows skin painting with DNFB. *J. Immunol.* **124,** 445–453.

688. Friedmann P. S. (1981) Disappearance of epidermal Langerhans cells during PUVA therapy. *Br. J. Dermatol.* **105,** 219–221.

689. Blum H. F. (1959) *Carcinogenesis by Ultraviolet Light.* (Princeton Univ. Press, Princeton, NJ).

690. Hersey P., Hasic E., Edwards A., Bradley M., Haran G., and McCarthy W. H. (1983) Immunological effects of solarium exposure. *Lancet* **1**, 545–548.

691. Hersey P., Haran G., Hasic E., and Edwards A. (1983) Alteration of T cell subsets and induction of suppressor T cell activity in normal subjects after exposure to sunlight. *J. Immunol.* **131**, 171–174.

692. Werkmeister J., McCarthy W., and Hersey P. (1981) Suppressor cell activity in melanoma patients. I. Relation to tumor growth and immunoglobulin levels in vivo. *Int. J. Cancer* **28**, 1–9.

693. Werkmeister J., Phillips G., McCarthy W., and Hersey P. (1981) Suppressor cell activity in melanoma patients. II. Concanavalin A-induced suppressor cells in relation to tumor growth and suppressor T-cell subsets. *Int. J. Cancer.* **28**, 11–15.

694. Ninnemann J. L. (1978) Melanoma-associated immunosuppression through B-cell activation of suppressor T cells. *J. Immunol.* **120**, 1573–1579.

695. Mukherji B., Wilhelm S. A., Guha A., and Ergin M. T. (1986) Regulation of cellular immune response against autologous human melanoma. I. Evidence for cell-mediated suppression of in vitro cytotoxic immune response. *J. Immunol.* **136**, 1888–1892.

696. Mukherji B., Nashed A. L., Guha A., and Ergin M. T. (1986) Regulation of cellular immune response against autologous human melanoma. II. Mechanism of induction and specificity of suppression. *J. Immunol.* **136**, 1893–1898.

697. Mukherji B., Ergin M. T., Guha A., Tatake R. T., and Nashed A. L. (1986) Suppressor cell activities in autologous human tumor systems. Suppression of tumor immunity. *Arch. Sur.* **121**, 1404–1408.

698. Hoon D. S. B., Bowker R. J., and Cochran A. J. (1987) Suppressor cell activity in melanoma-draining lymph nodes. *Cancer Res.* **47**, 1529–1533.

699. Gatter K. C., Morris H. B., Roach B., Mortimer P., Fleming K. A., and Mason D. Y. (1984) Langerhans cells and T cells in human skin tumors: An immunohistological study. *Histopathology* **8**, 229–244.

700. Uchida A. (1984) Generation of suppressor cells against natural killer cell activity by interferon administration, in *Natural Killer Activity and Its Regulation* (Hoshino T., Koren H. S., and Uchida A., eds.), Excerpta Medica, Amsterdam, pp. 263–269.

701. Uchida A., Yanagawa E., Kokoschka E. M., Michsche M., and Koren H. S. (1984) In vitro modulation of human natural killer cell activity by interferon generation of adherent suppressor cells. *Br. J. Cancer* **50**, 483–492.

702. Karavodin L. M. and Golub S. H. (1983/1984) Systemic adminis-

tration of human leukocyte interferon to melanoma patients. III. Increased helper:suppressor cell ratios in melanoma patients duirng interferon treatment. *Nat. Immun. Cell Growth Regul.* **3**, 193–202.

703. Koren H. S., Brandt C. P., Tso C. Y., and Laszlo J. (1983) Modulation of natural killing activity by lymphoblastoid interferon in cancer patients. *J. Biol. Resp. Modif.* **2**, 151–165.

704. Karavodin L. M., Giuliano A. E., and Golub S. H. (1981) T lymphocyte subsets in patients with malignant melanoma. *Cancer Immunol. Immunother.* **11**, 251–254.

705. Maluish A. E., Leavitt R., Sherwin S. A., Oldham R. K., and Herberman R. B. (1983) Effects of recombinant interferon-α on immune function in cancer patients. *J. Biol. Resp. Modif.* **2**, 470–481.

706. Ozer H., Gavigan M., O'Malley J., Thompson D., Dadey B., Nussbaum-Blumenson A., Snider C., Rudnick S., Ferraresi R., Norred S., and Han T. (1983) Immunomodulation by recombinant interferon-α₂ in a phase I trial in patients with lymphoproliferative malignancies. *J. Biol. Resp. Modif.* **2**, 499–515.

707. Ernstoff M. S., Fusi S., and Kirkwood J. M. (1983) Parameters of interferon action. I. Immunological effects of whole cell leukocyte interferon (IFN-Alpha) in phase I-II trials. *J. Biol. Resp. Modif.* **2**, 528–539.

708. Ernstoff M. S., Fusi S., and Kirkwood J. M. (1983) Parameters of interferon action. II. Immunological effects of recombinant leukocyte interferon (IFN-Alpha) in phase I-II trials. *J. Biol. Resp. Modif.* **2**, 540–547.

709. Silver H. K., Connors J. M., Karim K. A., Kong S., Spinelli J. J., deJong G., McLean D. M., and Salinas F. A. (1983) Effect of lymphoblastoid interferon on lymphocyte subsets in cancer patients. *J. Biol. Resp. Modif.* **2**, 428–440.

710. Gifford R. R. M., Ferguson R. M., and Voss B. V. (1981) Cimetidine reduction of tumour formation in mice. *Lancet* **1**, 638–640.

711. Osband M. E., Shen Y.-J., Shlesinger M., Brown A., Hamilton D., Cohen E., Lavin P., and McCaffrey R. (1981) Successful tumour immunotherapy with cimetidine in mice. *Lancet* **1**, 636–638.

712. Flodgren P., Borgström S., Jönsson P. E., Lindström C., and Sjögren H. O. (1983) Metastatic malignant melanoma: Regression induced by combined treatment with interferon [HuIFN-α (Le)] and cimetidine. *Int. J. Cancer* **32**, 657–665.

713. Tilden A. B. and Balch C. M. (1981) Indomethacin enchancement of immunocompetence in melanoma patients. *Surgery* **90**, 77–84.

714. Tilden A. B. and Balch C. M. (1982) Immune modulatory effects

of indomethacin in melanoma patients are not related to prosta-glandin E_2-mediated suppression. *Surgery* **92**, 528–532.

715. Modlin R. L., Meyer P. R., Ammann A. J., Rea T. H., Hofman F. M., Vaccaro S. A., Conant M. A., and Taylor C. R. (1983) Altered distribution of B and T lymphocytes in lymph nodes from homo-sexual men with Kaposi's sarcoma. *Lancet* **2**, 768–771.

716. Gottlieb M. S., Groopman J. E., Weinstein W. M., Fahey J. L., and Detels R. (1983) The acquired immunodeficiency syndrome. *Ann Intern. Med.* **99**, 208–220.

717. Lane H. C., Masur H., Edgar L. C., Whalen G., Rook A. H., and Fauci A. S. (1983) Abnormalities of B-cell activation and immuno-regulation in patients with the acquired immunodeficiency syn-drome. *N. Engl. J. Med.* **309**, 453–458.

718. Marmor M., Friedman-Kien A. E., Zolla-Pazner S., Stahl R. E., Rubinstien P., Laubenstein L., William D. C., Klein R. J., and Spigland I. (1984) Kaposi's sarcoma in homosexual men: A seroepidemiologic case control study. *Ann. Intern. Med.* **100**, 809–815.

719. Marinig C., Fiorini G., Boneschi V., Melotti E., and Brambilla L. (1985) Immunologic and immunogenetic features of primary Koposi's sarcoma. *Cancer* **55**, 1899–1901.

720. Fauci A. S., Macher A. M., Longo D. L., Lane H. C., Rook A. H., Masur H., and Gelmann E. P. (1984) Acquired immunodeficiency syndrome: Epidemiologic, clinical, immunologic and therapeutic considerations. *Ann. Intern. Med.* **100**, 92–106.

721. Laurence J., Gottlieb A. B., and Kunkel H. G. (1983) Soluble sup-pressor factors in patients with acquired immune deficiency syn-drome and its prodrome. Elaboration in vitro by T lymphocyte-adherent cell interactions. *J. Clin. Invest.* **72**, 2072–2081.

722. Laurence J. and Mayer L. (1984) Immunoregulatory lymphokines of T hybridomas from AIDS patients: Constitutive and inducible suppressor factors. *Science* **225**, 66–69.

723. Popovic M., Sarngadharan M. G., Read E., and Gallo R. C. (1984) Detection, isolation, and continuous production of cytopathic retroviruses (HTLV-III) from patients with AIDS and Pre-AIDS. *Science* **224**, 497–500.

724. Gallo R. C., Salahuddin S. Z., Popovic M., Shearer G. M., Kaplan M., Haynes B. F., Palker T. J., Redfield R., Oleske J., Safai B., White G., Foster P., and Markham P. D. (1984) Frequent detec-tion and isolation of cytopathic retroviruses (HTLV-III) from pa-tients with AIDS and at risk for AIDS. *Science* **224**, 500–503.

725. Klatzmann D., Barré-Sinoussi F., Nugeyre M. T., Dauguet C., Vilmer E., Griscelli C., Brun-Vezinet F., Rouzioux C., Gluckman J. C., Chermann J.-C., and Montagnier L. (1984) Selective tro-

pism of lymphadenopathy associated virus (LAV) for helper-inducer T lymphocytes. *Science* **225**, 59–63.

726. Kornblith P. L., Walker M. D., and Cassady J. R. (1985) Neoplasms of the central nervous system, in *Cancer Principles and Practice of Oncology* (DeVita V. T., Jr., Hellman S., and Rosenberg S. A., eds.), J.B. Lippincott, Philadelphia, pp. 1437–1510.

727. Brooks W. H., Netsky M. G., Normansell D. E., and Horwitz D. A. (1972) Depressed cell-mediated immunity in patients with primary intracranial tumors. Characterization of a humoral immunosuppressive factor. *J. Exp. Med.* **136**, 1631–1647.

728. Young H. F., Sakalas R., and Kaplan A. M. (1976) Inhibition of cell-mediated immunity in patients with brain tumors *Surg. Neurol.* **5**, 19–23.

729. Brooks W. H., Roszman T. L., Mahaley M. S., and Woosley R. E. (1977) Immunobiology of primary intracranial tumours. II. Analysis of lymphocyte subpopulations in patients with primary brain tumors. *Clin. Exp. Immunol.* **29**, 61–66.

730. Mahaley M. S., Brooks W. H., Roszman T. L., Bigner D. D., Dudka L., and Richardson S. (1977) Immunobiology of primary intracranial tumors. I. Studies of the cellular and humoral general immune competence of brain-tumor patients. *J. Neurosurg.* **46**, 467–476.

731. Roszman T. L., and Brooks W. H. (1980) Immunobiology of primary intracranial tumours. III. Demonstration of a qualitative lymphocyte abnormality in patients with primary brain tumours. *Clin. Exp. Immunol.* **39**, 395–402.

732. Braun D. P., Penn R. D., Flannery A. M., and Harris J. E. (1982) Immunoregulatory cell function in peripheral blood leukocytes of patients with intracranial gliomas. *Neurosurgery* **10**, 203–209.

733. Roszman T. L., Brooks W. H., and Elliott L. H. (1982) Immunobiology of primary intracranial tumors. VI. Suppressor cell function and lectin-binding lymphocyte subpopulations in patients with cerebral tumors. *Cancer* **50**, 1273–1279.

734. Wood G. W. and Morantz R. A. (1982) In vitro reversal of depressed T-lymphocyte function in the peripheral blood of brain tumor patients. *J. Natl. Cancer Inst.* **68**, 27–33.

735. Roszman T. L., Brooks W. H., Steele C., and Elliott L. H. (1985) Pokeweed mitogen-induced immunoglobulin secretion by peripheral blood lymphocytes from patients with primary intracranial tumors. Characterization of T helper and B cell function. *J. Immunol* **134**, 1545–1550.

736. Wood G. W., Neff J. E., and Stephens R. (1979) Relationships between monocytosis and T-lymphocyte function in human cancer. *J. Natl. Cancer Inst.* **63**, 587–592.

737. Romagnani S., Maggi E., Del Prete G., Biti G., Ponticelli P., and Ricci M. (1980) Short and long-term effects of radiation on T-cell subsets in peripheral blood of patients with Hodgkin's disease. *Cancer* **46**, 2590–2595.

738. Dillman R. O., Koziol J. A., Zavanelli M. I., Beauregard J. C., Halliburton B. L., Glassy M. C., and Royston I. (1984) Immunoincompetence in cancer patients. Assessment by in vitro stimulation tests and quantification of lymphocyte subpopulations. *Cancer* **53**, 1484–1491.

739. Schroff R. W., Gottlieb M. S., Prince H. E., Chai L. L., and Fahey J. L. (1983) Immunological studies of homosexual men with immunodeficiency and Kaposi's sarcoma. *Clin. Immunol. Immunopathol.* **27**, 300–314.

740. Hersh E. M., Patt Y. Z., Murphy S. G., Dicke K., Zander A., Adegbite M., and Goldman R. (1980) Radiosensitive, thymic hormone-sensitive peripheral blood suppressor cell activity in cancer patients. *Cancer Res.* **40**, 3134–3140.

741. Borzy M. S. and Ridgway D. (1985) The effects of thymic epithelial monolayer-conditioned medium on suppressor cell function following chemotherapy in pediatric patients. *Cancer Immunol. Immunother.* **19**, 154–157.

742. Pinsky C. M., El Domeiri A., Caron A. S., Knapper W. H., and Oettgen H. F. (1974) Delayed-hypersensitivity reactions in patients with cancer. *Recent Results Cancer Res.* **47**, 37–41.

743. Gardner R. J., Hart J. T., Sutton W. R., and Preston F. W. (1961) Survival of skin homografts in terminal cancer patients. *Surg. Forum* **12**, 167–168.

744. McCluskey R. T. and Bhan A. K. (1977) Cell-mediated reactions in vivo, in *Mechanisms of Tumor Immunity* (Creen I., Cohen S., and McCluskey R. T., eds.), Wiley Inc., New York. pp. 1–25.

745. Hesse D. G., Cole D. J., Van Epps D. E., and Williams R. C., Jr. (1984) Decreased T lymphocyte migration in patients with malignancy mediated by a suppressor cell population. *J. Clin. Invest.* **73**, 1078–1085.

746. Cole D., Van Epps D. E., and Williams R. C., Jr. (1986) Defective T-lymphocyte chemotactic factor production in patients with established malignancy. *Clin. Immunol. Immunopathol.* **38**, 209–221.

747. Burtin C., Scheinmann P., Salomon J. C., Lespinats G., Frayssinet C., Lebel B., and Canu P. (1981) Increased tissue histamine in tumor-bearing mice and rats. *Br. J. Cancer* **43**, 684–688.

748. Mavligit G. M., Calvo D. B. III, Patt Y. Z., and Hersh E. M. (1981) Immune restoration and/or augmentation of local xenogeneic graft versus host reaction by cimetidine in vitro. *J. Immunol.* **126**, 2272–2274.

749. Talpaz M., Medina J. E., Patt Y. Z., Goepfert H., Guillamondegui O. M., Wong W., and Mavligit G. M. (1982) The immune restorative effect of cimetidine administration in vivo on the local graft-versus-host reaction of cancer patients. *Clin. Immunol. Immunopathol.* **24,** 155–160.

750. Shore A., Dosch H.-M., and Gelfand E. W. (1978) Induction and separation of antigen-dependent T helper and T suppressor cells in man. *Nature* **274,** 586–587.

751. Mavligit G. M. and Wong W. L. (1982) Practical restoration of local GVH reaction in cancer patients by depletion of theophylline-sensitive suppressor T-cells. *Cancer* **49,** 2029–2033.

752. Minkes M., Stanford N., Chi M. M.-Y., Roth G. J., Raz A., Needleman P., and Majerus P. W. (1977) Cyclic adenosine 3′, 5′-monophosphate inhibits the availability of arachidonate to prostaglandin synthetase in human platelet suspensions. *J. Clin. Invest.* **59,** 449–454.

753. Davies P., Bonney R. J., Humes J. L., and Kuehl F. A., Jr. (1980) The synthesis of arachidonic acid oxygenation products by various mononuclear phagocyte populations, in *Mononuclear Phagocytes* (Van Furth B., ed.), Nijhoff, The Hague, pp. 1317–1350.

754. Fischer A., Durandy A., and Griscelli C. (1981) Role of prostaglandin E_2 in the induction of nonspecific T lymphocyte suppressor activity. *J. Immunol.* **126,** 1452–1455.

755. Santoro M. G., Philpott G. W., and Jaffe B. M. (1976) Inhibition of tumor growth in vivo and in vitro by prostaglandin E. *Nature* **263,** 777–779.

756. Panje W. R. (1981) Regression of head and neck carcinoma with prostaglandin-synthesis inhibitor. *Arch. Otolaryngol.* **107,** 658–663.

757. Al-Saleem T., Sabri Ali Z., and Qassab M. (1980) Skin cancers in xeroderma pigmentosum: Response to indomethacin and steroids. *Lancet* **2,** 264–265.

758. Stoll B. A. (1973) Indomethacin in breast cancer. *Lancet* **2,** 384.

759. Kauffman G. R., Bankhurst A. D., Goodwin J. S., and Williams R. C., Jr. (1978) Suppressor leukocytes in cancer patients. *Clin. Res.* **26,** 133A.

760. Vosika G. and Thies J. (1979) Indomethacin sensitive suppressor cells in the diagnosis of immunoincompetence. *Proc. Am. Assoc. Cancer Res.* **20,** 101.

761. Santos L. B., Yamada F. T., and Scheinberg M. A. (1985) Monocyte and lymphocyte interaction in patients with advanced cancer. Evidence for deficient IL-1 production. *Cancer* **56,** 1553–1558.

762. Hubbard W., Fukuda M., Pace R., and Wanebo H. (1979) Defective suppressor cell activity in cancer patients. A defect in immune regulation. *Proc. Amer. Assoc. Cancer Res.* **20**, 364.

763. Treves A. J., Heidelberger E., Feldman M., and Kaplan H. S. (1978) In vitro sensitization of human lymphocytes against histiocytic lymphoma cell lines. II. Characterization of two different effector activities and of suppressor cells. *J. Immunol.* **121**, 86–90.

764. Treves A. J., Heidelberger E., and Kaplan H. S. (1979) In vitro sensitization of human lymphocytes against histiocytic lymphoma cell lines. III. The activity of cultured-induced suppressor cells. *J. Immunol.* **122**, 643–647.

765. Maguire H., Berd D., Engstrom P., Paul A., and Mastrangelo M. (1981) Cyclophosphamide (Cy) increases the acquisition of T-cell immunity in patients with melanoma and colo-rectal cancer. *Proc. Amer. Assoc. Cancer Res.* **22**, 279.

766. Berd D., Mastrangelo M. J., Engstrom P. F., Paul A., and Maguire H. (1982) Augmentation of the human immune response by cyclophosphamide. *Cancer Res.* **42**, 4862–4866.

767. Berd D., Maguire H. C., Jr., and Mastrangelo M. J. (1984) Impairment of Concanavalin A-inducible suppressor activity following administration of cyclophosphamide to patients with advanced cancer. *Cancer Res.* **44**, 1275–1280.

768. Berd D. and Mastrangelo M. J. (1987) Effect of low dose cyclophoshamide on the immune system of cancer patients: Reduction of T-suppressor function without depletion of the CD8$^+$ subset. *Cancer Res.* **47**, 3317–3321.

769. Braun D. P. and Harris J. E. (1981) Effects of combination chemotherapy on immunoregulatory cells in peripheral blood of solid tumor cancer patients: Correlation with rebound overshoot immune function recovery. *Clin. Immunol. Immunopathol.* **20**, 193–214.

770. Braun D. P. and Harris J. E. (1984) Effect of cytotoxic antineoplastic chemotherapy on immunoregulatory leukocytes measured with monoclonal antibodies. *Clin. Immunol. Immunopathol.* **33**, 54–66.

771. Ben-Efraim S., Komlos L., Notmann J., Hart J., and Halbrecht I. (1985) In vitro selective effect of melphalan on human T-cell populations. *Cancer Immunol. Immunother.* **19**, 53–56.

772. Low T. L. K. and Goldstein A. L. (1979) Thymosin and other thymic hormones and their synthetic analogues. *Springer Semin. Immunopathol.* **2**, 169–186.

773. Trainin N., Pecht M., and Handzel Z. T. (1983) Thymic hor-

mones: inducers and regulators of T-cell system. *Immunol. Today* **4**, 16–21.

774. Chretien P. B., Lipson S. D., Makuch R. W., Kenady D. E., and Cohen M. H. (1979) Effects of thymosin in vitro in cancer patients and correlation with clinical course after thymosin immunotherapy. *Ann. NY. Acad. Sci.* **332**, 135–147.

775. Serrou B., Cupissol D., Caraux J., Thierry C., Rosenfeld C., and Goldstein A. L. (1980) Ability of Thymosin to decrease in vivo and in vitro suppressor cell activity in tumor bearing mice and cancer patients. *Recent Results in Cancer Res.* **75**, 110–114.

776. Friedman R. M. and Vogel S. N. (1983) Interferons with special emphasis on the immune system. *Adv. Immunol.* **34**, 97–140.

777. Mittelman A., Krown S. E., Cirrincione C., Safai B., Oettgen H. F., and Koziner B. (1983) Analysis of T cell subsets in cancer patients treated with interferon. *Am. J. Med.* **75**, 966–972.

778. Toge T., Yamada H., Aratani K., Kameda A., Kuroi K., Hisamatsu K., and Hattori T. (1985) Effects of intraperitoneal administration of OK-432 for patients with advanced cancer. *Jpn. J. Surg.* **15**, 260–265.

779. Jessup J. M., Kahan B. D., and Pellis N. R. (1982) Mechanisms of immunosuppression in tumor-bearing mice. A multifactorial analysis. *Cancer* **49**, 1158–1167.

780. Kedar E., Chriqui-Zeira E., and Mitelman S. (1984) Methods for amplifying the induction and expression of cytotoxic response in vitro to syngeneic and autologous freshly-isolated solid tumors of mice. *Cancer Immunol. Immunother.* **18**, 126–134.

781. Mizushima Y., Wepsic H. T., Yamamura Y., and Desilva M. A. (1984) Tumour-induced suppressor macrophages in rats: Differences in their suppressive effects on the Con A and PHA responses. *Clin. Exp. Immunol.* **57**, 371–379.

782. Pelus L. M. and Bockman R. S. (1979) Increased prostaglandin synthesis by macrophages from tumor-bearing mice. *J. Immunol.* **123**, 2118–2125.

783. Fujii T., Igarashi T., and Kishimoto S. (1987) Significance of suppressor macrophages for immunosurveillance of tumor-bearing mice. *J. Natl. Cancer Inst.* **78**, 509–517.

784. Young M. R. and Henderson S. (1982) Enhancement in immunity of tumor bearing mice by immunization against prostaglandin E_2. *Immunol. Commun.* **11**, 345–356.

785. Young M. R. and Dizer M. (1983) Enhancement of immune function of tumor growth inhibition by antibodies against prostaglandin E_2. *Immunol. Commun.* **12**, 11–23.

786. Young M. R., Newby M., and Wepsic H. T. (1987) Hematopoiesis and suppressor bone marrow cells in mice bearing large metastatic Lewis lung carcinoma tumors. *Cancer Res.* **47**, 100–105.

787. Caulfield M. J. and Cerny J. (1980) Cell interactions in leukemia-associated immunosuppression: Suppression of thymus-independent antibody responses by leukemia spleen cells (Moloney) in vitro is mediated by normal T cells. *J. Immunol.* **124**, 255–260.

788. Gatenby P. A., Basten A., and Creswick P. (1981) "Sneaking through": A T-cell-dependent phenomenon. *Br. J. Cancer* **44**, 753–756.

789. McBride W. H. and Howie S. E. M. (1986) Induction of tolerance to a murine fibrosarcoma in two zones of dosage—the involvement of suppressor cells. *Br. J. Cancer* **53**, 707–711.

790. Haubeck H.-D. and Kölsch E. (1986) Regulation of immune responses against the syngeneic ADJ-PC-5 plasmacytoma in BALB/c mice. IV. Tumor-specific T suppressor cells, induced at early stages of tumorigenesis, act on the induction phase of the tumor-specific cytotoxic T cell response. *Immunobiol.* **171**, 357–365.

791. Haubeck H.-D., Kloke O., and Kölsch E. (1986) Analysis of T suppressor cell mediated tumor escape mechanisms. *Curent Topics Microbiol. Immunol.* **126**, 225–230.

792. Brodt P. and Lala P. K. (1983) Changes in the host lymphocyte subsets during chemical carcinogenesis. *Cancer Res.* **43**, 4315–4322.

793. Brodt P. and Lala P. K. (1984) An analysis of host T-cell subsets based on Lyt antigenic markers during the development of spontaneous C3H mammary carcinomas. *Cell Immunol.* **84**, 427–432.

794. Yoshida K. and Tachibana T. (1985) Studies on lymphatic metastasis. I. Primary immunoregulatory role of regional lymph nodes in the establishment of lymphatic metastases. *J. Natl. Cancer Inst.* **75**, 1049–1058.

795. Mullen C. A., Urban J. L., Van Waes C., Rowley D. A., and Schreiber H. (1985) Multiple cancers. Tumor burden permits the outgrowth of other cancers. *J. Exp. Med.* **162**, 1665–1682.

796. Roberts L. K. and Daynes R. A. (1980) Modification of the immunogenic properties of chemically induced tumors arising in hosts treated concomitantly with ultraviolet light. *J. Immunol.* **125**, 438–447.

797. Ingenito G. G. and Calkins C. E. (1981) Evidence for interaction between T cell populations of tumor-bearing and normal mice in immune suppression. *J. Immunol.* **127**, 1236–1240.

798. Ingenito G. G. and Calkins C. E. (1983) Lymphocyte subsets involved in tumor-activated nonspecific feedback suppression. *Cell Immunol.* **79**, 26–35.

799. Pope B. L. (1985) Activation of suppressor T cells by low-molecular-weight factors secreted by spleen cells from tumor-bearing mice. *Cell Immunol.* **93**, 364–374.

800. Almawi W. Y. and Pope B. L. (1985) Induction of suppression by a murine nonspecific suppressor-inducer cell line (M1-A5). *Cell Immunol.* **96**, 199–209.

801. Halliday W. J., Koppi T. A., and McKenzie I. F. C. (1982) Regulation of cell-mediated immunologic reactivity to Moloney murine sarcoma virus-induced tumors. III. Further characterization of tumor-specific serum blocking factors. *J. Natl. Cancer Inst.* **69**, 939–944.

802. Kuchroo V. K. and Halliday W. J. (1986) Cellular requirements for the suppression of leucocyte adherence inhibition reactions by serum from tumour-bearing mice. *Immunology* **57**, 545–552.

803. Koppi-Reynolds T. A. and Halliday W. J. (1984) A two-chain tumour-related suppressor factor specific for a sequenced antigen. *Immunol. Lett.* **8**, 219–225.

804. Koppi T. A. and Halliday W. J. (1983) Cellular origin of blocking factors from cultured spleen cells of tumor-bearing mice. *Cell Immunol.* **76**, 29–38.

805. Kuchroo V. K., Lee V. K., Hellström I., Hellström K. E., and Halliday W. J. (1987) Tumor-specific idiotopes on suppressor factors and supressor cells revealed by monoclonal anti-idiotope antibodies. *Cell Immunol.* **104**, 105–114.

806. Moser G., Tominaga A., Greene M. I., and Abbas A. K. (1983) Accessory cells in immune suppression. I. Role of I-A+ accessory cells in effector phase idiotype-specific suppression of myeloma function. *J. Immunol.* **131**, 1728–1733.

807. Maier T. and Levy J. G. (1982) Anti-tumor effects of an antiserum raised in syngeneic mice to a tumor-specific T suppressor factor. *Cancer Immunol. Immunother.* **13**, 134–139.

808. Maier T., Stammers A. T., and Levy J. G. (1983) Characterization of a monoclonal antibody directed to a T cell suppressor factor. *J. Immunol.* **131**, 1843–1848.

809. Steele J. K., Stammers A. T., Chan A., Maier T., and Levy J. G. (1985) Preliminary characterization of a soluble immunosuppressive molecule from DBA/2 spleen cells using monoclonal antibody immunoadsorbence. *Cell Immunol.* **90**, 303–313.

810. Strayer D. S. and Leibowitz J. L. (1986) Reversal of virus-induced immune suppression. *J. Immunol.* **136**, 2649–2653.

811. Bruley-Rosset M. and Payelle B. (1987) Deficient tumor-specific immunity in old mice: *in vivo* mediation by suppressor cells, and correction of the defect by interleukin 2 supplementation *in vitro* but not *in vivo*. *Eur. J. Immunol.* **17**, 307–312.

812. Haubeck H.-D. and Kölsch E. (1985) Isolation and characterization of in vitro and in vivo functions of a tumor-specific T suppressor cell clone from a BALB/c mouse bearing the syngeneic ADJ-PC-5 plasmacytoma. *J. Immunol.* **135**, 4297–4302.

813. Koyama S., Yoshioka T., Sakita T., and Fujimoto S. (1985) Generation of T cell growth factor (TCGF)-dependent splenic lymphoid cell line with cell-mediated immunosuppressive reactivity against syngeneic murine tumor. *Eur. J. Cancer Clin. Oncol.* **21**, 257–261.

814. Steele J. K., Stammers A. T., and Levy J. G. (1985) Isolation and characterization of a tumor-specific T suppressor factor from a T cell hybridoma. *J. Immunol.* **134**, 2767–2778.

815. Swartz R. P. (1986) Suppression of delayed-type hypersensitivity to radiation [UV, 280–320 nm (UVB)]-induced tumor cells with serum factors from UVB-irradiated mice. *J. Natl. Cancer Inst.* **76**, 1181–1184.

816. Palaszynski E. W. and Kripke M. L. (1983) Transfer of immunological tolerance to ultraviolet-radiation-induced skin tumors with grafts of ultraviolet-irradiated skin. *Transplantation* **36**, 465–467.

817. Roberts L. K. (1986) Characterization of a cloned ultraviolet radiation (UV)-induced suppressor T cell line that is capable of inhibiting anti-UV tumor-immune responses. *J. Immunol.* **136**, 1908–1916.

818. Bursuker I. and North R. J. (1985) Suppression of generation of concomitant antitumor immunity by passively transferred suppressor T cells from tumor-bearing donors. *Cancer Immunol. Immunother.* **19**, 215–218.

819. Dent L. A. and Finlay-Jones J. J. (1985) In vivo detection and partial characterization of effector and suppressor cell populations in spleens of mice with large metastatic fibrosarcomas. *Br. J. Cancer* **51**, 533–541.

820. North R. J. (1985) Down-regulation of the antitumor immune response. *Adv. Cancer Res.* **45**, 1–43.

821. North R. J. and Dye E. S. (1985) Ly 1^+2^- suppressor T cells down-regulate the generation of Ly 1^-2^+ effector T cells during progressive growth of the P815 mastocytoma. *Immunology* **54**, 47–56.

822. Bear H. D. (1986) Tumor-specific suppressor T-cells which inhibit the in vitro generation of cytolytic T-cells from immune and early tumor-bearing host spleens. *Cancer Res.* **46**, 1805–1812.

823. North R. J. (1986) Radiation-induced, immunologically mediated regression of an established tumor as an example of successful therapeutic immunomanipulation. Preferential elimination of suppressor T cells allows sustained production of effector T cells. *J. Exp. Med.* **164**, 1652–1666.

824. Kurashige S., Akuzawa Y., and Mitsuhashi S. (1985) Synergistic anti-suppressor effect of mini cells prepared from Salmonella typhimurium and mitomycin C in EL4-bearing mice. *Cancer Immunol. Immunother.* **19**, 127–129.

825. Potter M., Wax J. S., Anderson A. O., and Nordan R. P. (1985) Inhibition of plasmacytoma development in BALB/c mice by indomethacin. *J. Exp. Med.* **161**, 996–1012.

826. Pope B. L. (1985) The effect of indomethacin on the activation and effector function of suppressor cells from tumor-bearing mice. *Cancer Immunol. Immunother.* **19**, 101–108.

827. Gorczynski R. M., Kennedy M., and Ciampi A. (1985) Cimetidine reverses tumor growth enhancement of plasmacytoma tumors in mice demonstrating conditioned immunosuppression. *J. Immunol.* **134**, 4261–4266.

828. Nagarkatti M., and Kaplan A. M. (1985) The role of suppressor T cells in BCNU-mediated rejection of a syngeneic tumor. *J. Immunol.* **135**, 1510–1517.

829. Chen Y.-H., Anderson A. B., and Williams K. G. (1985) Splenic immune effector and suppressor cells in mice bearing a growing plasmacytoma. *Cancer Res.* **45**, 5473–5479.

830. Comoglio P. M., Prat M., and Bretti S. (1985) Enhancement of immunity against RSV-induced sarcomas by generation of hapten-reactive helper T lymphocytes. *Immunology* **54**, 289–295.

831. Fujiwara H., Moriyama Y., Suda T., Tsuchida T., Shearer G. M., and Hamaoka T. (1984) Enhanced TNP-reactive helper T cell activity and its utilization in the induction of amplified tumor immunity that results in tumor regression. *J. Immunol.* **132**, 1571–1577.

832. Kaymakcalan Z., Spitalny G. L., and Bursuker I. (1987) *In vitro* expression of secondary antitumor immunity by *in vivo* tumor-sensitized T cells: Inhibition by tumor-induced suppresor T cells. *Cancer Immunol. Immunother.* **25**, 69–74.

833. DiGiacomo A. and North R. J. (1986) T cell suppressors of antitumor immunity. The production of Ly-1^{-}, 2^{+} suppressors of delayed sensitivity precedes the production of suppressors of protective immunity. *J. Exp. Med.* **164**, 1179–1192.

834. Greenberg P. D., Kern D. E., and Cheever M. A. (1985) Therapy of disseminated murine leukemia with cyclophosphamide and immune Lyt-1^{+}, 2^{-} T cells. Tumor eradication does not require

participation of cytotoxic T cells. *J. Exp. Med.* **161**, 1122–1134.

835.   Shu S. and Rosenberg S. A. (1985) Adoptive immunotherapy of newly induced murine sarcomas. *Cancer Res.* **45**, 1657–1662.

836.   Kloke O., Haubeck H.-D., and Kölsch E. (1986) Evidence for a T suppressor cell-inducing antigenic determinant shared by ADJ-PC-5 plasmacytoma and syngeneic BALB/c spleen cells. *Eur. J. Immunol.* **16**, 659–664.

837.   Tilkin A. F., Gomard E., Begue B., and Levy J.-P. (1984) T cells from naive mice suppress the in vitro cytotoxic response against endogenous Gross virus-induced tumor cells. *J. Immunol.*, **132**, 520–526.

838.   Tilkin A.-F., Begue B., Gomard E., Levy J.-P. (1985) Natural suppressor cell inhibiting T killer responses against retroviruses: A model for self tolerance. *J. Immunol.* **134**, 2779–2782.

839.   Rich S. S. and Rich R. R. (1974) Regulatory mechanisms in cell-mediated immune responses. I. Regulation of mixed lymphocyte reactions by alloantigen-activated thymus-derived lymphocytes. *J. Exp. Med.* **140**, 1588–1603.

840.   Von Roenn J., Harris J. E., and Braun D. P. (1987) Suppressor cell function in solid tumor cancer patients. *J. Clin. Oncol.* **5**, 150–159.

841.   Saxon A., Stevens R. H., and Golde D. W. (1979) Helper and suppressor T-lymphocyte leukemia in ataxia telangiectasia. *N. Engl. J. Med.* **300**, 700–704.

842.   Raziuddin S., Madan A., and Danial B. H. (1987) Unique immunological behaviour of CD8+ (suppressor T cell) leukaemia cells. *Scand. J. Immunol.* **26**, 487–493.

843.   Kronenberg M., Siu G., Hood L. E., and Shastri N. (1986) The molecular genetics of the T-cell antigen receptor and T-cell antigen recognition. *Ann. Rev. Immunol.* **4**, 529–591.

844.   Marrack P. and Kappler J. (1987) The T cell receptor. *Science* **238**, 1073–1079.

845.   Brenner M. B., McLean J., Dialynas D. P., Strominger J. L., Smith J. A., Owen F. L., Seidman J. G., Ip S., Rosen F., and Krangel M. S. (1986) Identification of a putative second T-cell receptor. *Nature* **322**, 145–149.

846.   Bank I., DePinho R. A., Brenner M. B., Cassimeris J., Alt F. W., and Chess L. (1986) A functional T3 molecule associated with a novel heterodimer on the surface of immature human thymocytes. *Nature* **322**, 179–181.

847.   Pardoll D. M., Fowlkes B. J., Bluestone J. A., Kruisbeek A., Maloy W. L., Coligan J. E., and Schwartz R. H. (1987) Differential expression of two distinct T-cell receptors during thymocyte development. *Nature* **326**, 79–81.

848. Bluestone J. A., Pardoll D., Sharrow S. O., and Fowlkes B. J. (1987) Characterization of murine thymocytes with CD3-associated T-cell receptor structures. *Nature* **326**, 82–84.

849. Chien Y.H., Iwashima M., Kaplan K. B., Elliott J. F., and Davis M. M. (1987) A new T-cell receptor gene located within the alpha locus and expressed early in T-cell differentiation. *Nature* **327**, 677–682.

850. Kranz D. M., Saito H., Heller M., Takagaki Y., Haas W., Eisen H. N., and Tonegawa S. (1985) Limited diversity of the rearranged T-cell γ gene. *Nature* **313**, 752–755.

851. Weiss A., Imboden J., Hardy K., Manger B., Terhorst C., and Stobo J. (1986) The role of the T3/antigen receptor complex in T-cell activation. *Ann. Rev. Immunol.* **4**, 593–619.

852. Saito T., Weiss A., Miller J., Norcross M. A., and Germain R. N. (1987) Specific antigen-Ia activation of transfected human T cell expressing murine Tiαβ-human T3 receptor complexes. *Nature* **325**, 125–130.

853. Littman D. R., Newton M., Crommie D., Ang S.-L., Seidman J. G., Gettner S. N., and Weiss A. (1987) Characterization of an expressed CD3-associated Tiγ-chain reveals Cγ domain polymorphism. *Nature* **326**, 85–88.

854. Tada T. and Okumura K. (1979) The role of antigen-specific T cell factors in the immune respone. *Adv. Immunol.* **28**, 1–87.

855. Blanckmeister C. A., Yamamoto K., Davis M. M., and Hämmerling G. J. (1985) Antigen-specific, I-a-restricted suppressor hybridomas with spontaneous cytolytic activity. Functional properties and lack of rearrangement of the T cell receptor β chain genes. *J. Exp. Med.* **162**, 851–863.

856. De Santis R., Givol D., Hsu P.-L., Adorini L., Doria G., and Appella, E. (1985) Rearrangement and expression of the α- and β-chain genes of the T-cell antigen receptor in functional murine suppressor T-cell clones: *Proc. Natl. Acad. Sci. USA* **82**, 8638–8642.

857. Modlin R. L., Brenner M. B., Krangel M. S., Duby A. D., and Bloom B. R. (1987) T-cell receptors of human suppressor cells. *Nature* **329**, 541–545.

858. Hedrick S. M., Germain R. N., Bevan M. J., Dorf M., Engel I., Fink P., Gascoigne N., Heber-Katz E., Kapp J., Kaufmann Y., Kaye J., Melchers F., Pierce C., Schwartz R. H., Sorensen C., Taniguchi M., and Davis M. M. (1985) Rearrangement and transcription of a T-cell receptor β-chain gene in different T-cell subsets. *Proc. Natl. Acad. Sci. USA* **82**, 531–535.

859. Kronenberg M., Goverman J., Haars R., Malissen M., Kraig E., Phillips L., Delovitch T., Suciu-Foca N., and Hood L. (1985) Rear-

rangement and transcription of the β-chain genes of the T-cell antigen receptor in different types of murine lymphocytes. *Nature* **313,** 647–653.

860.   Mori I., Lecoq A. F., Robbiati F., Barbanti E., Righi M., Sinigaglia F., Clementi F., and Ricciardi-Castagnoli P. (1985) Rearrangement and expression of the antigen receptor α, β, and γ genes in suppressor antigen-specific T cell lines. *EMBO J.* **4,** 2025–2030.

Appendix
List of Acronyms

ADCC	Antibody dependent cellular cytotoxicity
AIDS	Acquired immunodeficiency syndrome
ALL	Acute lymphoblastic leukemia
APC	Antigen presenting cell
ATG	Antilymphocytic globulin
ATL	Adult T cell leukemia
ATS	Anti thymocyte serum
B-ALL	B cell ALL
B cell	Bursal equivalent derived cell
BCG	Bacillus Calmette-Guérin
BCGcw	BCG cell walls
B-CLL	B cell CLL
BCNU	1,3-bis(2-chloroethyl)-1-nitrosourea
BFU-E	Erythroid burst-forming unit
B-PLL	B cell prolymphocytic leukemia
C	Complement
c-ALL	Common ALL
CAR	Carrageenan
CFA	Complete Freund's adjuvant
CFU-E	Erythroid colony-forming unit
CLL	Chromic lymphocytic leukemia
CML	Chronic myelogenous leukemia
CNS	Central nervous system
Con A	Concanavalin A
C. parvum	Corynebacterium parvum
CSF	Colony stimulating factor
Cy	Cyclophosphamide
DEAE	Diethylaminoethyl
DNBS	Dinitrobenzene sulfonic acid
DNCB	Dinitrochlorobenzene
DTH	Delayed type hypersensitivity

EAC-RFC	Cells forming rosettes with sheep erythrocytes coated with IgM antisheep erythrocytes antibody and C3 from human serum
EA-RFC	Cells forming rosettes with human type O/Rh positive erythrocytes coated with human anti-D immunoglobulin
EA rosettes	Cells producing rosettes with antibody coated erythrocytes
EBV	Epstein-Barr virus
E^+ cells, E rosettes, or E-RFC	Cells forming rosettes with sheep erythrocytes
FACS	Fluorescence-activated cell sorter
FCS	Fetal calf serum
FLV	Friend leukemia virus
FLV-P	Polycythemic variant of FLV
FPLC	Fast protein liquid chromatography
GVHR	Graft vs host reaction
HD	Hodgkin's disease
HPGPC	High-performance gel permeation chromatography
HTLV	Human T cell leukemia/lymphoma virus
Ig	Immunoglobulin
IL-1	Interleukin-1
IL-2	Interleukin-2
INF	Interferon, usually referring to α-INF
JRA	Antibody found in the serum of patients with active juvenile rheumatoid arthritis
KLH	Keyhole limpet hemocyanin
LAI	Leukocyte adherence inhibition
LDA	Limiting dilution assay
LGL	Large granular lymphocytes
LLC	Lewis lung carcinoma
LPS	Lipopolysaccharide
MAF	Macrophage activating factor
MBP	Myelin basic protein
MCA	Methylcholanthrene
MER	Methanol extract residue
MHC	Major histocompatibility complex
MIF	Migration inhibitory factor
MLC	Mixed lymphocyte culture

MLR	Mixed lymphocyte reaction
MM	Multiple myeloma
MMC	Mitomycin C
M-MuLV	Moloney murine leukemia virus
MNC	Mononuclear cells
MSV	Murine sarcoma virus
MuLV	Murine leukemia virus
NC cells	Natural cytotoxic cells
NHL	Non-Hodgkin's lymphoma
NK ·	Natural killer
PBL	Peripheral blood-lymphocytes
PEC	Peritoneal exudate cells
PFC	Plaque forming cells
PG	Prostaglandin, usually referring to PGE_2
PHA	Phytohemagglutinin
pIEF	Preparative isoelectric focussing
pITP	Preparative isotachophoresis
PMA	Phorbol myristate acetate
PMN	Polymorphonuclear leukocytes
Poly I:C	Polyinosinic-polycytidilic acid
PPD	Purified protein derivative
PWM	Pokeweed mitogen
RBC	Red blood cells
SDS	Sodium dodecyl sulphate
SDS-PAGE	Sodium dodecyl sulphate polyacrylamide gel electrophoresis
SF	Suppressor factor
SRBC	Sheep red blood cells
Tac	Human IL-2 receptor
T-ALL	T cell ALL
TBH	Tumor bearing host
T cell	Thymus derived cell
T-CLL	T cell CLL
TCR	T cell receptor
Tg	T cell bearing a receptor to the Fc portion of IgG
Tg-LPD	Tg-lymphoproliferative disease
Th:Ts	Helper T cell: suppressor T cell ratio
TIL	Tumor infiltrating lympocytes
T-LL	T cell lymphoblastic lymphoma
Tm	T cell bearing a receptor to the Fc portion of IgM

TNCB	Trinitrochlorobenzene
T non g cells	T cells depleted of Tg cells
TNP	Trinitrophenyl
TPA	12-0-tetradecanoylphorbol-13-acetate
T-PLL	T cell prolymphocytic leukemia
TSTA	Tumor-specific transplantation antigen
UV	Ultraviolet

Index